Slavery, Disease, and Suffering in the Southern Lowcountry

On the eve of the Revolution, the Carolina lowcountry was the wealthiest and unhealthiest region in British North America. *Slavery, Disease, and Suffering in the Southern Lowcountry* argues that the two were intimately connected: both resulted largely from the dominance of rice cultivation on plantations using imported African slave labor. This development began in the coastal lands near Charleston, South Carolina, around the end of the seventeenth century. Rice plantations spread north to the Cape Fear region of North Carolina and south to Georgia and northeast Florida in the late colonial period. The book examines perceptions and realities of the lowcountry disease environment; how the lowcountry became notorious for its "tropical" fevers, notably malaria and yellow fever; how people combated, avoided, or perversely denied the suffering they caused; and how diseases and human responses to them influenced not only the lowcountry and the South, but the United States, even helping secure American independence.

Peter McCandless received his Ph.D. in history from the University of Wisconsin-Madison in 1974. He joined the faculty of the College of Charleston that year and retired in 2008 as Distinguished Professor of History. He won the Distinguished Teaching Award and was selected as a South Carolina Governor's Distinguished Professor. He has traveled extensively in the United Kingdom, Europe, and Turkey. He is the author of *Moonlight, Magnolias, and Madness: Insanity in South Carolina from the Colonial Period to the Progressive Era*; an associate editor of the *South Carolina Encyclopedia*; and author of numerous articles and other writings in historical journals. He is currently a member of the American Association for the History of Medicine and the Eighteenth-Century Scottish Studies Society; and he serves on the executive board of the Waring Library Society in Charleston, South Carolina, which is devoted to the collection and restoration of materials related to the history of medicine.

CAMBRIDGE STUDIES ON THE AMERICAN SOUTH

Series Editors

Mark M. Smith
University of South Carolina, Columbia

David Moltke-Hansen
*Center for the Study of the American South,
University of North Carolina at Chapel Hill*

Interdisciplinary in its scope and intent, this series builds upon and extends Cambridge University Press's long-standing commitment to studies on the American South. The series not only will offer the best new work on the South's distinctive institutional, social, economic, and cultural history but also will feature works in national, comparative, and transnational perspectives.

Other Titles in the Series

Robert E. Bonner, *Southern Slaveholders and the Crisis of American Nationhood*

Slavery, Disease, and Suffering in the Southern Lowcountry

PETER MCCANDLESS

College of Charleston

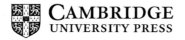

CAMBRIDGE
UNIVERSITY PRESS

CAMBRIDGE UNIVERSITY PRESS
Cambridge, New York, Melbourne, Madrid, Cape Town,
Singapore, São Paulo, Delhi, Tokyo, Mexico City

Cambridge University Press
32 Avenue of the Americas, New York, NY 10013-2473, USA

www.cambridge.org
Information on this title: www.cambridge.org/9781107004153

First published 2011

Printed in the United States of America

A catalog record for this publication is available from the British Library.

Library of Congress Cataloging in Publication data
McCandless, Peter.
  Slavery, disease, and suffering in the southern Lowcountry / Peter McCandless.
    p. cm. – (Cambridge studies on the American South)
  Includes bibliographical references and index.
  ISBN 978-1-107-00415-3 (hardback)
  1. Diseases – Social aspects – South Carolina – History. 2. Diseases and history – South
  Carolina – History. 3. Plantation life – South Carolina – History. 4. Environmental health
  – South Carolina – History. 5. South Carolina – Social conditions. 6. Charleston Region
  (S.C.) – Social conditions. 7. South Carolina – Economic conditions. 8. Charleston Region
  (S.C.) – Economic conditions. 9. South Carolina – History – Colonial period,
  ca. 1600 – 1775. 10. South Carolina – History – 1775–1865. I. Title II. Series.
  RA418.3.U6M35 2011
  362.109757–dc22   2010051694

ISBN 978-1-107-00415-3 Hardback

For Alastair and Colin

Where wouldn't they go for pepper! For a bag of pepper they would cut each other's throats without hesitation, and would forswear their souls, of which they were so careful otherwise: the bizarre obstinacy of that desire made them defy death in a thousand shapes; the unknown seas, the loathsome and strange diseases; wounds, captivity, hunger, pestilence, and despair. It made them great! By heavens! It made them heroic; and it made them pathetic, too, in their craving for trade with the inflexible death levying its toll on young and old.

Joseph Conrad, *Lord Jim*, 1900

Contents

Figures

Maps

Preface

Here was a thin neck in the hourglass of the Afro-American past, a place where individual grains from all along the West African coast had been funneled together, only to be fanned out across the American landscape with the passage of time.

Peter Wood, *Black Majority*

Slavery, Disease, and Suffering in the Southern Lowcountry examines the impact of disease in the region known as the South Atlantic lowcountry. The book focuses primarily on South Carolina and its metropolis, Charleston, from 1670 to 1860.[1] Because this area was in many ways the seedbed for much of subsequent southern and American culture, the story told here has a much wider significance. In the mid-eighteenth century, the rice and indigo plantations that dominated the region spread north into the Cape Fear region of North Carolina and south to the coastal lands of Georgia. After 1763, they moved into northern Florida. In the late eighteenth century, the lowcountry plantation regime began to move into the Carolina backcountry, though cotton replaced rice as the most important crop. In the nineteenth century, lowcountry folk spread their plantations and diseases westward throughout much of the South.[2] What a small number of settlers began in 1670, where the Ashley and Cooper Rivers come together to form the Atlantic Ocean (a local joke), had a huge influence on the history of the South and the United States. The Carolina lowcountry became the wealthiest region in late colonial North

---

[1] Charleston was officially called "Charles Town" from 1670 until 1783, but for convenience and to avoid confusion, I have generally used "Charleston" throughout the book except in quotations. It should also be noted here that the name "Carolina" originally referred to both South and North Carolina. The two did not become fully separate colonies until the 1720s.

[2] Joyce Chaplin, *An Anxious Pursuit: Agricultural Innovation and Modernity in the Lower South, 1730–1815* (Chapel Hill: University of North Carolina Press, 1993); Rachel N. Klein, *Unification of a Slave State: The Rise of the Planter Class in the South Carolina Backcountry, 1760–1808* (Chapel Hill: University of North Carolina Press, 1990); Jack P. Greene, *Pursuits of Happiness: The Social Development of Early Modern British Colonies in the Formation of America* (Chapel Hill: University of North Carolina Press, 1988).

America. It also became the unhealthiest, and the book argues that the two were intimately connected. *Slavery, Disease, and Suffering in the Southern Lowcountry* examines how the lowcountry became such an unhealthy place; how people tried to cope with the suffering it caused; and how their actions, experiences, and responses affected a culture that enormously influenced the development of the South and the United States.

Writing this tale would have been impossible without the path-breaking work of many other historians. My indebtedness to them will become abundantly clear from the notes, but a few works related to this one should be mentioned here. In the 1960s, Joseph Waring produced two volumes on medicine in South Carolina between 1670 and 1900 that remain an essential starting point for anyone exploring the historical epidemiology of the state and region. This is also true of John Duffy's *Epidemics in Colonial America*, written in the 1950s. Another old work, by St. Julien Ravenel Childs, *Malaria and Colonization in the Carolina Low Country, 1526–1696*, is a goldmine of information on the early history of that disease in the region. Albert Cowdrey's more recent *This Land, This South* contains a seminal chapter on the relationship between the southern environment and southern diseases. Cowdrey stressed the mixing of European and African microbes and the friendliness of the southern climate and topography to diseases of tropical origins. Two books in particular helped inspire and inform the present volume: Peter Wood's *Black Majority* and Peter Coclanis's *Shadow of a Dream* – both remarkable for their path-breaking scholarship and engaging style. Other authors whose works proved invaluable to me along the way include Joyce Chaplin, Margaret Humphreys, Todd Savitt, William Dusinberre, Sharla Fett, Philip Morgan, Judith Carney, Daniel Littlefield, Max Edelson, and Elizabeth Fenn. A book published just after I completed the manuscript, but in time for me to incorporate some of its information and insights, is J. R. McNeill's *Mosquito Empires*. It focuses on the relationship between war, yellow fever, and malaria in the Caribbean region and includes a chapter on the lowcountry. Prior to its appearance, I had benefited greatly from McNeill's earlier articles on yellow fever.[3] The present work builds on and complements but does not replicate any of these works.

---

[3] Joseph I. Waring, *A History of Medicine in South Carolina, 1670–1825* (Charleston: Medical Society of South Carolina, 1964) and *A History of Medicine in South Carolina, 1825–1900* (Charleston: Medical Society of South Carolina, 1967); John Duffy, *Epidemics in Colonial America* (Baton Rouge: Louisiana State University Press, 1953); St. Julien Ravenel Childs, *Malaria and Colonization in the Carolina Low Country, 1526–1696* (Baltimore: Johns Hopkins University Press, 1940); Albert E. Cowdrey, *This Land, This South: An Environmental History*, Revised Edition (Lexington: The University Press of Kentucky, 1996); Peter Wood, *Black Majority: Negroes in Colonial South Carolina from 1670 through the Stono Rebellion* (New York: W.W. Norton, 1975); Peter A. Coclanis, *The Shadow of a Dream: Economic Life and Death in the South Carolina Low Country, 1670–1920* (New York and Oxford: Oxford University Press, 1989); Chaplin, *An Anxious Pursuit*; Todd Savitt, *Medicine and Slavery: The Diseases and Health Care of Blacks in Antebellum Virginia* (Urbana: University of Illinois Press, 1978); Margaret Humphreys, *Yellow Fever and the South* (Baltimore: Johns Hopkins University Press, 1992); Margaret Humphreys, *Malaria: Poverty, Race, and Public Health in*

It is not a history of medicine, but medical theories, practice, and personnel form an important part of the story. It is a history not of epidemics but of the impact of infectious diseases – especially those of tropical origin – on the region. It is not an environmental history, but the epidemiological reality described here cannot be fully understood without discussing its connection to both the natural environment and human interventions in it. It is not a study of the lowcountry economy, but discussion of its effects is essential to the book's overall argument.

Slavery, Disease, and Suffering in the Southern Lowcountry is divided into two parts of seven chapters each. Part I, Talk about Suffering, looks at the disease environment and its human impact. It focuses on differing perceptions of the environment and tries to assess the reality by looking at the effects of disease and the experiences of individuals, ethnic and professional groups, residents and newcomers. Part II, Combating Pestilence, focuses on therapeutic, preventive, and restorative measures people used to reduce the impact of disease. Specific chapters deal with healers and the arts of healing, regular and irregular; religious and other forms of prophylactics including inoculation and vaccination for smallpox; quarantine and sanitary measures; and the migratory strategies elites used to avoid local fevers.

The evidence used for this study derives almost entirely from contemporary documents and accounts written by residents, travelers, and visitors. Inevitably, the book is somewhat skewed toward the experiences, actions, and ideas of white elites – planters, merchants, officials, and physicians – because they produced the bulk of the sources. The voices of African Americans – who were a majority of the population during much of the period covered by this volume – and poor whites are more muted and filtered through the elite's writings than I would like. The letters and other writings of the wealthy planters, merchants, officials, and doctors – along with accounts of travelers and immigrants – reveal much about the sufferings of Africans and poor whites, often unintentionally. The elite generally overlooked or looked away from those sufferings. In 1880, the Charleston city yearbook listed the names of every citizen who had died between 1808 and 1880 who allegedly had lived at least eighty years. The aim was a familiar one in the history of the lowcountry: to

the United States (Baltimore and London: Johns Hopkins University Press, 2001), 28; William Dusinberre, *Them Dark Days: Slavery in the American Rice Swamps* (Athens: University of Georgia Press, 2004); Philip D. Morgan, *Slave Counterpoint: Black Culture in the Eighteenth-Century Chesapeake and Lowcountry* (Chapel Hill: University of North Carolina Press, 1998); Sharla M. Fett, *Working Cures: Healing, Health, and Power on Southern Slave Plantations* (Chapel Hill: University of North Carolina Press, 2002); S. Max Edelson, *Plantation Enterprise in Colonial South Carolina* (Cambridge, MA: Harvard University Press, 2006); Judith Carney, *Black Rice* (Cambridge, MA: Harvard University Press, 2001); Daniel Littlefield, *Rice and Slaves: Ethnicity and the Slave Trade in Colonial South Carolina* (Urbana and Chicago: University of Illinois Press, 1991), Elizabeth Fenn, *Pox Americana: The Great Smallpox Epidemic of 1775–1782* (New York: Hill and Wang, 2001); J. R. McNeill, *Mosquito Empires: Ecology and War in the Greater Caribbean, 1640–1914* (Cambridge: Cambridge University Press, 2010).

counter charges that people rarely lived long there. The authors added that the list was surely incomplete: "many have doubtless escaped notice, especially among the colored population."[4] That was surely true and the admission is significant. Many things happened among that population that escaped the notice of the white elite, among them blacks' massive suffering from disease. Many things have undoubtedly escaped my notice as well. Despite the limitations of the sources, I have tried to re-create the human encounter with these diseases and its broader impact to the best of my ability. The reader must judge how well I have succeeded.

Note on Capitalization, Punctuation, and Spelling

For consistency and ease of reading I have modernized capitalization, punctuation, and sometimes spelling in quotations from original sources.

---

[4] City of Charleston, *Yearbook*, 1880.

Acknowledgments

Books of this sort can never have just one author. Many people contributed to its germination and fruition. Some know how they helped; others are probably unaware of their contribution or have forgotten it (if not me), so long did it take me to get this far. At various points in the saga, conversations and exchanges with other scholars, friends, and family helped me enormously. Among those I would like to thank for their encouragement, advice, thoughts, insights, and shared information are Chris Boucher, David Brown, Jason Coy, William Dalrymple, Max Edelson, Walter Edgar, Elizabeth Fenn, Gerald Grob, Margaret Humphreys, John McNeill, Ron Numbers, Bill Olejniczak, Todd Savitt, Lester Stephens, John Tone, and Maarten Ultee. Student assistants Jason Farr and Chris Willoughby unearthed some highly useful information. Sheridan Hough, Alastair McCandless, and Colin McCandless read the original shaky manuscript with great care and, beside pointing out many mistakes and making excellent suggestions for improvement, convinced me that I wasn't entirely crazy to write it. Lew Bateman, senior editor for history and political science at Cambridge University Press in New York, was highly supportive from the first, as was his editorial assistant, Anne Lovering Rounds. The Press's readers and David Moltke-Hansen, coeditor of this series, saved me from some egregious mistakes as well as helped and encouraged me to make the book more broadly relevant. I am also greatly indebted to the copyediting team at PETT Fox, Inc., for their careful work on the manuscript. Any remaining errors are mine.

The research and writing of this book were greatly aided by two summer fellowships from the Institute for Southern Studies at the University of South Carolina and several grants from the College of Charleston Research and Development Fund. Archivists and librarians could not have been nicer to this often bumbling researcher. The staff of the College of Charleston Library, particularly at Reference, Interlibrary Loans, and Special Collections, was unfailingly helpful over the many years of this project. I received enormous help at the Waring Historical Library at the Medical University of South Carolina, South Carolina Historical Society, South Carolina Department of Archives and History, and the Caroliniana Library, University of South Carolina. The same is true of the National Archives of the United Kingdom at Kew, Wellcome Library, British Library, Edinburgh University Special Collections, National Archives of Scotland (formerly Scottish Record Office), and Aberdeen Library Special Collections. I would like to extend particular thanks to Jane Brown, Kay Carter, Henry Fulmer, Susan Hoffius, Chuck Lesser, and Mike Phillips for their assistance. Above all, I want to thank Nalan for her love, patience, and support.

List of Abbreviations Used in Notes

BPRO/SC	British Public Record Office, Records re South Carolina
CO	Colonial Office Records, National Archives, Kew, United Kingdom
COCSC	College of Charleston Special Collections
FP	Family Papers
HLP	*The Papers of Henry Laurens*
JCHA	Journals of the Commons House of Assembly of South Carolina (manuscript)
JCHA	*Journals of the Commons House of Assembly of South Carolina* (printed)
MSM	Medical Society of South Carolina, Minutes, Waring Historical Library, Medical University of South Carolina, Charleston
NGP	*The Papers of Nathanael Greene*
PRO	Public Record Office, National Archives, Kew, United Kingdom
SCDAH	South Carolina Department of Archives and History, Columbia
SCG	*South Carolina Gazette*
SCHM	*South Carolina Historical Magazine*
SCHS	South Carolina Historical Society, Charleston
SCL	South Caroliniana Library, Columbia
SHC	Southern Historical Collection, Chapel Hill
SPG	Papers of the Society for the Propagation of the Gospel, London
SRO	Scottish Record Office (National Archives of Scotland), Edinburgh
Stats.	*Statutes at Large of South Carolina*
WHL	Waring Historical Library, Medical University of South Carolina, Charleston
WO	War Office Records, National Archives, Kew, United Kingdom

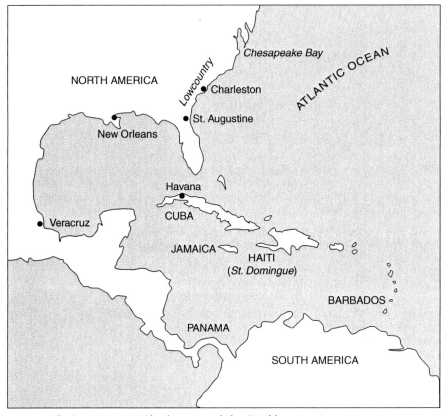

MAP 1. The Lowcountry, Charleston, and the Caribbean region.

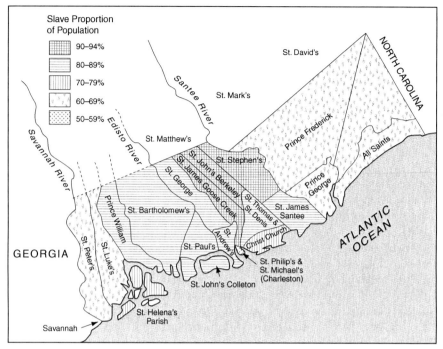

MAP 2. The South Carolina lowcountry, showing Anglican parishes and slave proportion of population, c. 1760s.

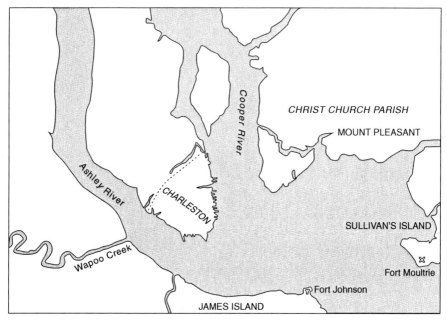

MAP 3. Charleston Harbor, based on a British map, c. 1780.
Source: Based on a contemporary map published in London.

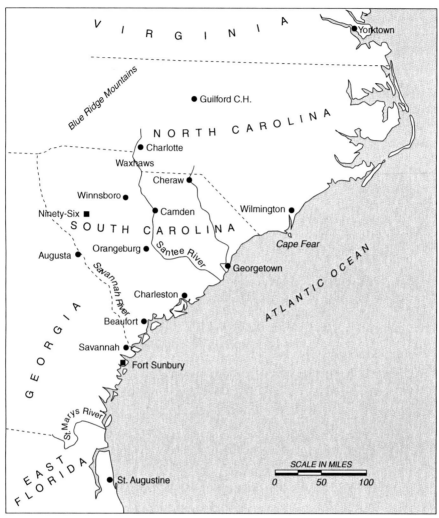

MAP 4. The Revolutionary War in the South.

PART I

TALK ABOUT SUFFERING

Talk about suffering here below,
And talk about loving Jesus.
Talk about suffering here below
And let's keep following Jesus.
                    Traditional Spiritual

Those who want to die quickly, go to Carolina

                    Eighteenth-century proverb

Many are dead. Many are running away to new settlements. The country is very sickly; I buried eight people the first nine weeks after I came to my parish. Forty two is looked upon to be the common age of man.

                    Robert Stone, 1750

Rhetoric and Reality

Black and white all mixed together,
Inconstant, strange, unhealthful weather
Burning heat and chilling cold
Dangerous both to young and old
Boisterous winds and heavy rains
Fevers and rheumatic pains
Agues plenty without doubt
Sores, boils, the prickling heat and gout
Mosquitoes on the skin make blotches
Centipedes and large cockroaches...
Water bad, past all drinking
Men and women without thinking...
Many a widow not unwilling
Many a beau not worth a shilling
Many a bargain if you strike it,
This is Charles-town, how do you like it?

Capt. Martin,
captain of a Man of War, 1769

[Charleston] is a noble monument of what human avarice can effect; its soil is a barren burning sand; with a river on either side, overflowing into pestilential marshes, which exhale a contagion so pernicious as to render sleeping a single night within its influence, during the summer months, an experiment of the utmost hazard ... But what will not men do, and bear, for money? These pestilential marshes are found to produce good rice, and the adjacent alluvions cotton; true, it is, no European frame could support the labour of cultivation, but Africa can furnish slaves, and thus amid contagion and suffering, both of oppressors and oppressed, has Charleston become a wealthy city – nay a religious one, too; to judge by the number of churches built, building, and to be built.

Francis Hall, 1817

Every day for years, the carriages passed my office on Glebe Street. Clop, clop, plop, plop, the horses went by, dragging their loads of tourists eager to hear about historic Charleston and the local plantation country. I often wondered what the drivers, adorned with gray Confederate caps and pants set off by bright red sashes, were telling them. Was it the sanitized version of local history I had heard so many times, or did the drivers tell the passengers how much people suffered to produce this unique slice of Old South ambience? Did they talk about the diseases that constantly assailed and thinned the population: yellow fever, malaria, dysentery, and smallpox? Did they explain how so much of the suffering from disease derived from the economy of plantation slavery, that gone-with-the-wind world of moonlight and magnolias? Perhaps they did talk about these things on another part of the trip, but what I overheard was more geared to fans of Scarlett and Rhett. The odor of horse dung and urine that occasionally wafted my way conveyed more truth about the past than the words I heard. Those odors, multiplied exponentially, and supplemented by the smells of cesspits, hog and cattle pens, slaughterhouses, dead dogs, cats, and humans, would have been a part of the ambient history of this place (see Figure 1.1). That was not unique to Charleston, of course; it would have been true of every town before exhaust fumes replaced those organic odors in the twentieth century. Perhaps the carriage drivers talked about Old Charleston's noxious smells; after all, such things are an endless source of amusement in our sanitized culture. But killer diseases? Maybe; some people can extract titillation even from deadly epidemics; for example, professors like me trying to keep students awake with jokes about microbes – "the gift that keeps on giving." Some years ago, a website specializing in satirical jabs at the "Holy City" (a local nickname for Charleston, along with the more apt "City of Disasters") lamented that tourists were not getting the complete lowcountry experience. To get a full taste of Historic Charleston, it was necessary to bring back the old diseases: malaria, cholera, and especially yellow fever, once known as "strangers' disease" because so many of its victims came "from off." The article reminded me of the quip that it's never safe to be nostalgic about anything until you're certain it can't come back. If yellow fever were around today, it might be known as "tourist's disease." But then if yellow fever were around, tourists would be few in number.[1]

As odd as it may seem, hearing and seeing these things helped prod me into writing this book. While researching an earlier book on the history of madness in South Carolina, I began to realize the immense role disease has played in the history of the Southern lowcountry, a region that extends from about Cape Fear in North Carolina to northern Florida, and inland from the Atlantic about 70 to 80 miles.[2] Having lived in Charleston for many years, I was vaguely aware that the lowcountry had once been an unhealthy place. But only immersing myself in eighteenth- and nineteenth-century sources brought

---

[1] The website was called "Upchuck." The "chuck" derives from a local slang term for Charleston, "Chucktown." The remark about nostalgia came from journalist Bill Vaughan.

[2] Peter McCandless, *Moonlight, Magnolias, and Madness: Insanity in South Carolina from the Colonial Period to the Progressive Era* (Chapel Hill: University of North Carolina Press, 1996).

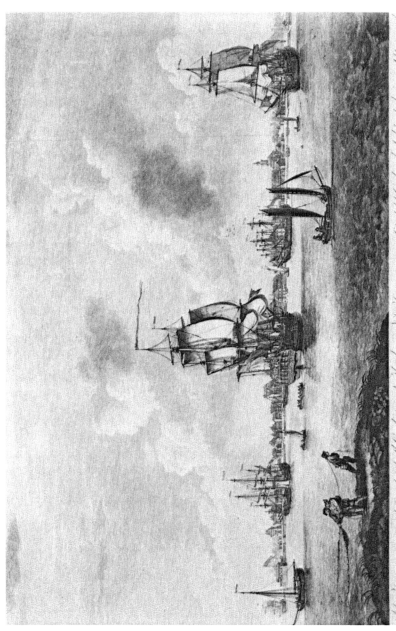

FIGURE 1.1. A View of Charles Town, the Capital of South Carolina in North America, 1768, Pierre Charles Canot (Library of Congress).

home to me just how unhealthy it had been. Other experiences brought me
personally and uncomfortably close to some of the truth about the region's
past. At the most basic level, the stifling heat and humidity for several months
a year made me wonder why anyone would want to settle there in the pre-air
conditioning age unless they could live on the beach. Summer trips to old rice
plantations taught me what it meant to be assaulted by clouds of voracious
mosquitoes, what one colonial planter aptly called devils in miniature. In
many former rice plantation areas, mosquitoes remain in control for months
at a time: Whenever I exited my car, thousands descended on me in seconds.
Like the elite planters of past times, I learned to visit the rice plantations in
the colder months. But even that might not be enough. A couple of years ago,
I was repeatedly attacked by mosquitoes on New Year's Day while walking in
an old rice-producing area. Perhaps this was just a result of global warming or
an unusually warm winter. Long before that experience, however, I concluded
that I could not have lasted long here in the plantation era and wondered how
anyone could have. Yet I knew that people had survived here, people who
must have been much stronger and tougher than I.

Today, many descendants of those people still live in the lowcountry, but
they also live all over the United States. It is estimated that about 40 percent
of today's African Americans descend from enslaved people who entered the
country through the port of Charleston. Sullivan's Island, at the entrance to
the harbor, is often called the Ellis Island of black America. Most Europeans
came voluntarily, drawn by the hope of becoming rich, or to escape poverty
or religious persecution. Their descendants, too, spread across America, especially the Lower South, spreading their plantation system, culture, and diseases. Many of the immigrants – European and African – died from those
diseases, too many and too young. The lowcountry was the deadliest disease
region on the North American mainland in the eighteenth and early nineteenth centuries. It was no country for old men, or rather for men who wished
to become old. Observers often noted how quickly people aged and died. In
the 1780s, traveler Johan David Schoepf declared that lowcountry residents –
white and black – seldom lived to an old age because their constitutions
were ruined by "the numerous fevers which every summer and autumn so
generally prevail."[3]

Many diseases contributed to the high mortality and morbidity rates of the
lowcountry. The region was a convention center for the diseases of the tropical
and temperate world. People living there had a "value-added" disease environment, with features of a wide spectrum of diseases from Africa, Europe, and
North America. As a result, it had higher mortality rates than more microbi-
ally deprived regions to the north. Among the most common and dangerous
diseases were malaria, yellow fever, smallpox, dysentery, respiratory disorders, numerous helminthic (worm) infestations, and tetanus. Yaws, a type

---

[3] Johann David Schoepf, *Travels in the Confederation, 1783–1784* (Reprint, New York: Burt
  Franklin, 1968), 216–217.

of nonvenereal syphilis, was common and often disfiguring but rarely fatal. These diseases were abetted occasionally by epidemics of measles, diphtheria, whooping cough, scarlet fever, and mumps. Many of the latter diseases were no more common in the lowcountry than in other parts of America, and are not singled out for particular attention here, although they formed a part of the overall disease matrix. For example, this book does not focus on cholera, a highly significant disease in many parts of the world. The reason is that cholera did not arrive in the region until very late in the story, in the 1830s, and did not have the impact it had on highly industrialized and urbanized regions. Two other major infectious diseases that I have largely ignored, typhoid and typhus, were surely present in the lowcountry at times, but do not appear to have affected the region more than other parts of British North America. On the other hand, I have devoted considerable space to smallpox, which was also probably no worse in the lowcountry than elsewhere in America. Smallpox is important to the story in part because Charleston was one of the first places in the West, in 1738, to use inoculation on a mass scale. This story has never been told in detail, unlike its earlier use in Boston in 1721, which has been recounted many times. Smallpox, like yellow fever, sometimes had an immense economic impact. Epidemics would virtually shut down the trade that was the lifeblood of the region. Smallpox, along with yellow fever, was a major focus of quarantine laws, which were highly contentious due to their effects on commerce. Much of the debate over inoculation was also concerned with its economic impact, and the connection between the economy and disease is central to the book's argument.

Slavery, Disease, and Suffering in the Southern Lowcountry focuses heavily on the impact of so-called tropical diseases. In 1768, British naval surgeon James Lind wrote that the danger of tropical fevers in South Carolina was far greater than in the colonies to the north, and was similar to that of the West Indies. Epidemiologically, as in many other ways, the lowcountry resembled the tropical and subtropical regions of the Americas, notably the plantation regions of the Caribbean and Brazil. The lowcountry is often referred to as the northern rim of the Caribbean. All these plantation lands were renowned for their slave majorities, wealth, and destruction of human life. They also shared many diseases of African origin: yellow fever, *falciparum* malaria, guinea worm, filariasis, and others. The lowcountry was unhealthier than some of these places. Barbados, for example, was virtually malaria free. The lowcountry also had epidemiological affinities with the rice-producing regions of southern Asia and West Africa, although the latter was deadlier.[4]

[4] James Lind, *An Essay on Diseases Incidental to Europeans in Hot Climates* (London, 1768), 36–37, 132–133, 148; J. R. McNeill, *Mosquito Empires: Ecology and War in the Greater Caribbean, 1640–1914* (New York: Cambridge University Press, 2010); Alfred W. Crosby, *Ecological Imperialism: The Biological Expansion of Europe, 900–1900* (Cambridge: Cambridge University Press, 2004), chapter 6; Richard S. Dunn, *Sugar and Slaves: The Rise of the Planter Class in the British West Indies, 1624–1713* (Chapel Hill: University of North Carolina Press, 2000); Richard B. Sheridan, *Sugar and Slavery: An Economic History of the*

Lowcountry rice plantations – abetted by a warm wet climate – provided an especially welcoming environment for diseases transmitted by mosquitoes and water-borne parasites. Mosquito-borne diseases – particularly malaria and yellow fever – and water-borne dysentery were the main diseases that gave the lowcountry its deadly reputation. Other mosquito-borne illnesses such as filariasis – the cause of elephantiasis – and dengue were common, if not endemic. These diseases thrived in its warm and wet climate, but nature was not the only culprit. Human migration – voluntary and forced – brought disease-causing microbes from Africa, Europe, and the Caribbean. A human invention, the rice plantation, helped keep them in circulation and spread them. The cultivation of rice provided large bodies of standing fresh water for malarial mosquitoes to breed in and large numbers of human bodies for them to bite. Microorganisms causing dysentery and other diarrheal diseases thrived in the region's warm waters. Parasitic worm infestations such as hookworm and guinea worm were ubiquitous in the countryside.[5] As a major importer of slaves, Charleston also got regular imports of yellow fever and other tropical diseases. The city's warm climate provided a pleasant home for the mosquitoes that carry yellow fever and dengue. By the 1690s at the latest, yellow fever had come, and it returned often until the 1870s. The other major ports of British North America – all in the north – also suffered yellow fever epidemics, but not as many as Charleston. Moreover, in the early nineteenth century, yellow fever retreated from the northern ports. Charleston proved to be a better host than those places, in part because it was warmer and closer to centers of endemic yellow fever in the Caribbean. No other disease became so identified with the city and so influenced its lifestyle, image, and culture. During the nineteenth century, as lowcountry people and their plantations moved west, yellow fever became a frequent visitor to southern ports and came to be seen as a southern problem. It also became a serious obstacle to commerce and immigration.[6]

British West Indies, 1623–1775 (Baltimore: Johns Hopkins University Press, 1974); David Watts, *The West Indies: Patterns of Development, Culture, and Environmental Change since 1492* (Cambridge: Cambridge University Press, 1987); Philip D. Curtin, *The Rise and Fall of the Plantation Complex* (New York: Cambridge University Press, 1990); Philip D. Curtin, *Death by Migration: Europe's Encounter with the Tropical World in the Nineteenth Century* (Cambridge and New York: Cambridge University Press, 1989); David Arnold, ed., *Warm Climates and Western Medicine: The Emergence of Tropical Medicine, 1500–1900* (Amsterdam: Rodopi, 1996); Peter A. Coclanis, *Time's Arrow, Time's Cycle: Globalization in South-East Asia over the Longue-Duree* (Singapore: Institute of South-East Asian Studies, 2006).

[5] E. Chernin, "The Disappearance of Bancroftian Filariasis from Charleston, South Carolina," *American Journal of Tropical Medicine and Hygiene* 37 (1987): 111–114; Todd Savitt, *Race and Medicine in Nineteenth- and Early Twentieth-Century America* (Kent, OH: Kent State University Press, 2007), 7–15. On human migration and the spread of disease microorganisms, see William H. McNeill, *Plagues and Peoples* (Garden City, NY: Anchor Press, 1976); Alfred W. Crosby, *Germs, Seeds and Animals: Studies in Ecological History* (Armonk, NY: M. E. Sharpe, 1994); Crosby, *Ecological Imperialism*.

[6] Margaret Humphreys, *Yellow Fever and the South* (Baltimore: Johns Hopkins University Press, 1992).

Ironically, the diseases that flourished in the lowcountry sometimes proved to be allies of the European settlers. Many Old World diseases struck Native Americans almost simultaneously and reduced their numbers exceedingly fast. The Indian nations that lived near the coast virtually disappeared within a few decades of the establishment of the Carolina colony, helped along by war and enslavement. As a result, they were not as much of an obstacle or threat to the new colony as they might have been. As an early governor put it, God had thinned their number to benefit the English. Disease, especially smallpox, greatly reduced the populations of the larger nations further inland as well, the Catawba and Cherokee. But they managed to survive as coherent groups into our own time, in part because they lived well back from the feverish coastal lowlands.

The role of Old World disease in reducing Native Americans numbers everywhere in the Americas is widely recognized today. Few people, however, are likely to be aware that lowcountry fevers helped the United States become independent. Of course, soldiers on both sides suffered higher casualties from disease than enemy action, as they always did before the twentieth century. Smallpox may have hurt the patriots more than the British before General Washington ordered a general inoculation of the Continental Army.[7] But British and Loyalist forces were severely mauled by fevers during the crucial southern campaign in the summer and fall of 1780. The following year, fear of further losses from disease was one of the main reasons Lord Cornwallis cited for his decision to march north to Virginia, where he lost the decisive Battle of Yorktown. The British faced many other obstacles during the southern campaign, notably a determined partisan resistance and a smaller number of Loyalist supporters than they had expected. Moreover, the presence of a French fleet at Yorktown made that encounter decisive by preventing British reinforcement or escape by sea. Nevertheless, the diseases of the Lower South greatly hindered British aims and actions and played an important role in deciding the outcome of the Revolutionary War.

Today, many people are vaguely aware that the Southern lowcountry was once a deadly region for whites. But they often think that blacks were wholly or largely immune to the diseases that killed so many whites, and that is why the planters chose them to work on the plantations. In the antebellum era, the real and alleged immunities of blacks to yellow fever and malaria became one of the justifications for slavery. In reality, people of all hues, including the oft-forgotten mixed-race folk, died in huge numbers from lowcountry diseases. But it was profitable and perhaps comforting to argue that Providence had graciously designed African bodies for the purpose of doing work for which whites were allegedly physically unsuited.[8]

---

[7] Elizabeth Fenn, *Pox Americana: The Great Smallpox Epidemic of 1775–1782* (New York: Hill and Wang, 2001); Ann Marie Becker, "Smallpox in Washington's Army: Strategic Implications of the Disease during the American Revolutionary War," *The Journal of Military History* 68 (2004): 381–430.

[8] Another example of the convenience of racial concepts is the idea that blacks felt, smelled, and sounded different from whites, and that whites could identify blacks through the senses

An argument of this sort was unnecessary in the first days of slavery in Carolina and perhaps inconceivable. The adoption of African slavery was not a response to an unhealthy environment. It was a major cause of it, along with human alterations of the landscape required for rice cultivation. White settlers did not bring African slaves to Carolina initially because they believed Africans were immune to local diseases, any more than people in colonies to the north enslaved Africans for that reason. Many of the earliest English settlers came from the sugar island of Barbados and they brought Africans with them as a matter of course. Sugar plantations using enslaved labor – white and black – had existed for centuries in the eastern Mediterranean, and planters from Portugal and Spain transferred that model to the New World. The Dutch, French, and English soon adopted it as well. On Barbados, white workers greatly outnumbered blacks at first. In 1638, indentured white laborers numbered about 2,000, blacks about 200. With the expansion of sugar cultivation, the demand for labor greatly increased. Barbadian planters decided that African slaves were easier to get, easier to manage, and cheaper to maintain than indentured white Britons. Disease surely helped speed the transformation. In 1647, yellow fever struck Barbados, probably the first epidemic in the New World. It killed far more whites than blacks, and Africans gradually replaced whites in the labor force. By 1670, when the Carolina colony was founded, Barbados contained about 30,000 blacks and 20,000 whites.[9]

No doubt the Barbadian planters believed black bodies were constitutionally more suited to labor in hot climates than white ones. It was a common European view. But – and this is an important point to be elaborated later – the white settlers who came to South Carolina in the 1670s did not believe they were going to a sickly environment. The colony's early rulers, the Lords Proprietors, published pamphlets praising it as a healthy and temperate location, indeed a paradise for English bodies. The authors of the pamphlets exaggerated, as promoters do, but the colony was not particularly unhealthy during its first decade. Nor did the white settlers arrive with a plan to set up the

---

of touch, smell, and hearing. Such claims became important in the antebellum period because of the increasing numbers of mixed-race people, and of "blacks" that looked "white." As with ideas about black immunities, they survived emancipation to provide support for segregation. See Mark M. Smith, *How Race is Made: Slavery, Segregation, and the Senses* (Chapel Hill: University of North Carolina Press, 2006).

[9] Stuart B. Schwartz, *Sugar Plantations in the Formation of Brazilian Society: Bahia, 1550–1835* (Cambridge: Cambridge University Press, 1985), chapter 1; Herbert S. Klein, *African Slavery in Latin America and the Caribbean* (Oxford and New York: Oxford University Press, 1986), chapters 1–3; Robin Blackburn, *The Making of New World Slavery* (London and New York: Verso, 1997), 229–232; Jack P. Greene, *Imperatives, Behaviors, and Identities: Essays in Early American Cultural History* (Charlottesville: The University Press of Virginia, 1992), chapter 2; Sheridan, *Sugar and Slavery*; Dunn, *Sugar and Slaves*; Walter Edgar, *South Carolina: A History* (Columbia: University of South Carolina Press, 1998), 35–38; Richard Waterhouse, *A New World Gentry: The Making of a Merchant and Planter Class in South Carolina, 1670–1770* (New York and London: Garland Publishing, Inc., 1989); Karen O. Kupperman, "Fear of Hot Climates in the Anglo-American Colonial Experience," *William and Mary Quarterly*, 3rd ser., 41 (1984): 213–240.

labor-intensive rice and indigo plantations that came to dominate the region's economy in the eighteenth century, supplemented by cotton in the nineteenth. The adoption of rice cultivation based on African slave labor emerged only after several decades of experiment with different crops, as indicated by the names of two early plantations, "Silk Hope" and "Rice Hope." The plantation system continued to evolve in various ways throughout the colonial and early national periods. The proportion of Africans in Carolina was much smaller in the first three decades of settlement than it later became – perhaps one-fourth to one-third of the several hundred settlers. They worked mainly at cattle herding, lumbering, and hunting for food.

The Africans were not alone as slaves. From an early period, the colonists enslaved Native Americans as well. Carolinians were the most active Indian slave traders in British North America. They exported Indian slaves to the northern and Caribbean colonies and sold them to local planters. In 1708, Native Americans made up about one-third of the slave labor force, 1,400 out of 4,300. But the rapid decline of local Indian populations left the field of labor open to slaves of African origin. Old World diseases helped ensure that the lowcountry, like the New World generally, would have a predominately Old World population. They also helped ensure that a large majority of the population would be of African descent into the twentieth century[10]

By 1700, rice had become a profitable staple and in the following decades the demand for enslaved labor increased greatly. By 1710, blacks constituted a majority of South Carolina's population. By 1730, the population was two-thirds black. A large immigration of whites into the backcountry from the late 1750s quickly narrowed the gap in the colony, and during the 1770s, whites constituted almost half of its population. But in the lowcountry, the black majority increased during the same period to more than 3 to 1. In most parishes, slaves constituted 70 percent or more of the population. In several, the proportion was as high as 9 to 1. Between 1790 and 1810, whites made up a slight majority of the state's population. During this period, however, the plantation system began to move into the upper country. Slave imports soared shortly before the legal slave trade was ended in 1808. By 1820, blacks were again the majority in South Carolina, a position they would retain until the early twentieth century. South Carolina was by far the largest importer of slaves among the mainland British colonies.[11]

---

[10] Peter Wood, *Black Majority: Negroes in Colonial South Carolina from 1670 through the Stono Rebellion* (New York: W.W. Norton, 1975); Peter A. Coclanis, *The Shadow of a Dream: Economic Life and Death in the South Carolina Low Country, 1670–1920* (New York and Oxford: Oxford University Press, 1989); Robert Weir, *Colonial South Carolina: A History* (Columbia: University of South Carolina Press, 1997; 1983), 26–27.

[11] Wood, *Black Majority*, 6–25, 131, 142–147, 151–152; Philip D. Morgan, *Slave Counterpoint: Black Culture in the Eighteenth-Century Chesapeake and Lowcountry* (Chapel Hill: University of North Carolina Press, 1998), 79, 95–96; Daniel Littlefield, *Rice and Slaves: Ethnicity and the Slave Trade in Colonial South Carolina* (Urbana and Chicago: University of Illinois Press, 1991), 116; Coclanis, *Shadow of a Dream*, 64–68; Edgar, *South Carolina*, 35–39, 78, 327.

The main reason the lowcountry became such a sickly place was the plantation economy the colonists created, and later defenses of the plantation system involved perverse distortion and denial of the epidemiological reality. As in many other parts of the Americas, the desire to produce staples in demand in an emerging global market created and drove the plantation system. The system produced enormous wealth for a small group: the merchant and planter elite. It also produced its own nemesis: the deadliest environment in North America, which in the long run helped undermine the economy of the region and even the prosperity of its elite. In the short and long run, it produced immense suffering for all the inhabitants, rich and poor, black and white. As large numbers of South Carolinians migrated westward in the nineteenth century, their diseases as well as their economic system influenced the culture, politics, and outlooks of the South and the nation. That influence remains strong.[12]

Between the late seventeenth and the early nineteenth century, the lowcountry received migrants from many disease regions. The pursuit of wealth brought together populations from different parts of Africa, the Americas, and Europe to work in the plantation lands. Unwittingly, the creators and enablers of the plantation system set in motion a global microbial migration. Along with the human migrants came their microbes, funneled through the tiny Charleston peninsula into the continent like an injection from a hypodermic needle. Alfred Crosby famously declared that "man and his migrations are the chief cause of epidemics." Sometimes people migrate to diseases; sometimes they migrate with them; sometimes they create them by the way they alter the environment.[13] In the case of the lowcountry, all three occurred. The eventual selection of rice as the main cash crop made things worse by providing ideal conditions for breeding the local mosquito vector of malaria. An English visitor to the region in 1817 succinctly summed up the results: "thus, amid contagion and suffering, both of oppressors and oppressed, has Charleston become a wealthy city."[14]

Of course, it is too simple to ascribe the disease environment of the lowcountry to greed alone, pervasive as it often was. Many of the colonists were fleeing religious persecution, notably French Huguenots, Scots and Scots-Irish Presbyterians, English Dissenters, German and Swiss Protestants. Others wished to escape from poverty or a fear of destitution. They had to find some way of making a living. Moreover, the decision of many of these people to

---

[12] Coclanis, *Shadow of a Dream*; Peter Coclanis, "Tracking the Economic Divergence of the North and the South," *Southern Cultures* 6.4 (2000), 82–103; Greene, *Pursuits of Happiness*, esp. 1–5, 142–151; Jeffrey Robert Young, *Domesticating Slavery: The Master Class in Georgia and South Carolina, 1670–1837* (Chapel Hill and London: University of North Carolina Press, 1999).

[13] Alfred W. Crosby, "Conquistador y Pestilencia: The First New World Pandemic and the Fall of the Great Indian Empires," *The Hispanic American Historical Review* 47 (1967): 322; McNeill, *Plagues and Peoples*.

[14] Francis Hall, *Travels in Canada and the United States in 1816 and 1817* (Boston, 1818), 245.

focus on crops like rice and later indigo was not entirely a matter of their own choosing. Despite the American myth of the self-made man, they were caught in a web of economic interdependence resulting from the emergence of a global economy. The lowcountry rice plantation was an outgrowth of the so-called Atlantic System, of which South Carolina became a small but not insignificant part. Its British overlords expected it to produce staples that could benefit the home country directly or through re-export to other countries. It was perhaps inevitable that the early settlers would look for economic models in places with similar climates and topographies, such as sugar plantations in the Mediterranean, eastern Atlantic, the Caribbean, Brazil, and the tobacco plantations in the Chesapeake regions of Virginia and Maryland. The mercantilist policies of the British government also encouraged such an outcome. But as noted earlier, rice emerged as the staple of choice only after decades of experimentation, and benefited from the presence of Africans with knowledge of its cultivation. In the 1740s, many planters added an upland crop, indigo, after the British government began to pay a bounty for its cultivation. Following the Revolution, the planters lost the bounty, and it took time for them to settle on cotton as a viable replacement. The choice was once again a response to external demand – in this case the needs of the mechanized British cotton industry.[15]

The early planters could not know that the economy they helped establish would have such ghastly epidemiological consequences. They were actors in a tragedy they had only partly helped write. This does not absolve them or their successors of responsibility for many aspects of the performance. The epidemiological consequences of their actions became increasingly clear in the late colonial and early national periods, even if they did not fully understand the processes that had produced this result. By then, some of them knew that the slave trade and rice cultivation were sources of deadly diseases. Their actions and sometimes their words prove it. But by then, they had also invested so much in the cultivation of rice and other staples with African labor that most of them found change inconceivable. Instead, they tended to deny or minimize the epidemiological effects, on Africans in particular.[16]

At the time the Carolina colony was founded, the Lords Proprietors, to whom Charles II granted the land, were concerned that disease might be a

---

[15] Weir, *Colonial South Carolina*, 61–65, 76–77; Wood, *Black Majority*; Coclanis, *Shadow of a Dream*; Littlefield, *Rice and Slaves*; Joyce E. Chaplin, *An Anxious Pursuit: Agricultural Innovation and Modernity in the Lower South, 1730–1815* (Chapel Hill: University of North Carolina Press, 1993); Judith Carney, *Black Rice* (Cambridge, MA: Harvard University Press, 2001); S. Max Edelson, *Plantation Enterprise in Colonial South Carolina* (Cambridge, MA: Harvard University Press, 2006); Lacy K. Ford, *The Origins of Southern Radicalism: The South Carolina Upcountry, 1800–1860* (New York: Oxford University Press, 1991).

[16] Coclanis, *Shadow of a Dream*; Coclanis, "Economic Divergence of the North and the South"; William Dusinberre, *Them Dark Days: Slavery in the American Rice Swamps* (Athens: University of Georgia Press, 2004); Young, *Domesticating Slavery*; Greene, *Imperatives, Behaviors, and Identities*, especially chapters 2–4.

problem. The reports of those they sent to explore it praised its healthiness, however, and the first colonists do not seem to have suffered much from disease. Promotional pamphlets from the early 1680s continued to emphasize the salubrious nature of Carolina, but around the middle of that decade, settlers began to die from infectious disease in large numbers. During the eighteenth century, the reputation of the region as a remarkably unhealthy place became well established. Despite mounting evidence that a virulent disease environment had developed, the colony's promoters developed a strategy that local boosters continued to employ well into the nineteenth century. They minimized the impact of disease and explained it as an anomaly, the result of personal imprudence, or a temporary problem that would soon be solved or resolve itself. Their denials and claims were sometimes perverse and produced perverse results. Their rhetoric ultimately redounded to the discredit of the region because it clashed glaringly with the lived experience of many people. Promoters of Carolina gained a reputation for mendaciousness, a reputation that later boosters of the region came to share. By minimizing or denying the danger of disease, they produced a huge credibility gap between rhetoric and reality.

Contemporary descriptions of the lowcountry disease environment both hide and reveal. Like shifting sands, they sometimes obscure the reality of immense human suffering beneath and sometimes provide a fleeting glimpse of it. Here and there, a strong wind blows and the reality is exposed in horrific detail. What we see, however, depends not on the movement of sand but on the vagaries of human records and how carefully we look at them. The suffering the rice plantation economy produced was obscured by elites who did not want to expose it and the illiteracy of most of those who suffered. But some people left detailed and revealing accounts of the impact of disease. From these accounts we can reconstruct something of the pestilent reality – and the perversity – that derived from the pursuit of prosperity. An example is the letters Francis Le Jau sent to the Society for the Propagation of the Gospel between 1706 and 1717.

Le Jau was a French Huguenot who had become a Church of England minister. The Society for Propagation of the Gospel (SPG), founded in 1701, sent him to South Carolina as a missionary. The colony was in turmoil when he arrived in 1706. The inhabitants had recently driven off a combined French and Spanish attack, and expected another. Protestant Dissenters and Anglicans were feuding furiously over the passage of an act making the Church of England the established church. More important for our story, Charleston was in the midst of a virulent yellow fever epidemic. The casualties included the first and until then the only SPG missionary in the colony, Samuel Thomas. Local officials immediately took Le Jau to his country parish, St. James Goose Creek, away from sickly Charleston. Despite this ominous beginning, Le Jau was cautiously optimistic about his chances for good health. He had been told that most newcomers suffered a bout of sickness during their first warm season in the region. People called it "the seasoning." It sounded like one was being preserved like a piece of meat, which, in a way, was true. "When I am seasoned to the country," Le Jau reflected, "I hope I'll do well." A few months after his arrival, his fibers braced by the pleasantly cool air of December, he was exuberant: "[T]his is the finest climate I ever saw, the soil produces every thing without much trouble, and at this time the weather is finer than in April with you in England." It was like paradise: "I am in health and well contented in this province, the climate and soil are admirable, the products may be improved with little trouble: any thing can grow here, we had a ravishing winter season; in January we had asparagus; in February roses and the woods full of flowers very fine and unknown to Europe; in March green peas and beans.... I hear only of three months wherein some days may be very hot; our springs are fine." He was equally pleased by the hospitality he had received from the local gentry, and impressed by their standard of living: "[F]or gentility, politeness and a handsome way of living this colony exceeds what I have seen. Poor families may come here and live very well; I don't talk of getting easily great estates which desire should never be in the heart of a Christian, but I mean they shall have a plenty of things necessary for life if they be industrious." He encouraged other clergymen to come to Carolina, where "they will find matters as I say, and much better."

In his early letters, Le Jau often sounds very much like a Carolina promoter. Before long, he began to rethink his positive assessment of both climate and people, and his altered perception of both was linked. During the summer of 1707, he became seriously ill for the first time. He was not unduly alarmed at first. Good soldier that he was, he blamed overwork in the heat and his own sins. His family arrived that summer and all of them quickly became sick. But had he not been told that a seasoning illness was "to be expected?" Carolina, he insisted, was "healthy enough," and he was sure recovery would come quickly. Instead, he remained almost constantly sick for more than a year with fevers and fluxes (dysentery or severe diarrhea). For months at a time, he was too ill to attend to his clerical duties. The summers turned out to be much hotter and longer than his parishioners had led him to expect, and his seasoning was agonizing and seemingly endless.

Notes of disillusionment crept into his letters. He began to sound as if he had been betrayed. Many of the white settlers were not the honest, sincere Christians he had first thought them to be. They were not content to live moderately well through honest industry but desired to become rich quickly and easily. They would "do any thing for money." Their religious profession was "often but a cloak" of hypocrisy covering grievous sins, notably mistreatment of slaves and Indians (some of whom were also slaves). Le Jau did not condemn slavery; indeed, he had several enslaved servants. His complaint was about the religious, moral, and physical abuse of the slaves. Many planters refused him permission to preach to their slaves and did nothing to prevent slaves' promiscuous cohabitation. Planters overworked them and punished them with hellish cruelty. Traders fomented war between Indian tribes and then bought war captives as slaves.

Le Jau's enthusiasm waned further when his wealthy parishioners failed to support him in his time of need. Few had honored their pledges of financial support, and inflation eroded what little he did receive. They had promised him a house and a church, which they never seemed able to finish. His fellow missionaries experienced similar problems: "I don't find that any of us can rely upon what is promised." As things stood, he could no longer encourage other clergymen to come to the colony. He urged the Society for the Propagation of the Gospel to be frank with any minister who desired to fill one of the vacant parishes, especially if he had a family: If such men "be your friends" they should be told that they "must prepare to suffer great hardships and crosses." Applicants for vacant parishes should not expect much generosity or honesty from the planters: "[T]hey deceived me more than I dare say."[17]

The writings of Le Jau and other disease sufferers are central to this book. When I began the research, my goal was to uncover the reality of disease's impact in the lowcountry. I soon began to doubt that it was possible to accomplish that goal, given the idiosyncratic nature of the historical record. The sources are mostly impressionistic; they are overwhelmingly focused on the white elite population; and statistics are patchy and sometimes of questionable validity. Finally, descriptions of the disease environment are often contradictory: The economic, political, or religious motives of the describers render many reports suspect. At one point, I decided to refocus the book around analyzing perceptions of disease rather than the reality. But that turned out to be unsatisfactory as well. Underneath layers of competing perceptions, I decided, one could glimpse some features of the reality. Despite contradictions and gaps in the historical record, a thorough examination of that record reveals not only immense suffering but an explanation for much of that suffering: One can call it greed or, more prosaically, economic forces, local and global, that produced the plantation system and ultimately a perverse denial of its epidemiological consequences.

These consequences eventually affected a far larger region than the lowcountry, and seldom in a good way. In the nineteenth century, many planters moved west, and their diseases moved with them, helping shape the culture of the American South and ultimately of the United States. Malaria became a fixture of life in many parts of the South until the early twentieth century. Yellow fever, once a scourge of northern ports, became a predominantly southern disease during the early nineteenth century. It not only attacked southern ports; it often moved well into the interior by water or railway lines. In terms of absolute numbers killed, the nation's worst yellow fever epidemic took place in Memphis, Tennessee, in 1878. The disease was not eradicated in the United States until the early twentieth century.[18] The "tropical" fevers affected

---

[17] Frank J. Klingberg, ed., *The Carolina Chronicle of Francis Le Jau* (Berkeley: University of California Press, 1956), 16–62, 88–89, 108–111.
[18] Margaret Humphreys, *Malaria: Poverty, Race, and Public Health in the United States* (Baltimore and London: Johns Hopkins University Press, 2001); Humphreys, *Yellow Fever*

settlement patterns, demographics, commerce, religion, education, and racial ideology. They helped make the South different from the rest of the nation, and because the South is a vitally important part of the United States – despite often being relegated to "Southern Studies" – they also influenced national culture, politics, economics, education, and religion.[19]

and the South; Ann Carrigan, *The Saffron Scourge: A History of Yellow Fever in Louisiana, 1796–1905* (Lafayette: University of Southwestern Louisiana Press, 1994); Khaled Bloom, *The Mississippi's Great Yellow Fever Epidemic of 1878* (Baton Rouge: Louisiana University Press, 1993); John H. Ellis, *Yellow Fever and Public Health in the New South* (Lexington: University of Kentucky Press, 1992).

[19] Todd L. Savitt and James H. Young, eds., *Disease and Distinctiveness in the American South* (Knoxville: University of Tennessee Press, 1988); Ronald L. Numbers and Todd L. Savitt, eds., *Science and Medicine in the Old South* (Baton Rouge: Louisiana State University Press, 1989); Stephen M. Stowe, *Doctoring the South: Southern Physicians and Everyday Medicine in the Mid-Nineteenth Century* (Chapel Hill: University of North Carolina Press, 2004), 5.

2

From Paradise to Hospital

A person with 500 pounds ... prudently managed in Carolina shall in a few years, live in as much plenty, yea more, than a man of 300 pounds a year in England; and if he continue careful ... shall increase to great wealth ... As to the air, it is serene and exceeding pleasant, and very healthy.

John Archdale, 1707

Myrtle Grove a terrestrial paradise? Let me see what paradisial objects present themselves to your mere corporeal view.... charming walks but ... they resemble the paths to the heavenly more than the walks to the earthly Garden of Eden.

George Ogilvie, 1774

An opinion generally prevails that South Carolina is unhealthy. This is neither correctly true nor wholly false.

David Ramsay, 1809

"THE SINK OF THE EARTH"

In the 1780s, German traveler Johan David Schoepf coined one of the most frequently quoted descriptions of South Carolina, when he wrote that "Carolina is in the spring a paradise, in the summer a hell, and in the autumn a hospital."[1] By "Carolina," Schoepf essentially meant the lowcountry. Schoepf's emphasis on the unhealthiness of the region was not unusual. By the time of the Revolution, the lowcountry was reputed the unhealthiest place in British North America. The anonymous author of *American Husbandry*, analyzing South Carolina a few years earlier, wrote "that the maritime part of the country is in one of the unhealthiest climates in the world cannot be doubted." The "excessive heat" of the climate, working on vast wetland areas of marsh, swamp, and rice fields, produced a deadly miasma: "from the mud

[1] Johann David Schoepf, *Travels in the Confederation, 1783–1784* (New York: Burt Franklin, 1968), 172, 216–217.

18

of these stinking sinks and sewers the heat exhales such putrid effluvia as must necessarily poison the air." The lowcountry was "the sink of the earth."[2] In 1800, Mary Inglis Hering compared the region to Jamaica, where she had lived, in terms of the ravages of fever, heat, and insects: "I must admit," she wrote to her newly arrived daughter, "that your first entre does not give you the most favorable opinion of [the lowcountry], visited as it is with a malignant fever, the weather so uncommonly hot for the time of year, and the abominable insects by which you and your children are almost devoured, is so like what I suffered in Jamaica, that I know exactly how you feel."[3] These images persisted well into the nineteenth century. In the 1840s, a British visitor proclaimed that the countryside near Charleston was "so unhealthy much of the year that the traveler who sleeps there but for one night a mile out of town, is almost sure to be attacked by the country fever [malaria]."[4]

The opinion was common. George Washington told a prospective British immigrant in the 1790s that the seaboard of the Carolinas and Georgia was such a sickly region that he would not choose to live there, and consequently would not say "anything that would induce others" to do so.[5] What would, and did, induce people to settle in the region, Washington knew, was the prospect of amassing great wealth. The author of *American Husbandry* asked rhetorically why people would choose to live in such an unhealthy place, and adduced two causes: the proximity to "ports and trade" and "the necessity of swamps for cultivating their grand staple, rice." If these incentives were removed, it was likely that "all of the inhabitants would flock backwards" into the much healthier backcountry.[6]

By the late colonial period, South Carolina was the wealthiest colony in British North America, with a booming economy based primarily on the staple production of rice and indigo. Its capital and main port, Charleston, glittered with wealth. In the 1770s, John G. W. De Brahm called Charleston "the most eminent and by far the richest city in the southern district of North America," replete with numerous stately homes, elegant churches, and opulent public buildings. Josiah Quincy of Massachusetts found the city "magnificent ... in grandeur, splendor of buildings, decorations, equipages, numbers, commerce, shipping, and indeed in almost every thing, it far surpasses all I ever saw, or ever expected to see in America ... All seems, at present, to be trade, riches, and magnificence."[7]

[2] Harry J. Carman, ed., *American Husbandry* (Port Washington, NY: Kennikat Press, Inc., 1964; originally published in London, 1775), 264.

[3] Mary Inglis Hering to Mrs. Henry Middleton, Jan. 8, 1800, SCHS, 43/0034.

[4] George Lewis, *Impressions of America and the American Churches* (Edinburgh, 1845), 112, quoted in Joseph I. Waring, *A History of Medicine in South Carolina, 1825–1900* (Charleston: Medical Society of South Carolina, 1967), 36.

[5] *The Writings of George Washington*, ed. John C. Fitzpatrick (Washington, DC: United States Government Printing Office, 1940), 35: 326.

[6] Carman, *American Husbandry*, 265.

[7] C. J. Weston Plowden, *Documents Connected with the History of South Carolina* (London, 1856), 195; *Memoir of Josiah Quincy*, quoted in *Yearbook, City of Charleston* (Charleston, 1880), 256.

Beginning in the late colonial period, many observers drew a direct connection between the lowcountry's wealth and its virulent disease environment. De Brahm argued that dams constructed to hold back water for use in rice fields had produced opulence but also deadly miasmas: "the corrosive vapours of these stagnant waters evaporating and mixing with the air become prejudicial to health by cloaking the stomachs of the inhabitants with slime, and corrupt their blood." The result was ubiquitous fevers and other disorders that tormented and killed both Europeans and Africans.[8] Dr. George Milligen declared that the planters were more concerned with acquiring "splendid fortunes" than preserving their health.[9] The observation was a common one in the late colonial period and after. Benjamin West remarked that the planters' "love of riches" trumped their "fear of death." How else could one explain their living in the swamps or on the riverbanks? To the author of *American Husbandry*, the planters' obsession with "the grand staple" of rice was so misguided as to be almost criminal. Farming the mephitic swamps could only be done at great human cost.[10] Francis Hall, a British officer who visited the region in the early nineteenth century, argued that the region's poor health was the direct consequence of its profitable economic system. Charleston, with its glittering mansions and impressive public edifices, was "a noble monument of what human avarice can effect." The city and its environs were so unhealthy that only the lure of large profits could explain their habitation: "But what will not men do, and bear, for money? These pestilential marshes are found to produce good rice, and the adjacent alluvions cotton."[11]

COMING TO PARADISE

Many people ascribed the unhealthiness of the lowcountry to its topography and climate. In 1779, Alexander Hewatt argued that the low-lying, swampy terrain and hot, humid climate differed so markedly from that of Northern Europe that the earliest colonists must have experienced extremely high mortality due to disease.[12] Evidence from the first years of English settlement does not support this view. Before the 1680s, most descriptions of Carolina stressed its remarkable healthiness. Soon after Charles II granted the territory

[8] John G. W. De Brahm, *Report of the General Survey in the Southern District of North America* ed. by Louis De Vorsey, Jr. (Columbia: University of South Carolina Press, 1971), 79. De Brahm's first name is sometimes listed as William.

[9] Chapman J. Milling, ed., *Colonial South Carolina: Two Contemporary Descriptions by Governor James Glen and Dr. George Milligen-Johnston* (Columbia: University of South Carolina Press, 1951), 44–45.

[10] *Life in the South, 1778–1779: Letters of Benjamin West*, ed. James S. Schoff (Ann Arbor, MI: The William Clements Library, 1963), 2; Carman, *American Husbandry*, 276–277; J. F. D. Smyth, *A Tour in the United States of America*, 2 vols. (London, 1784), 2: 53–54; Newton D. Mereness, ed. *Travels in the American Colonies* (New York, 1916), 399.

[11] Francis Hall, *Travels in Canada and the United States in 1816 and 1817* (Boston, 1818), 244–245.

[12] Alexander Hewatt, *An Historical Account of the Rise and Progress of the Colonies of South Carolina and Georgia*, 2 vols. (London, 1779) 1: 49–50, 2: 136–137.

to eight of his political allies, the "Lords Proprietors," in 1663, they began to sponsor promotional literature designed to attract settlers to the colony.[13] There was nothing unusual in this. All colonial ventures – just like all real estate developments today – had their promoters. The Carolina promotional pamphlets were unremarkable, too, in that they stressed the healthiness of the region. They declared that it was highly suitable to "English constitutions."[14] It was a slice of paradise located on the same latitude as the sunny, warm places of the Levant such as Palestine, Egypt and Syria. The author of one of the pamphlets admitted that he had never been to Carolina, but that did not prevent him from assuring prospective settlers that they would find a "serene air" which prevented infections of any kind. Extremes of heat were unknown in this temperate climate, upon which the heavens shone "the sovereign ray of health."[15] Another author declared that the colony's air was "of so serene a temper, that the Indian natives prolong their days to an extremity of old age."[16] One pamphlet designed to encourage Scottish immigrants called Carolina the healthiest of the king's territories in North America. Others repeated similar messages, including some written in French in a bid to attract Huguenot exiles to the new colony.[17]

Some pamphlets conceded that disease did occur, but insisted that it was a minor problem. In the summer, the settlers sometimes endured brief and mild "touches" of fever and ague.[18] One author explained that people who settled near large marshes sometimes suffered from agues, but added that was also true of people who lived near marshes in England. Those who inhabited areas more remote from marshes or standing waters were "exceedingly healthy." For those concerned about the next generation, the pamphlets stressed that the women were "very fruitful" and the children had ruddy, "fresh sanguine complexions."[19]

[13] On the promotional literature, see H. Roy Merrens, "The Physical Environment of Early America: Images and Image Makers in Colonial South Carolina," *Geographical Review* 59, No. 4 (Oct. 1969): 529–556; William S. Powell, "Carolina in the Seventeenth Century: An Annotated Bibliography of Contemporary Publications," *North Carolina Historical Review* 41 (Jan. 1964): 74–104.

[14] Alexander S. Salley, Jr., *Narratives of Early Carolina, 1650–1708* (New York: Barnes & Noble, 1967), 33, 45, 65–70; John Ogilby, *America: Being the Latest, and Most Accurate Description of the New World* (London, 1671), 205–212; Powell, "Carolina in the Seventeenth Century," 86–87.

[15] [Robert Ferguson], *The Present State of Carolina with Advice to the Settlers* (London, 1682).

[16] Salley, *Narratives*, 138–141; Powell, "Carolina in the Seventeenth Century," 92–93.

[17] [John Crafford], *A New and Most Exact Account of the Fertiles and Famous Colony of Carolina* (Dublin, 1683), title page; *Carolina Described More Fully then Heretofore* (Dublin, 1684). On the promotional literature directed toward Huguenots, see Bertrand van Ruymbeke, *From New Babylon to Eden: the Huguenots and Their Migration to Colonial South Carolina* (Columbia: University of South Carolina Press, 2006), 33–42; Powell, "Carolina in the Seventeenth Century."

[18] Salley, *Narratives*, 141.

[19] Salley, *Narratives*, 138–141, 168–169. See also *Carolina Described More Fully Then Heretofore* (Dublin, 1684), 2–5; Powell, "Carolina in the Seventeenth Century," 92–93.

It is easy to be skeptical about such claims. But if we can believe the words of the English settlers who arrived in the early 1670s, the Carolina colony initially enjoyed good health. Colonists' letters from this period stress the absence of serious illness.[20] Some of the letters sound like advertising and probably were. One from the early 1670s evokes comparisons of Carolina to Eden and the Promised Land. The colony's excellent climate, abundant vegetable and animal life, and location along the same latitude as Canaan and many other "healthy, fertile, and prosperous" lands, made it more like "a garden" than "an untilled place." Summers were warm but not so hot as to corrupt the air with "contagious infections." Carolina compared favorably with any place in the world "for health, pleasure, profit or delight." None of the 200 settlers had died thus far except the octogenarian Governor William Sayle.[21] Despite the exaggerated praise in the letters, if epidemics had struck the colony in the 1670s, it is unlikely that the fact could have been hidden. Epidemics of the 1680s and 1690s certainly were not. Carolina began its transformation from paradise to hospital.

A HOSPITAL IN THE MAKING

In 1680, Maurice Matthews, a large landowner and colonial official, described Carolina in much the same terms as the promotional pamphlets. The inhabitants enjoyed remarkably good health. Sometimes they suffered from "fever and ague" in the summer, but the illnesses were seldom fatal.[22] Mortal or not, any reports of fever concerned the Lords Proprietors, and they instructed local officials to establish port towns further up the rivers, in higher, drier locations than the current settlements.[23] Their concern proved well-founded. In 1684, they revealed that many people had told them that Charleston was in an unhealthy location; so many settlers were becoming sick that "it brings a disreputation upon the whole country." A few months later, they ordered the courts in Charleston shut down from June 10 to October 10, "so that men may not be obliged to come into so unhealthy a place at that time of the year." They suggested that newcomers be encouraged to settle far from the sea and that the seat of government be moved to a healthier location farther inland. Every effort should be made to minimize the need for the inhabitants to come to "sickly Charles Town"[24] Needless to say, this information did not appear in the promotional pamphlets.

The Proprietors were responding to the colony's first epidemiological crises. During the mid-1680s, more settlers left the colony than arrived,

[20] *Collections of the South Carolina Historical Society*, 5 vols. (Charleston, 1897) 5: 180, 185, 193, 197, 200–203.
[21] *Collections of South Carolina Historical Society*, 5: 307–309.
[22] Maurice Matthews, "A Contemporary View of Carolina in 1680," *SCHM*, 55 (1954), 153, 157.
[23] BPRO/SC, 1: 143, 149, 221.
[24] BPRO/SC, 2: 4–5, 35–36.

according to the colonial council.[25] Although the causes of discouragement were numerous – they included a fear of Spanish attacks, famine, and a hurricane – virulent disease was one of the most important.[26] Newly arrived settlers suffered especially heavily. In October 1684, 148 Scots led by Lord Cardross and William Dunlop arrived in Charleston on their way to establish a settlement at Port Royal. Despite a difficult ten-week voyage, only one of them had died so far. Once ashore, a raging disease in the town quickly killed many of them and demoralized others, who abandoned the expedition. In November, remnants of the group, many still ill, went on to Port Royal. They established Stuart Town on a stretch of bluff land away from "swamps and marshes" about twenty miles from the sea.[27] The losses continued. In a letter of 1686, Dunlop noted that he had lost eight of twenty-two people he had brought with him from Scotland, and seven other white indentured servants he had bought since. Most of the settlers who had arrived in a ship the previous year had also died. Nevertheless, he refused to believe that the country was unhealthy and resolved to go on "so long as we have six men alive."[28] Spanish attacks and disease in the summer of 1686 ended his dream. Only a handful of the Scots were able to bear arms, presumably because most of them were incapacitated by disease.[29]

Huguenot settlers who arrived in the 1680s received a similar epidemiological shock. In 1687, a Huguenot refugee in Boston recorded the arrival of two of his co-religionists from South Carolina, who declared that they had "never before seen so miserable a country, nor an atmosphere so unhealthy." Fevers prevailed throughout the year and were frequently mortal. Shortly before they left Charleston, a ship arrived from London with 130 passengers and crew. All but fifteen died from "malignant fevers" soon after landing. The informants reported that about eighty other Huguenots were coming from Carolina to settle in Massachusetts or New York.[30] About the same time, another Huguenot set out to counter the glowing reports of the promotional pamphlets. The author of *Remarques sur la Nouvelle Relacion de la Carolina par un Gentilhomme Francais* (1686) argued that the topography and climate

---

[25] "Spanish Depredations, 1686," *SCHM* 30 (1929), 84–86.

[26] *The Diary of Samuel Sewell, 1674–1729*, ed. by M. Halsey Thomas, 2 vols. (New York: Farrar, Strauss, & Giroux, 1973) 1:77.

[27] "Arrival of the Cardross Settlers," *SCHM* 30 (1929), 72–73.

[28] William Dunlop to James Montgomerie, undated [E], Letters of William Dunlop to James Montgomerie, photocopies of originals in Scottish Record Office, with handwritten transcripts, SCDAH.

[29] William Dunlop to James Montgomerie, July 15, 1686 [B], 1686 [before Aug. 17] [G], Oct. 21, 1686 [C], July 13, 1687 [F], Letters of William Dunlop to James Montgomerie; "Spanish Depredations, 1686" *SCHM* 30 (1929): 82; Charles H. Lesser, *South Carolina Begins: The Records of a Proprietary Colony, 1663–1721* (Columbia: South Carolina Department of Archives and History, 1995).

[30] Charles Washington Baird, *History of the Huguenot Emigration to America*, 2 vols. (New York, 1885) 1: 393. Baird's source was "A Narrative of a French Protestant Refugee in Boston, 1687,"in Bibliotheque de Geneve, Collection Court, No. 17, tome I, folios 71–76.

of Carolina – flat terrain, damp air, and heavy rains – made it an unhealthy place. As proof, he offered the "frequent sickness and great mortality which have reigned there." Charleston was a "charnel house." The bad publicity Carolina received from these accounts may explain a decline in Huguenot immigrants to the colony after 1686.[31]

The epidemics of the mid-1680s justified the Proprietors' forebodings. The colony was indeed acquiring a "disreputation." Added to real or perceived dangers from the Spanish, Indians, pirates, heat, hurricanes, earthquakes, rattlesnakes, and alligators, disease was proving to be a major bar to immigration. This was a matter of serious concern to the Proprietors who could not hope to make much profit off a sparsely inhabited colony. It was equally troubling to the existing settlers who needed reinforcement for military as well as economic reasons, given the proximity of the Spanish in Florida and the outbreak of war with France in 1689. The bleak prospect of the settlement was worsened by religious and political dissensions among the colonists themselves, especially between Anglicans and Dissenters, the first fighting for the establishment of the Church of England and the second struggling to maintain the religious toleration the Proprietors had promised to all settlers. In 1690, the Proprietors warned that religious factionalism would discourage potential newcomers, which the colony could ill afford because "[m]en will die in Carolina for some time faster than they are born or grow up, and if none come to you your numbers will by degrees [be] so diminished, that you will be easily cut off by the Indians or pirates."[32] When the Proprietors appointed Quaker John Archdale governor of the province in 1694, they urged him to establish towns in places that were healthy "and commodious for commerce" and to promote the draining of marshes – a truly Herculean assignment.[33]

New settlers may have made the situation sound worse than it was, because they had been encouraged by promotional literature to believe that they were going to paradise. The extravagant hopes the colony aroused in newly arrived settlers emerges from letters of 1690 from Scot John Stewart to William Dunlop, former leader of the short-lived Scottish colony near Port Royal. By this time, Dunlop had returned to Scotland. Stewart had remained and urged Dunlop to return, reminding him that he was once a stout advocate of the province's bounty and potential: "Remember, Dear Major, Jerusalem's parallel latitude ... did you not at my first arrival here ... comfort me with the plaudits of pleasant Carolina [where] ... the most clownish and poorest planter may justly hope for an earl's estate?... a climate the very phoenix

[31] No copy of the French original of *Remarques* has apparently survived, but William Gilmore Simms reviewed it in "South Carolina in 1686," in *The Magnolia; or, Southern Apalachian,* Oct. 1842, 226–229; see also, Van Ruymbeke, *From New Babylon to Eden,* 43–44, 48; Powell, "Carolina in the Seventeenth Century," 102–103; *Transactions of the Huguenot Society of South Carolina,* 1, no. 5 (1897): 88–90.

[32] James W. Rivers, *A Sketch of the History of South Carolina to the Close of the Proprietary Government* (Charleston, 1856), 415.

[33] BPRO/SC, 3:140–141.

of the universe, liable to no extremes, salubrious ... to a miracle." Stewart sounded as if he was being sarcastic – he had previously mentioned that he had recently suffered from "the greatest load of sickness and despondency in my life" – but perhaps he wasn't. He went on to declare that Carolina could be turned into a highly profitable country, and was "the paradise of America." He also declared that Charleston was now healthy and that in his vicinity along the upper Cooper River, no white person had died for nineteen months except for a woman of seventy years of age.[34]

Stewart may not have been exaggerating, at least not much. By the early 1690s, the colony had emerged from its first epidemiological crisis. For several years, none of the sources report any epidemic disease. The colony may also have momentarily shed its disreputable image, to judge by the instructions that a group of prospective migrants from Massachusetts brought with them in 1697. They were told to observe the country carefully and make an accurate report about its character, including its disease environment: "We would have you curious in informing yourselves how the country is for health: and whether the climate does agree well with the bodies of New England people." This passage indicates that the mortality of the 1680s had not fatally injured Carolina's reputation in New England. But the New Englanders did not share the utopian outlook of settlers fed on a diet of promotional pamphlets. They firmly downplayed anticipations of paradise: It was "vanity" to expect "that any country on this side [of] heaven should have a writ of ease and security against disease or death." They merely wanted to be sure that the country was not much unhealthier than their own; they also had heard that Carolina water was not pure. The New Englanders arrived at an opportune time, or so it seemed. In 1697, local officials informed the Proprietors that the colony was extremely healthy and growing in population and wealth.[35]

That soon changed. Between 1698 and 1700, smallpox and yellow fever ravaged the population. The smallpox lasted for nine or ten months and killed hundreds of settlers and slaves. Some colonists managed to find a silver lining. Smallpox had devastated the Indians to such an extent, officials reported, that they would not present a danger to the colonists for years to come. Affra Coming related that one nearby nation had been virtually extinguished, except for a few who "ran away and left their dead unburied lying on the ground for vultures to devour." Governor John Archdale viewed the epidemic as part of the divine plan: "[T]he hand of God was eminently seen in thinning the Indians, to make room for the English." Providence had graciously spared the English the necessity of killing off the Indians themselves, permitting them to avoid the cruelties the Spanish had inflicted on such inconvenient people. Archdale did not mention – perhaps did not realize – that the colonists had

---

[34] "Letters from John Stewart to William Dunlop," *SCHM* 32 (1931), 4–5, 20, 23.

[35] "Instructions for Emigrants from Essex County, Massachusetts, to South Carolina," 1697, in *Yearbook, City of Charleston* (Charleston, 1899), 150–152; *Commissions and Instructions from the Lords Proprietors of Carolina to the Public Officials of South Carolina, 1685–1715,* ed. by A.S. Salley, Jr. (Columbia, 1916), 102.

helped spread the epidemic, especially traders involved in the Indian slave trade and the trade in deerskins.[36] Smallpox and other Old World diseases, along with war and enslavement, thinned the Indians numbers so rapidly by the early eighteenth century that most of the small coastal tribes had disappeared as organized communities. By the mid-eighteenth century, only a few hundred of the Indians survived.[37] Indian losses may have temporarily removed any danger from that quarter, but they also hurt the lucrative deerskin trade. In fact, the epidemics virtually stopped all kinds of trade for more than a year. They also struck a severe blow at the colony's image and discouraged new settlers for a time. Coming wrote to her sister in England, advising her not to come to Carolina until "you can hear [of] better times ... for the whole country is full of trouble and sickness."[38]

Following the yellow fever epidemic of 1699, Boston's Samuel Sewall recorded "amazing news of the dismal mortality in Charlestown," with people dying so fast that they were being taken to the grave piled up in carts.[39] Sewall's source, Hugh Adams, was a recent immigrant from New England, who described the epidemic as "dreadful and astonishing ... a tempest of mortality ... worse by far than the Great Plague of London, considering the smallness of the town. Shops shut up for six weeks; nothing but carrying medicines, digging graves, carting the dead; to the great astonishment of all beholders."[40] In addition to the pestilence, a major fire burned down a large section of Charleston and it was struck by an earthquake. Stunned officials – many of them replacements for ones who had died – informed the Proprietors that these disasters had greatly disheartened the settlers. The provincial assembly did not meet between November 1698 and October 1700. In desperation, the council appealed to their lordships to find some means of encouraging new settlers.[41]

[36] Anne Simons Deas, *Recollections of the Ball Family of South Carolina* (Charleston, 1909), 29–30; John Lawson, *A New Voyage to Carolina*, ed. by Hugh T. Lefler (Chapel Hill: University of North Carolina Press, 1967), 231–232; Salley, *Narratives*, 285; Paul Kelton, "The Great Southeastern Smallpox Epidemic, 1696–1700," in *The Transformation of the Southeastern Indians, 1540–1760*, ed. by Robbie Ethridge and Charles Hudson (Jackson: University Press of Mississippi, 2002), 21–37.

[37] James H. Merrell, *The Indians' New World* (Chapel Hill: University of North Carolina Press, 1989), 18–21, 97–98, 136–137, 193–196; Kelton, "Southeastern Smallpox Epidemic," 36–37; Peter H. Wood, "The Changing Population of the Colonial South: An Overview by Race and Region, 1685–1790," in Gregory A. Waselkov, ed., *Powhatan's Mantle: Indians in the Colonial Southeast* (Lincoln and London: University of Nebraska Press, 1989), 35–65; Gene Waddell, *Indians of the South Carolina Lowcountry, 1562–1751* (Columbia, SC: Southern Studies Program, 1980), 8–15.

[38] *Commissions and Instructions from the Lords Proprietors*, 103; Anne Simons Deas, *Recollections of the Ball Family of South Carolina* (Charleston, 1909; reprint, 1978), 29–30.

[39] *The Diary of Samuel Sewell, 1674–1729*, ed. M. Halsey Thomas, 2 vols. (New York: Farrar, Strauss, & Giroux, 1973), 1: 415.

[40] Massachusetts Historical Society, *Collections*, 5th ser., 6: 11–12; Petrona Royall McIver, "Wappetaw Congregational Church," *SCHM* 58 (1957), 40–41.

[41] *Commissions and Instructions from the Lords Proprietors*, 103, 129, 131, 135, 145, 148; Salley, *Narratives*, 199–200; BPRO/SC, 4: 58.

For a few years after 1700, the colony was relatively healthy, and immigrants once again began to come. It was merely a reprieve. In 1706, yellow fever killed hundreds in Charleston.[42] The pattern continued. Between 1710 and 1712, the young colony was extremely sickly, as several disorders swept it simultaneously. The sources list smallpox, pleurisies, bloody flux, pestilential fevers, and dry belly-ache. Never had the town experienced "a more sickly or fatal season," exclaimed Gideon Johnston. Hardly anyone had been spared: "[T]he town looks miserably thin and disconsolate, and there is not one house in twenty that has not considerably suffered and still labours under this general calamity." Few people came to church. Some people shut themselves up in their houses to avoid infection. Others were too busy nursing the sick to go to church or anywhere else. Francis Le Jau added that the mortality struck every family in his parish at Goose Creek, some fifteen miles upriver from the capital. An "abundance of newcomers" had recently died.[43] Mary Stafford ascribed the deaths to heat: "We have been as if we were baked in an oven and multitudes of people died."[44]

CONTESTED TERRAIN

To counter the colony's growing reputation for unhealthiness, promoters gradually adopted a new strategy. True, some continued to portray it as a land of milk and honey, where only the stupid, lazy, or immoral could fail to achieve great wealth. John Lawson, hired by the Proprietors as surveyor-general of North Carolina, published a book based on his travels through the Carolinas in 1700. Lawson repeated the effusive praise of many of the earlier promotional tracts. Carolina was "a delicious country, being placed in that girdle of the world which affords wine, oil, fruit, grain, and silk, with other rich commodities, besides a sweet air, moderate climate, and fertile soil … blessings … that spin out the thread of life to its utmost extent, and crown our days with the sweets of health and plenty." The inhabitants lived "an easy and pleasant life."[45]

After the early 1700s, however, it was difficult for promoters to completely ignore the problem of disease. Instead, they tended to describe it as exaggerated or avoidable by prudent conduct. John Archdale denied that the region

[42] BPRO/SC, 5: 107, 161–162, 203–204; *Commissions and Instructions from the Lords Proprietors*, 189, 273; Frank Klingberg, ed., *The Carolina Chronicle of Francis Le Jau, 1706–1717* (Berkeley and Los Angeles: University of California Press, 1956), 16–18.

[43] Frank J. Klingberg, ed., *Carolina Chronicle: The Papers of Commissary Gideon Johnston, 1710–1716* (Berkeley and Los Angeles: University of California Press, 1946), 34–37, 71, 75–77, 98–104; Klingberg, *Le Jau*, 103–115; Benjamin Dennis, Feb. 26, 1711/12, SPG, A7: 402–403; Frank Klingberg, "Commissary Johnston's Notitia Parochialis," *SCHM* 48 (1947), 26–34; *Stat.* 2: 382; JCHA, Oct. 26, 1711, SCDAH; John Duffy, "Eighteenth-Century Carolina Health Conditions," *Journal of Southern History* 18 (1952): 289–302; John Duffy, "Yellow Fever in Colonial Charleston," *SCHM*, 52 (1951), 192.

[44] "A Letter Written in 1711 by Mary Stafford to her Kinswoman in England," *SCHM* 81 (1980), 2–3, 6.

[45] Lawson, *New Voyage to Carolina*, 86, 93.

was naturally unhealthy. The first planters, he noted – correctly – had seldom
had any "raging sickness." Archdale conceded the obvious: In late summer,
fevers were endemic and often dangerous to newcomers. But like some of the
early pamphlets, he described the most common diseases as "gentle touches
of fever and ague." The malignant epidemic diseases (yellow fever and smallpox) that had recently scourged the colony were not native but imported, or
arose from intemperate living.[46] Other promoters echoed Archdale's main
arguments. In 1712, John Norris conceded that people living in the lowest
marshlands often suffered from fever and ague, especially if they were newcomers. After their "seasoning," they were generally very healthy if they lived
temperately and resided on high, dry land. Many chronic diseases common in
Europe, such as gout and stone, were rare.[47] In the 1730s, Jean-Pierre Purry
used similar arguments to lure Swiss settlers to the inland townships he was
promoting near the Savannah River. Unlike Archdale, Purry claimed that the
first English settlers had "very fatal beginnings." But now people who lived
prudently were healthy and rich.[48]

They could also live long lives, according to the *South Carolina Gazette*.
The *Gazette*, established in 1731, often disputed Carolina's reputation for
unhealthiness. In 1734, it published the obituary of Elizabeth Baker, who died
at age 104. Baker had been in the colony for 54 years, had 12 children, 25
grandchildren, and 43 great-grandchildren. On other occasions, the newspaper cited the deaths of superannuated locals as proof that Carolinians could
live as long as in other parts of the world. In 1735, the *Gazette* reported the
death of Captain Anthony Matthews at 73. Like Mrs. Baker, he had been in
Carolina since 1680. But what the paper emphasized was that his coffin was
carried by six "ancient inhabitants" whose combined ages were about 400
years. When the *Gazette* reported the death of Colonel Miles Brewton in 1745
at age 70, it commented that "this instance joined to many others, that might
be produced of ancient settlers ... might be urged as a pretty strong argument
to remove a too common prejudice entertained by our northern neighbours
against us ... that grey-hairs would not flourish in this climate."[49]

The reference to northern prejudices is an early example of a regional defen-
siveness that would become more pronounced in the nineteenth century. But
as many locals knew, it was more than prejudice. Anglican minister Robert
Stone wrote that in his parish, "forty-two is looked upon to be the common
age of man." Moreover, in a region with a majority black slave population, it
was considered crucial to attract white immigrants. One way to do that was

---

[46] Salley, *Narratives*, 290–308.

[47] Jack P. Greene, ed., *Selling a New World: Two Colonial South Carolina Promotional Pamphlets by Thomas Nairne and John Norris* (Columbia: University of South Carolina Press, 1989), 92.

[48] B. R. Carroll, *Historical Collections of South Carolina* 2 vols. (New York: Harper & Brothers, 1836), 2: 128, 135–136.

[49] SCG, April 1, 1751, July 22, 1745; A. S. Salley, *Death Notices in the South Carolina Gazette, 1731–1775* (Charleston: Historical Commission of South Carolina, 1917), 8–10, 27, 31.

to convince prospective settlers that they had a good chance of longevity. The *Gazette's* editors made the case at every opportunity. Their efforts may have been seen as more necessary by the appearance in the 1730s and 1740s of pamphlets promoting the healthiness of the new colony to the south, Georgia. Emphasizing South Carolina's healthiness for whites, however, contradicted a key rationale for African slavery – that whites were unable to perform hard labor in such a climate. The contradiction continued throughout slavery times.[50]

Reports that the region's unhealthiness had been exaggerated lured some prospective settlers. James Steuart wrote to his father in 1749 on the eve of leaving for South Carolina that he was going "to a good climate – excepting two months as healthy a place as in the world."[51] In 1798, Charles Cotton, an English schoolteacher seeking his fortune in America, decided to head for Charleston after being told that it was "not so unhealthy as is generally thought." The local disorders generally arose "from intemperance and want of caution in exposing themselves to the night dews."[52] Settlers sometimes repeated benign descriptions of the disease environment after their arrival. A Scot who returned to his native country after about ten years in Virginia and Carolina told his doctor that he had always enjoyed perfect health in both places. His only illness during that period, he claimed, was a severe fever he contracted during a visit to his native Scotland.[53] Swiss Anthony Gondy wrote his brother in Lausanne in 1733 that the Carolina air was healthy. The country was "an earthly paradise" where nobody worked more than two months a year and anyone could get rich quickly. Gondy's letter echoed the early promotional pamphlets and was probably part of Purry's campaign to recruit Swiss settlers.[54]

Disillusionment came soon for many newcomers. When Cotton arrived in Charleston, he reported that it was "remarkably healthy."[55] But he quickly changed his tune. During his first summer in the city, he was tormented by heat, mosquitoes, and fevers. He was fortunate to avoid yellow fever, which killed hundreds of strangers that year, by fleeing Charleston for the rural hinterland, but there he contracted malaria. Deciding that the climate was extremely unhealthy, the following year he fled to Ontario, where he became minister to an Anglican Church.[56] Suffering newcomers sometimes denounced the colony's promoters as mendacious, in part because of their myopic descriptions of the region's healthiness. In the early 1700s, Anglican Commissary Gideon Johnston lamented that the colony had been "magnified to an uncommon

---

[50] Betty Wood, *Slavery in Colonial Georgia, 1730–1775* (Athens: The University of Georgia Press, 1984), 9–11.

[51] James Steuart to John Steuart of Dalguise, July 7, 8, Oct. 17, 1749, Steuart of Dalguise Muniments, SRO/GD38/2/9/15.

[52] "The Letters of Charles Caleb Cotton, 1798–1802," *SCHM* 51 (1950): 133.

[53] William Cullen MSS, Royal College of Physicians, Edinburgh, Vol. IX (1782) letter no. 143.

[54] R. W. Kelsey, "Swiss Settlers in South Carolina," *SCHM* 23 (1922): 86–88.

[55] "Cotton Letters," 217.

[56] "Cotton Letters," 140, 142, 217–218, 220, 223–226.

degree." Reading and hearing tales about the paradisiacal nature of Carolina made "a strange impression upon the fancy of a missionary when he is at London." The reality of the province was "poverty and diseases." Thus "deceived and disappointed," Johnston dubbed the Carolinians "the vilest race of men" on earth.[57]

Swiss immigrant Samuel Dyssli wrote home to friends and families in the 1730s warning them that Purry's pamphlet extolling Carolina as a paradise was a pack of lies. Dyssli had suffered from severe bouts of fever and bloody flux for several months, as well as "a great swelling" in his belly that made him feel as if he would burst. He told people back home that they should not think of coming to the region, "for diseases here have too much sway and people have died in masses." Carolina was "a damned fraud" and he was heading to Pennsylvania.[58] Wernhard Trachsler, another Swiss, agreed. He declared that everybody who came to the colony would "endure severe diseases, especially fevers, from which the most die." A Swiss publication of the time repeated a proverb then supposedly circulating in England: "Those who want to die quickly go to Carolina."[59] John Tobler, a German who settled in the Carolina backcountry in the 1750s, warned his countrymen not to go to Charleston in the hot months because of the "severe and dangerous contagious fevers which occasionally bring many people to the grave." Tobler attributed Charleston's unhealthiness to its role as a major seaport and importer of slaves: "The blame is placed on the many ships which land there, coming from all parts of the world, especially from Africa with blackamoor slaves, on whose arrival often yellow fever, smallpox, and other diseases follow, just as if they had brought them along."[60] Alexander Hewatt rejected what he saw as one of the most fundamental errors of the promotion literature: the claim that Carolina was as healthy as Palestine and Egypt because they shared the same latitude. Significant differences in climate and terrain, he argued, made Carolina one of the unhealthiest places in the world.[61]

The sense of betrayal many settlers felt provoked Governor James Glen to condemn the too optimistic language of the promotional literature. He wrote the Duke of Bedford in 1748 that he wished "that some honest plain account of Carolina was printed ... avoiding all false and flattering descriptions." The existing accounts made those that were "deluded by them think themselves

---

[57] Klingberg, *Johnston*, 22, 60–61.

[58] Kelsey, "Swiss Settlers in South Carolina," 89–91.

[59] Gilbert P. Vogt, "Swiss Notes on South Carolina," *SCHM* 21 (1920): 102; Merrens, "Physical Environment," 535. Merrens states that in Switzerland, it became common practice in the 1730s to publish counterarguments to pamphlets encouraging immigration to South Carolina. The descriptions of Dyssli and Trachsler may have been examples of this counterpromotion.

[60] "John Tobler's Description of South Carolina (1753)," ed. and trans. Walter L. Robbins, *SCHM* 71 (1970): 146; James Grant to Alex. Brodie, Sept. 22, 1757, James Grant Manuscripts, SCL.

[61] Alexander Hewatt, *An Historical Account of the Rise and Progress of the Colonies of South Carolina and Georgia* 2 vols. (London, 1779), 1: 79.

trepanned when they do not find the paradise that had been painted to them."[62] In 1751, Glen himself wrote an analysis of the colony that conceded its health dangers but also argued that its population was beginning to adjust to them. He referred to the settled white inhabitants as "an invaluable treasure." By this he meant that many of them had become "seasoned" to the lowcountry disease environment and had developed strategies to cope with its threats to health: "[M]any thousands must have died before such a number could have been established, so habituated to the climate ... acquainted with our seasons, their sudden changes, and the methods of guarding against them."[63] Glen was surely being honest, although he made the process sound less horrible than it was. On another occasion, he called the climate "pretty healthful."

During the late eighteenth and early nineteenth centuries, some South Carolina promoters followed Glen's advice, but their accounts were not entirely honest or plain. They sought to paint a picture of the disease environment that conceded some of its dangers without being so pessimistic as to stifle white immigration. They ascribed the local fevers, like Alexander Hewatt, largely to climate and terrain, but they rejected his view that Carolina was one of the unhealthiest places on earth. One of the most prominent of the promoters in this period was David Ramsay, who came to Charleston from his native Pennsylvania in 1774 (see Figure 2.1). Ramsay's descriptions of the region conceded that the terrain and climate produced potentially dangerous miasmas. In the swamps, bays, and low grounds, he declared, "the waters spread over the face of the country, and in consequence of heat and stagnation produce mephitic exhalations. Thick fogs cover the low lands throughout the night during the summer months.... In such a situation it is no matter of surprise that fevers prevail in places contiguous to fresh, and especially stagnant water ... when weeds and vegetables are rankest, and putrefaction is excited by the operations of heat and moisture, the atmosphere becomes deleterious."[64] Ramsay's contemporary, planter and governor John Drayton, said much the same thing: "Continually intersected by multitudes of swamps, bays, and low grounds; and having large reservoirs of water, and rice fields at particular times overflowed, the elasticity of the atmosphere is weakened; and its tonic power thereby reduced. Acted on by the rays of the sun, and indifferently exposed to the action of the winds, the waters, thus spread over the face of the country, become unfriendly to health, and acquire some degree of mephitic influence." The sun's heat acting on water and plants saturated the air with humidity, leading to heavy rains, dews, and fogs that planted the seeds of fevers.[65] Ramsay and Drayton did not conclude from this, however, that

[62] BPRO/SC, 23: 233; Milling, *Colonial South Carolina*, 39; BPRO/SC, 21: 403.
[63] Milling, *Colonial South Carolina*, 11, 16, 31; BPRO/SC, 24: 303–330, contains Glen's complete report.
[64] David Ramsay, *History of South Carolina* 2 vols. (Charleston, 1858; first published 1809), 2: 36.
[65] John Drayton, *A View of South Carolina as Respects her Natural and Civil Concerns* (Charleston, 1802), 16.

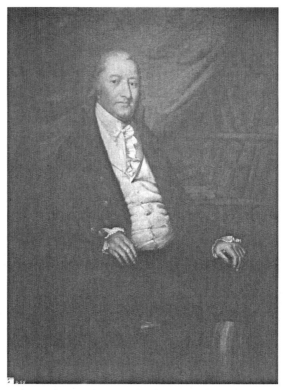

FIGURE 2.1. David Ramsay, M.D., medical writer, historian, patriot, and South Carolina booster (Courtesy of the Waring Historical Library, MUSC).

the region was inevitably unhealthy, only potentially so. Like Archdale, they declared that the prudent could live as healthily there as elsewhere in America. They also argued that the disease environment or climate was improving and would continue to improve as the result of human action, particularly agricultural development. The one thing they did not do was blame the rice plantation economy, even though by their time many people had posited a connection between rice cultivation and fevers.

One change that may have reduced the incidence of malaria somewhat in the late eighteenth century was the gradual switch from the cultivation of rice in swamps to a system of tidal cultivation. This involved cultivating fields along the banks of tidal rivers. The fields were protected by dikes and flood-gates that allowed planters to use the rising tide to flood the fields with fresh water and the falling tide to drain the fields. This method solved two major problems of swamp cultivation: weeding and irrigation. Inadvertently, it may have reduced the population of mosquito vectors because the alternate flood-ing and draining of the fields disrupted their breeding. Tidal cultivation also allowed some planters to move their houses away from the swamps, which were better suited to the breeding habits of the malarial mosquitoes. The adoption of tidal cultivation is unlikely to have brought a great reduction in the incidence of malaria, however. It did not become common until after the Revolution, and many planters continued swamp cultivation for long thereafter. Some antebellum observers thought the problem of malaria became worse after the Revolution.[66]

The idea of an improving disease environment did not begin with Ramsay and Drayton. The English naturalist Mark Catesby, who visited the region in the 1720s, declared that "where the country is opened and cleared of wood, the winds have a freer passage, and the air grows daily more healthy."[67] The idea that clearing forests was beneficial to health was common. Even Hewatt claimed that cultivation, especially in the interior, had made the climate more "salubrious and pleasant." In 1774, planter George Ogilvie rejected the view that his uncle's Santee plantation, Myrtle Grove, was "a terrestrial paradise" but predicted that in time it would become a pleasant and healthy place.[68]

After the Revolution, Ramsay became the greatest champion of the improving disease environment idea. Ironically, when he first came to Charleston, he had found the lowcountry repellent. Soon after he arrived, he informed Benjamin Rush that even the prospect of great wealth could not lure him to live permanently in such a sickly region. But as he settled in, married into the elite, and became one of Charleston's intellectual leaders, Ramsay wrote more optimistically about his adopted homeland. A staunch patriot, he argued that the state had been much healthier since independence. Perhaps in that he was right. The departure of the opposing armies and a temporary prohibition of the slave trade may have reduced the ravages of disease for a time. Surprisingly, Ramsay did not credit the suspension of the slave trade for the improvement because he had argued soon after moving there that the region's ubiquitous fevers were due more to slavery than the climate.[69] But he wrote nothing about that in subsequent years. Perhaps this was because any criticism of slavery was becoming increasingly hazardous, especially for those who had political ambitions, as he did. His marriage to Martha Laurens, whose father, Henry Laurens, a merchant-planter who had become immensely wealthy through the slave trade, may also have helped to alter his views. After the 1790s, Ramsay hardly mentioned slavery at all in his writings, and blacks largely disappeared from his view, too. It is difficult to escape the conclusion

[66] Randall M. Packard, *The Making of a Tropical Disease: A Short History of Malaria* (Baltimore: Johns Hopkins University Press, 2007), 59–60.

[67] Mark Catesby, *The Natural History of Carolina, Florida, and the Bahama Islands* 2 vols. (London: 1771), 1: i.

[68] Hewatt, *Historical Account*, 2: 135–137; George Ogilvie to Margaret Ogilvie, Nov. 22, 1774, Ogilvie-Forbes of Boyndlie Papers, University of Aberdeen Archives; McNeill, *Mosquito Empires*, 30, 48.

[69] Robert L. Brunhouse, ed., *David Ramsay, 1749–1815: Selections from His Writings*, Transactions of the American Philosophical Society, N.S. 55, Part 4. (Philadelphia: American Philosophical Society, 1965), 99, 113.

that a desire to be accepted as a political and intellectual leader in his adopted state motivated his changes of opinion on the connection between slavery and disease. At the same time, and perhaps not coincidentally, he began to promote his adopted home. Most relevant here is that he began to dispute the widespread notion that the lowcountry was unhealthier than other parts of America. Some of his arguments sound like modern political spin: "Instead of saying, '[Charleston] is more sickly than other maritime towns of the United States,' it ought only to be said, 'that more care is necessary on the part of its inhabitants for the preservation of their health.'" But he could also be more direct. In 1790, he published an essay arguing that health conditions in the lowcountry were better than its reputation proclaimed and were improving all the time. He concluded that "Charleston is now more healthy than formerly, and likely to be more and more so.... I indulge the hope that our grandchildren will be less exposed to fevers than we are." Some Charlestonians would soon go much farther and claim that their city was the healthiest in America.[70] Much like rice had become the region's economic staple, a disjunction between its epidemiological reality and descriptions of that reality had become a staple of its thought.

Ramsay's work is significant in another way. Earlier promoters of the region had directed their arguments at prospective immigrants. Ramsay focused his also at lowcountry residents, as if trying to convince them – and perhaps himself – that their homeland was not as unhealthy as they thought. Perhaps he was trying to stem "white flight" to the backcountry and beyond. Everywhere he found reason for local folk to be optimistic about their epidemiological circumstances. The coastal pinelands, though unproductive, were healthy. In Charleston, the disease situation had improved and further improvement could be expected through increased attention to drainage and sanitation. Bilious remitting autumnal fevers (which probably included malaria, dengue, and yellow fever) in the city had "evidently declined" in recent years. Smallpox was now of little consequence thanks to inoculation. Pleurisies were now much less common and more easily curable. The dry belly ache, or dry gripes, was seldom a problem anymore. Yellow fever, a great danger until the 1740s, had disappeared. True, the city had suffered epidemics of a malignant fever in 1792 and 1794, which mimicked yellow fever in many of its characteristics, but Ramsay insisted that it was another disease, not contagious or dangerous to locals. A few years later, he conceded that

[70] David Ramsay, *A Dissertation on the Means of Preserving Health in Charleston, and the Adjacent Lowcountry* (Charleston, 1790), 31–32; David Ramsay, *A Sketch of the Soil, Climate, Weather, and Diseases of South Carolina* (Charleston, 1796), 25; Arthur H. Schaefer, *To Be An American: David Ramsay and the Making of the American Consciousness* (Columbia: University of South Carolina Press, 1991); Arthur H. Schaefer, "David Ramsay and the Limits of Revolutionary Nationalism," in David Moltke-Hansen and Michael O'Brien, eds., *Intellectual Life in Antebellum Charleston* (Knoxville: University of Tennessee Press, 1986), 47–84.

the disease in question was yellow fever, but maintained that it was no longer as dangerous as it once had been. Ramsay sometimes seemed inconsistent. In one place, he attributed improvements in health to the clearing and cultivation of land. The cutting down of trees had "destroyed their perspiration," making the "rich low grounds ... higher and drier." But elsewhere he stated that the "felling of trees, and the opening of avenues to the rivers," had helped to spread the "marsh miasmata" that caused fevers, and that "bilious remitting and intermittent fevers had increased in the countryside."[71]

Moreover, lurking elsewhere in one of Ramsay's works was a different, almost subversive picture. The appendix to his *History of South Carolina* (1809) contains epidemiological reports he had solicited from others. That by fellow doctor Isaac Auld reported that on Edisto Island, just south of Charleston, "the climate may be considered sickly." This reality, Auld added, should "excite no surprise." The marvel was that the inhabitants were not even unhealthier in such an environment. The marshes and ponds in the central parts of the island were extremely dangerous areas. Fresh water from the Edisto River penetrated these places during high tides and floods and then stagnated. Auld's description, as he acknowledged, fit many locations in the lowcountry, and the vital statistics he revealed were depressingly similar as well. More than three-fourths of the white inhabitants had died in the past fifteen years. The annual mortality rate for that period was one in twenty-two. In 1798, one white person in eight died of autumnal fevers. Of the twenty-four white deaths, seventeen were children under the age of five years. In 1802, dysentery had ravaged the island, killing many "respectable characters" as well as a large number of blacks. Since then, the island had been somewhat healthier. Nevertheless, the situation of white families was precarious. White females outnumbered males 135 to 111. Among the surviving children of thirty-eight white families in 1808, females outnumbered males seventy-two to forty-seven. Few people lived long. Only two whites on the island were older than seventy, both widows in poor health. White births had slightly exceeded deaths in recent years, but the white population was continuing to decline because many families were leaving the island. In contrast, the black population was increasing. In 1807, slaves outnumbered whites 11 to 1, 2,609 to 236 overall. Given this disparity, perhaps it is not surprising that Auld noted "a disposition among the [white] islanders to treat this patient and laborious race with indulgence and to meliorate their condition." Some planters were even contemplating supplying their slaves with more expensive "regular rations of beef or some other animal food" at least during the busiest times of the farming year.

In St. Stephens Parish on the Santee River, Ramsay's informant reported drily that "this district is not remarkable for the longevity of its inhabitants."

---

[71] Ramsay, *Soil, Climate, Weather, and Diseases*, pp. 8–9, 20–28; see also Ramsay, *History of South Carolina*, 2: 36, 40, 42, 54–56.

Only two of the white residents were older than sixty years. In Orangeburg District, Ramsay's sources reported that the healthiest people were those who lived on the high and open pinelands. People who lived in low areas, near stagnant ponds, fresh water bays, riverbanks, and mill ponds, were often afflicted with fevers. These places were the "scourge of country settlements." With no apparent sense of contradiction, the writers criticized local planters for not properly appreciating the profits they could make from farming the bogs and swamps. The juxtaposition illustrates how a concern with profit making could trump logic and reality. In the port of Georgetown, about sixty miles north of Charleston, Ramsay's informants were more optimistic, but why is hard to say. They claimed that the town had become healthier in recent years, but the evidence they presented was unconvincing. Between 1796 and 1808, there had been 399 deaths among the white population, which numbered only 624 in the latter year. Deaths averaged thirty-three per year, or a very high one in nineteen of the population. All through these reports in Ramsay's appendix runs a tension between a depressing reality and an attempt to spin it into something less grim. Moreover, Ramsay's summary was much more optimistic than the evidence of his informers.

Ramsay's views were echoed in a broadsheet of 1795 issued by the South Carolina Society. This elite group was promoting immigration to the new state. Ramsay was then vice president of the society. They admitted that the swampy areas of the lowcountry could not be cultivated by white men without danger to health and life. But the swamps had given the entire state an undeserved reputation for unhealthiness. Swamps made up a small part of the state. Whites could live healthily in Charleston, in the pinelands, or in the backcountry.[72] John Drayton repeated these views in *A View of South Carolina* (1802). He conceded that bilious, remitting, and intermitting fevers were common in the swampy regions. But such a situation was probably temporary, and the state possessed many healthy areas in its pine-barrens and interior uplands. Some planters spent the fever months in Charleston, but the majority continued to reside on their country plantations and many of them were as healthy as people anywhere in the world. Yellow fever was confined to Charleston and did not appear every year. Moreover, natives of the city and long-term residents were seldom hurt by this disorder. Its victims were newcomers and they could take precautions to avoid the fever.[73]

Boosterism is a historical constant. In the lowcountry, however, the consequences of minimizing the region's unhealthiness were particularly tragic. People who read only the promotional literature would not have felt

---

[72] Ramsay, *History of South Carolina*, 2: 278–286, 294, 299–303; *Information, To those who are disposed to migrate to South Carolina* (Charleston, 1795), in Early American Imprints, first series, no. 28411.

[73] Drayton, *View of South Carolina*, 16, 21, 24–28. See also, Robert Mills, *Statistics of South Carolina* (Charleston, 1826), 138–149.

unduly alarmed at the prospect of coming to the region. For many of those who did come, the result was an early death. Some prospective migrants may also have read works that presented a far less benign view of the disease environment. An example is a book by John Davis, an Englishman who – by happy chance – had been tutor to John Drayton's children. Davis found Drayton's claim that yellow fever was dangerous only to strangers no consolation: "The mortality among foreigners during the summer months at Charleston is incredibly great. Few Europeans escape.... The attack is always sudden, and lays hold of the strongest. He, whose veins glowed but yesterday with health, shall today be undergoing the agonies of the damned." Moreover, it appeared that Drayton did not fully believe his own rhetoric about yellow fever not being harmful to locals. In common with many other elite families, he moved his family to the beaches of nearby Sullivan's Island in the hot season to avoid this scourge "which every summer commits its ravages in Charleston." Drayton's seasonal relocations were not unusual. Elite South Carolinians, Davis declared, were some of the most migratory folk in the world. After leaving Sullivan's Island in the fall, Drayton took his family to Drayton Hall, his stately neo-Palladian mansion on the Ashley River. Soon afterward, Davis decided that he could no longer remain in "the tainted atmosphere that had dispatched so many of my countrymen" and he "left this charming family" to seek a healthier climate.[74] Two decades later, another English visitor repeated the connection so many observers had made between the region's prosperity and its unhealthiness. Isaac Holmes, like John Davis, highlighted the dangers to strangers and discussed the peregrinations of wealthy South Carolinians to avoid the lowcountry's diseases. In June of every year, he noted, nearly all of the whites who could afford it escaped to the North, or to other healthier locations within the state, to escape the local fevers. However, most of the migrants returned in late fall, "the prospect of wealth encouraging them to brave every danger."[75] As we shall see, "the prospect of wealth" – or at least jobs – also lured many unlucky strangers to an early death.

Some locals, however, continued to insist that the region had improved and would continue to improve in healthiness. In his *Statistics of South Carolina* (1826), architect Robert Mills predicted that the danger of fevers would recede with more extensive "cultivation and agricultural advancement."[76] Over the long term, this optimism would appear to have been justified. Killer diseases like malaria, yellow fever, and smallpox did decline and then disappeared from the region during the next century or so. But predictions of a distant healthy future were probably of little consolation to many inhabitants and even less to prospective settlers. In 1815, Alice Izard concluded that Carolina would be a

[74] John Davis, *Travels of Four Years and a Half in the United States of America, 1798–1802* (London, 1803), 112, 114–115.
[75] Isaac Holmes, *An Account of the United States of America* (London, 1823), 277.
[76] Mills, *Statistics*, 140.

healthy country in 50 or 100 years. But in the meantime she added, Candide-like, "We must endeavour to make the best of our situation."[77] How people tried to make the best of their situation, and how disease and their efforts to combat it shaped their world and beyond, is the subject of the remainder of this book.

---

[77] A. Izard to Mrs. Manigault, Feb. 9, 1815, Manigault FP, SCL.

3

"A Scene of Diseases"

At Midnight when the Fever rag'd
By Physick Art still unasswag'd,
And tortur'd me with Pain:
When most it scorch'd my aching Head,
Like sulph'rous Fire, or liquid Lead,
And hiss'd through every Vein.

> *South Carolina Gazette,*
> July 28, 1732

I was ill with fever in Purrysburg about three months and afterwards in Georgia at Savannah ... I had the bloody flux for six months. Also a great swelling befell me. My whole belly was swollen so that I might have burst.

> Samuel Dyssli, 1737

I am heartily tired of Carolina and dread the approach of summer which I am afraid will renew my intermittent complaint, from which I have never been thoroughly free since August last.

> John Murray of Murraywhat, 1763

"A COMPLICATION OF DISORDERS"

In 1711, Gideon Johnston, Anglican Commissary in Charleston, described his body as "a scene of diseases." The phrase could have been a metaphor for the lowcountry, for it encapsulated the experience of much of the population. Another Anglican missionary aptly summed up the situation when he wrote that he had endured "a complication of disorders."[1] Many people suffered almost continually from one disease or another, sometimes several at once. It is not always possible to determine what people suffered or died

---

[1] Klingberg, *Johnston*, 35; Petition of William Langhorne to the Archbishop of Canterbury, Nov. 20, 1751, quoted in John Duffy, "Eighteenth-Century Carolina Health Conditions," *Journal of Southern History* 18 (1952), 296.

from in particular cases, but we can identify the major culprits. The most visible suffering was that caused by deadly epidemics, mainly smallpox and yellow fever but also other epidemics from time to time. Such "malignant" epidemics were part of the public sphere: Official documents and newspapers (after 1731) often discussed them, at least once they could no longer be denied to exist. Harder to detect in public sources are the endemic disorders that claimed numerous victims every year. Any disease can be endemic or epidemic, depending on its degree of frequency and regularity within a given community. For example, smallpox was endemic in large European cities but epidemic in the Americas. Malaria became endemic in the lowcountry during the colonial period but could also become epidemic under certain conditions. Endemic diseases were the disease equivalent of background noise. They were regularly present but rarely caused a ripple in the public sphere, unless their victim was someone of importance. In the long run, however, they caused more suffering and death than the epidemics. The diaries, letters, and journals of eighteenth-century visitors and residents are filled with laments about various fevers, respiratory disorders, dysentery, and other excruciating maladies. Nearly everyone suffered to some degree from these disorders, regardless of color, origins, or wealth.[2]

In 1776, Lionel Chalmers (see Figure 3.1) published a two-volume study on the relationship between weather and diseases in South Carolina. He classified the diseases into those of spring, summer, autumn, and winter. His system was flawed but his chapters provide a litany of the myriad diseases that afflicted the lowcountry. Just as it hosted a huge variety of flora and fauna, to the great delight of naturalists, it also provided a comfortable residence for microbes and parasites of many regions. The most common warm-weather diseases were fevers (malaria, yellow fever, dengue, and perhaps typhoid), fluxes (dysentery and severe diarrhea), worm infestations, and the dry belly ache or dry gripes (a form of colic due to lead poisoning). The main winter diseases were respiratory and throat infections: pleurisies and peripneumonies (such as pneumonia and bronchitis), catarrhal fevers (such as influenza), and quinsies (severe throat disorders such as diphtheria and scarlet fever).[3] In 1789, Dr. Samuel Miller, who practiced in the rice-producing areas along the lower Santee River, wrote that he "had more business than I could rightly manage." His patients suffered most frequently from "remittents, called here the fall fever, dysentery, malignant sore throat, diarrhea, putrid and nervous fevers, and in the winter season peripneumonia." Worm infestations were common among children.[4]

[2] Francis Hall, *Travels in Canada and the United States in 1816 and 1817* (Boston, 1818), 245.
[3] Lionel Chalmers, *An Account of the Weather and Diseases of South-Carolina* 2 vols. (London, 1776) 1: 66, 2: 10, 21–55, 65; George Milligen-Johnston, *A Short Description of the Province of South Carolina* (London, 1770), 43; John Duffy, *Epidemics in Colonial America* (Baton Rouge: Louisiana State University Press, 1953), 125–134, 180–181, 189–193, 214–222; Oscar Reiss, *Medicine in Colonial America* (Lanham, MD: University Press of America, 2000), 330.
[4] Samuel Miller to William Cullen, Oct. 6, 1789, Cullen Mss., Royal College of Physicians, Edinburgh.

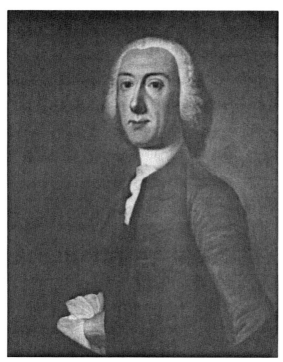

FIGURE 3.1. Lionel Chalmers, M.D., author of *Weather and Diseases of South Carolina* (London, 1776) (Courtesy of the Waring Historical Library, MUSC).

Of the endemic disorders, dysentery was one of the biggest causes of suffering and death. Dysentery can be caused by an amoeba, by bacteria, and sometimes by worms. The main symptoms are severe diarrhea, blood or mucus in the feces, and sometimes vomiting of blood. Separating dysentery from other diarrheal disorders and malaria, however, can be difficult. People frequently complained of enduring flux and fever together and they probably did. But malaria sometimes produces dysentery-like symptoms, so it is often difficult to be sure when both or only one is at work. References to fluxes abound in correspondence and diaries. In 1710, Gideon Johnston reported that the flux had been "fatal to a great many this year ... I dread it more than any other disease." It had killed several of his colleagues.[5]

Malaria was the king of the endemic disorders, and the one that did most to give the region its unhealthy reputation. It was known by many names: ague and fever or simply ague, intermittent fever, remittent fever, bilious fever, nervous fever, and country fever. In the 1780s, Francisco de Miranda declared the lowcountry so "infested with the ague" that if one asked a native how they were they would often answer, "teeth chattering with cold of the ague, 'Pretty

⁵ Klingberg, *Johnston*, 34–63.

well, only the fever!'"[6] Malaria provoked much less public discussion than yellow fever and smallpox, probably because it was so common. It was also less likely to kill, at least right away. But its impact in terms of morbidity and mortality was greater than either. Whereas yellow fever and smallpox tended to erupt in spectacular but relatively short-lived epidemics, and yellow fever was confined largely to Charleston before the nineteenth century, malaria quietly and steadily eroded the lives and energy of a large part of the population. It continued to plague the region and much of the South throughout the eighteenth and nineteenth centuries. It did not recede completely from South Carolina until the 1950s.

The most common symptoms of malaria are fever, chills, and aches. In classic cases, malarial fevers are intermittent, with paroxysms of chills and fever at regular intervals; but the classic patterns are seldom evident except in "virgin" or first cases of the disease, and do not occur in the deadly *falciparum* type. Lionel Chalmers emphasized this lack of regularity in the 1770s: "intermitting fevers ... are sometimes so irregular, as to be scarcely reducible to any class, which hitherto hath been described; for the fits are of unequal continuance, and the intermissions as uncertain as to time."[7] In severe cases malaria may produce vomiting, severe headaches, anemia, convulsions, rashes, hemorrhaging, hypoglycemia (low blood sugar), liver dysfunction, enlargement of the spleen, kidney failure, and excess fluid in the lungs. Chalmers described the onset of malarial fevers as follows: "they commence with a sensible or even a severe horror; and [are] attended with bilious vomitings; and a violent head-ache or a stupor will accompany fevers, more especially if the belly be bound, as it now generally is ... a painful lassitude, head-ache, sickness at the stomach, thirst, as well as a hard and too quick pulse."[8]

Malaria was well known in the ancient world. It remains one of the greatest causes of sickness and death on earth, accounting for about 1–2 million deaths and hundreds of millions of debilitating infections per year. It is particularly dangerous among young children and pregnant women. The maternal deaths, abortions, miscarriages, stillbirths, and neonatal deaths malaria caused the lowering of the lowcountry's birth rate. The many fatalities among children greatly lowered the average life span. Because it mimics other diseases and lowers the body's ability to fight them off, malaria was probably responsible, directly and indirectly, for a great proportion of illness and death ascribed to other disorders.[9] Malaria infections generally began in the early summer and

---

[6] Francisco de Miranda, *The New Democracy in America, 1783–1784*, trans. by Judson P. Wood and ed. by John S. Ezell (Norman: University of Oklahoma Press, 1963), 33.

[7] Chalmers, *Weather and Diseases*, 1: 178–179, 2: 6–7; Margaret Humphreys, *Malaria: Poverty, Race, and Public Health in the United States* (Baltimore and London: Johns Hopkins University Press, 2001), 28.

[8] Chalmers, *Weather and Diseases*, 2: 62–63.

[9] Leonard Jan Bruce-Chwatt, *Essential Malariology*, 2d edition (New York: John Wiley and Sons), 62–65; Herbert M. Gilles and David A. Warell, *Bruce-Chwatt's Essential Malariology*, 3d edition (New York: Oxford University Press, 1993), 36–49; Humphreys, *Malaria*, 28;

continued into the late autumn or early winter, often ending only with a sharp frost. A case contracted in the fall might linger into the winter, weakening resistance to respiratory disorders. Relapses often occurred in the spring. Depending on the type, the effects of malaria could last months or even years. Reinfections were common, but had one advantage for those determined or forced to stay in the region: They provided partial immunity or resistance in survivors.

Malaria was often misdiagnosed as something else, including dengue (break-bone) fever, yellow fever, dysentery, pneumonia, worms, influenza, and even tuberculosis. Margaret Humphreys notes that "twentieth-century physicians had trouble diagnosing malaria with certainty into the 1940s, so retrospective diagnosis to the colonial era should be made with both care and humility." The fact that patients can harbor more than one malaria infection at a time further complicates identification of the disease.[10] Diagnostic confusion in the past was increased by the various names used to denote malaria, which themselves were often inconsistently used. It should be stressed that not all illnesses labeled with these names were necessarily malaria. Almost any spell of fever with chills might be called fever and ague. Any fever with remissions might be termed an intermittent or a remittent. Any fever contracted in rural areas during warm weather might be denoted country fever. Remittent fever might denote malaria or some other fever with an intermission, such as dengue. Bilious (or bilious remittent) fever could mean malaria, dengue, yellow fever, or something else that affected the liver. From around 1800, South Carolinians often used the term "country fever" to distinguish what we call malaria from yellow fever, which was largely an urban disease.

Malaria is a parasitic infection caused by protozoa known as plasmodia and transmitted by anopheline mosquitoes, which are abundant in the low-country. The main local vector, *A. quadrimaculatus*, is not the most efficient transmitter of the plasmodium, but in the lowcountry, it made up for this by its ubiquity. Avoiding mosquito bites during the warm weather months was virtually impossible, especially for anyone living on rice plantations. When George Ogilvie sought to disabuse his sister of the notion that a lowcountry plantation was "a terrestrial paradise," he asked her to picture "swarms of mosquitoes … drawing blood at every pore."[11] Two types of malaria became prevalent in the lowcountry: *Plasmodium vivax* and *Plasmodium falciparum*. A third form, *Plasmodium malariae*, may also have been present, but was much less important. For reasons that are not entirely clear, *vivax* tends to be a disease of the early summer and midsummer, *falciparum* of the late summer and fall. It is impossible to pinpoint the exact moment of arrival the various

Randall M. Packard, *The Making of a Tropical Disease: A Short History of Malaria* (Baltimore: Johns Hopkins University Press, 2007).

[10] Humphreys, *Malaria*, 26–28; Bruce-Chwatt, *Essential Malariology*, 38.

[11] George Ogilvie of Auchiries to Margaret Ogilvie, Nov. 22, 1774, Ogilvie-Forbes of Boyndlie Papers, University of Aberdeen Archives.

forms of malaria in the lowcountry, but *vivax* and *falciparum* were both present by the 1690s. *Vivax*, the less virulent of the two, probably came from England in the 1670s. *Vivax* was endemic in marshy areas of the British Isles and occasionally epidemic in London and other areas in the seventeenth and eighteenth centuries, even as far north as Scotland.[12]

The fact that fevers were reputedly a minor problem before the 1680s indicates that *falciparum* was not yet present. The lack of an effective vector may also have kept the incidence of malaria low. During the 1670s, most of the population remained close to the seacoast and its salt marshes. The main local vector of malaria, *A. quadrimaculatus*, prefers to breed in fresh and still water. Another local mosquito, *A. crucians*, can transmit malaria and does breed in salt marshes, but it is both less susceptible to infection and not an effective vector. As people moved up the rivers, they entered into fresh water areas more hospitable to *A. quadrimaculatus*. The deadly *falciparum* parasite probably arrived in the early 1680s. In 1683 and 1684, pirates raided Vera Cruz and other Spanish possessions where malaria and yellow fever were endemic. Among their booty was a large number of Africans, and they sold about two hundred of them in Charleston. The first major health crisis of the colony followed quickly.[13] The causes of the mortality of the mid-1680s cannot be identified with any certainty. Yellow fever, typhoid, or typhus may have contributed to it, but *falciparum* is likely to have become a problem around this time. Unlike *vivax*, it was to be largely restricted to the southern parts of North America because the plasmodium needs an extended period of warm temperatures to complete the mosquito phase of its development.[14]

---

[12] Mary Dobson, "Mortality Gradients and Disease Exchanges: Comparisons from Old England and Colonial America," *Social History of Medicine* 2 (1989) 261–272, 280; St. Julien Ravenel Childs, *Malaria and Colonization in the Carolina Low Country, 1526–1696* (Baltimore: Johns Hopkins University Press, 1940), 125–127; Kirsty Duncan, "The Possible Influence of Climate on Historical Outbreaks of Malaria in Scotland," *Proceedings of the Royal College of Physician of Edinburgh* 23 (1993) 55–62; Jon Kukla, "Kentish Agues and American Distempers: The Transmission of Malaria from England to Virginia in the Seventeenth Century," *Southern Studies* 25 (1986): 135–147; Gerald Cates, "'The Seasoning': Disease and Death Among the First Colonists of Georgia," *Georgia Historical Quarterly* 64 (1980): 146–158.

[13] Jill Dubisch, "Low Country Fevers: Cultural Adaptations to Malaria in Antebellum South Carolina," *Social Science Medicine* 21 (1985): 642; Humphreys, *Malaria*, 12; Peter Coclanis, *The Shadow of a Dream: Economic Life and Death in the South Carolina Low Country* (New York: Oxford University Press, 1989), 41; Packard, *Making of a Tropical Disease*, 56–57; K. David Patterson, "Disease Environments of the Antebellum South," in Ronald Numbers and Todd Savitt, eds., *Science and Medicine in the Old South* (Baton Rouge: Louisiana State University Press, 1989), 160; Childs, *Malaria and Colonization*, 197–198, 205, 207; Peter Wood, *Black Majority: Negroes in Colonial South Carolina from 1670 through the Stono Rebellion* (New York: W.W. Norton, 1975), 87; BPRO/SC, 1: 293, 2: 4–5, 35–36.

[14] Wood, *Black Majority*, 86–87; Kukla, "Kentish Agues," 135–147; Humphreys, *Malaria*, 24; Judith A. Carney, *Black Rice: The Origins of Rice Cultivation in the Americas* (Cambridge, MA and London: Harvard University Press, 2001), 84. The exact date at which rice cultivation began is debated, with historians arguing for various dates between the 1670s and 1700.

The low, swampy terrain and the warm, humid climate of the lowcountry made it friendly to malarial parasites and their local vectors. But the planters made things much worse by cultivating rice with enslaved African labor. Rice cultivation, anopheline mosquitoes, and malaria have gone hand in hand historically. The planters brought *falciparum* to the region by purchasing Africans as slaves. Using this labor force, they created abundant breeding sites for the mosquito vector by cutting down trees and building rice ponds and reservoirs. *A. quadrimaculatus* thrives in sunlight and standing water. Removal of forest cover, together with hunting, also reduced the number of birds that fed on mosquitoes. A desire to secure quick returns on investments aggravated the situation. In the 1760s, the author of *American Husbandry* claimed that planters did not wait to clear the stumps of the removed trees, but immediately planted rice among them. Tree stumps provided well-protected breeding places for the mosquito vector.[15] The adoption of rice cultivation in turn led to increased reliance on enslaved African labor. The planters especially valued people from coastal rice-producing areas for their experience in rice cultivation. In these areas, *falciparum* was endemic or hyperendemic, and African captives and white sailors transported it to the Americas in their bodies. Similar developments took place several decades later in Georgia, founded in 1732. Slavery was not legalized there until 1750, but by 1776, Georgia had 16,000 slaves and 17,000 whites. As in South Carolina, slavery, deforestation, and rice cultivation produced a deadly malarial environment in the Georgia lowcountry.[16]

With the benefit of hindsight and modern microbiology, we can see what the planters at first did not, namely that malaria was an enemy they had themselves largely created. Despite its marshy topography and warm, humid climate, the lowcountry environment was not naturally especially unhealthy. It is not so today. Human action made it so. The planters could not know that the disease was caused by a plasmodium transmitted by mosquitoes. Many people noted that the mosquito and fever seasons coincided, but viewed the mosquitoes as an annoying corollary to the season, not its cause. The main cause, most educated people believed, was the climate and terrain, which blanketed the region with fever-inducing miasmas during the warm, rainy months of summer and fall.[17] The climate differed so markedly from that of Northern Europe, wrote

---

Carney argues that rice was cultivated in South Carolina in the 1670s and emerged as an export crop in the 1690s. By the 1720s, it was the colony's leading export.

[15] Harry J. Carman, ed., *American Husbandry* (Port Washington, NY: Kennikat Press, Inc., 1964; originally published in London, 1775), 275.

[16] Packard, *Making of a Tropical Disease*, 55–61; Cates, "'The Seasoning,'"146–158; George Fenwick Jones, *The Georgia Dutch* (Athens and London: The University of Georgia Press, 1992), 233–234, 165–174; Robin Blackburn, *The Making of New World Slavery* (London and New York: Verso, 1997), 464–465.

[17] H. Roy Merrens and George D. Terry, "Dying in Paradise: Malaria, Mortality, and the Perceptual Environment in Colonial South Carolina," *Journal of Southern History* 50 (1984), 533–550.

Alexander Hewatt, that it was natural for many newcomers to "sicken and die by the change" soon after they arrived. During the hot months, the body's fibers were "relaxed" by perpetual perspiration, and it became "feeble and sickly," an easy prey to intermittent fevers, putrid fevers, and dysentery. In the winter and spring, the survivors of fevers and fluxes were often vulnerable to pleurisies and peripneumonies. Lionel Chalmers attributed the high incidence of disease to the frequent "alterations our bodies are made to undergo from the weather, in several seasons of the year." Many of them would not occur, he claimed, if the climate was less changeable. His colleague Alexander Garden agreed. Sudden changes of weather produced "autumnal intermittents and winter inflammatory diseases." The lowcountry climate was one of the "most changeable, and consequently most unhealthy" in the world.[18]

FEVERED BODIES

The toll taken by fevers and fluxes was written on the bodies of many lowcountry inhabitants. If we can believe numerous observations of the time, the white settlers were a ghastly-looking bunch. Lionel Chalmers claimed that people were prematurely aged by their constant battle with sickness: "Few live above sixty years; and the bald or hoary and wrinkled appearances of old age, often shew themselves at the age of thirty years; or even earlier, more especially on those who dwell in the country." From an early age, their bodies were often marked by swelling and hardness of the spleen and obstructions of the liver, both common results of malaria. Chalmers attributed these conditions to the long hot summers, especially in those who had suffered from intermittents, which meant almost everybody. He estimated that two people out of five showed enlarged and often hard and painful spleens. "Ague cake," as the condition was often called, was especially common among those who dwelt in the countryside. In Charleston, fewer people had enlarged spleens, which indicates that malaria was less common there than in the country.[19] Newcomers frequently remarked on the pale, sallow, or tawny skin, and enfeebled and prematurely aged constitutions of the residents. An Anglican missionary who arrived in July 1769 declared that a forty-year-old man looked "as old as one of 60." When Lutheran pastor Henry Melchior Muhlenberg arrived from Philadelphia in 1774, he was struck by the faces of the residents: "sallow, pale, or yellow, as if they had come out of the graves or the lazaretto." An English visitor who came the same year commented that most of the women had "pale sickish languid complexions." In 1802, French botanist Francois Andre Michaux remarked that "[t]he extreme unwholesomeness of the climate is

[18] Alexander Hewatt, *An Historical Account of the Rise and Progress of the Colonies of South Carolina and Georgia* 2 vols. (London, 1779) 2: 136–137; see also, 1: 49–50; Chalmers, *Weather and Diseases*, 2: 215; James E. Smith, *A Selection of the Correspondence of Linnaeus and Other Naturalists* 2 vols. (New York: Arno Press, 1978) 1: 552.

[19] Chalmers, *Weather and Diseases*, 1: 38, 2: 21–22.

clearly demonstrated by the pale and livid countenances of the inhabitants." Such observations were common.[20]

The ubiquitous diseases also affected mental states. Gideon Johnston reported that he was often mentally confused and "distracted" by the suffering of his parishioners as well as his own. Visiting the numerous sick and dying was not only physically demanding but extremely unpleasant, especially when one was seriously ill oneself. It involved exposure to "filth, nauseous smells, and ghastly sights."[21] When the English naturalist John Ellis reproached Dr. Alexander Garden for not being more energetic in studying the local life forms, Garden replied that Ellis did not understand the enervating effects of the climate. If Ellis spent two or three summers in Carolina, the sun would sweat out most of his "good English blood and animal spirits ... instead of fire and life of imagination, indifference and graceful despondency would overwhelm your mind."[22]

"AN INHUMAN AND UNCHRISTIAN PRACTICE"

In the summer of 1769, Charleston residents complained to Governor Charles Montagu that their noses and health were endangered by the decomposing bodies of dead Africans who had been thrown from slave ships into the Cooper River:

It has been represented to me that a large number of dead negroes who have been thrown into the river, are driven upon the marsh opposite of Charles Town, and the noisome smell arising from their putrefaction may become dangerous to the health of the inhabitants of this province: In order to prevent such an inhuman and unchristian practice, I think fit, by the advice of his Majesty's council, to issue this my proclamation strictly forbidding this same: And I do hereby offer a reward of ONE HUNDRED POUNDS to be paid on the conviction of the offender to any person that will inform against any one person who shall be guilty of such practice.[23]

The "burial" of these Africans was not unusual. Neither were their deaths. For them, as for many white immigrants, death often came soon after arrival

---

[20] *The Fulham Papers in the Lambeth Palace Library; American Colonial Section Calendar and Indexes*, compiled by William W. Manross (Oxford: Clarendon Press, 1965), nos. 204–205; *The Journals of Henry Melchior Muhlenberg* 3 vols. (Philadelphia: The Muhlenberg Press, 1945), 3: 566; "Charleston in 1774 as Described by an English Traveler," *SCHM* 47 (1945), 180; Francois Andre Michaux, *Travels to the West of the Alleghany Mountains* (London, 1805), in Reuben Gold Thwaites, ed., *Travels West of the Alleghanies* (Cleveland, 1904), 296; Elkanah Watson, *Men and Times of the Revolution; or Memoirs of Elkanah Watson*, ed. by Winslow C. Watson (New York, 1856), 56; A. Izard to Mrs. Manigault, Oct. 19, 1815, Manigault FP, SCL; William Mylne, *Travels in the Colonies, 1773–1775*, ed. Ted Ruddock (Athens: University of Georgia Press, 1993) 44–45.

[21] Klingberg, *Johnston*, 21, 35, 40–42, 75–76, 90–91, 98–99.

[22] Alexander Garden to John Ellis, April 20, 1759, Collinson MSS, Linnaean Society Archives, quoted in Edmund and Dorothy Smith Berkeley, *Dr. Alexander Garden of Charles Town* (Chapel Hill: University of North Carolina Pres, 1969), 125.

[23] *SCG*, June 8, 1769.

in the new country. It is difficult to measure how much their sicknesses were due to weeks or months crammed into unsanitary ships and how much to their new environment. After the rigors of a long voyage, worsened by dietary deficiencies, newcomers were likely to be highly vulnerable to local diseases. Henry Laurens reported of one cargo of 140 Angola slaves that when they landed, most were severely ill of "the flux, which ... could not be stopped by the most able of our physicians." Thirteen had already died and the rest were severely ill or "in a poor and meager condition."[24]

Immigrants from Europe sometimes suffered similar experiences, especially if they were poor. An Anglican missionary who arrived in the late 1760s recorded that half of the people he came over with died on shipboard and most of the rest had died since arriving. A ship full of Scots-Irish that year suffered high mortality both during and after the voyage. Some of the survivors later sued the captain, claiming that he had packed them too tightly and starved and abused them. That many of them died months after arrival indicates that local diseases may have been responsible for their deaths.[25] The following year, the overseers of the poor reported many of about 300 Irish immigrants who had recently arrived in the port were ill with a "cruel flux and fever." They had been placed in the town barracks, where their condition had quickly deteriorated. The overseers were appalled by what they found: "We saw in several rooms two and three corps[es] at a time – many dying – some deprived of their senses – young children lying entirely naked, whose parents had expired but a few days ago, and they themselves reduced by sickness to a situation beyond any description."[26]

The long voyages were worse for the enslaved. In the 1750s, Alexander Garden, who served as one of the port physicians inspecting slave ships for contagious disease, wrote that most of them "have had many of their cargoes thrown overboard; some one-fourth, some one-third, some lost half; and I have seen some that have lost three-fourths of their slaves." All the ships he had visited had smelled "most offensive and noisome." They were so filthy and foul from "putrid dysenteries (which is their common disorder) it is a wonder any escape with life."[27] More than 200,000 Africans were imported to the lowcountry legally between the late seventeenth century and the federal abolition of the

[24] *HLP*, 2: 91.
[25] Manross, *Fulham Papers*, nos. 204–205; Richard J. Hooker, ed., *The Carolina Backcountry on the Eve of the Revolution: The Journal and Other Writings of Charles Woodmason, Anglican Itinerant* (Chapel Hill: University of North Carolina Press, 1953), 4–9, 84–87, 191–192, 200–201; *HLP*, 5: 198, 165; *Death Notices in the South Carolina Gazette*, 34–35; *Register of St. Philip's Parish, Charles Town, South Carolina, 1754–1810*, ed. by A.S. Salley, Jr. (Charleston, 1904), 313–322; Journals of His Majesty's Council of South Carolina, July 7, Sept. 8, 1767, SCDAH.
[26] *SCG*, June 22–29, 1767; BPRO/SC, 30: 234.
[27] Alexander Garden to Stephen Hales, undated, c. 1758–1760, quoted in Berkeley, *Alexander Garden*, 124; Robin Blackburn, *The Making of New World Slavery* (London and New York: Verso, 1997), 392–393.

trade in 1808. The trade was slowed or interrupted – but never totally shut off – by war, high duties, or prohibitions on imports. But in each instance, the damming of imports was followed by a flood. More than 120,000 slaves were legally and illegally imported into South Carolina and Georgia between 1783 and 1807, nearly 100,000 through Charleston alone. How many of them died before being sold is a matter of conjecture. Eighteenth-century sources indicate heavy losses from smallpox, scurvy, and dysentery on slave ships. Mortality rates generally averaged between 9 and 18 percent. British slavers managed to reduce it to 3–5 percent by the late 1790s, probably due to improved diet, ventilation, and sanitation and smallpox inoculation.[28]

Africans who survived the Atlantic crossing often died soon after they arrived. About one-third of the enslaved landed in South Carolina died within a year of arrival.[29] How many died from diseases contracted during the voyage, while sitting in port, or after sale is impossible to say. But many people agreed that slaves brought from Africa were more vulnerable to local diseases than those born in the lowcountry. A doctor explained to readers of the Charleston *Courier* in 1806 that "New Negroes" required "more nursing, more tenderness, and more indulgence, than country-born Negroes, until they become accustomed to the change of climate and the difference in their mode of living." The greatest danger to new slaves, he argued, was dysentery.[30]

The mortality of imported Africans could be greatly increased by the long periods they sometimes remained on board ships after arriving in port, either in quarantine or waiting to be sold. If slavers arrived at the wrong time of year, if too many ships arrived at the same time, if an epidemic was raging in Charleston, or if the Africans were considered a "poor parcel," they might languish on the ships for weeks or months. This was more than a "marketing problem." Many of the Africans died of dysentery, typhus, or some other disease. The ship's masters did not squander profits on funeral formalities. They simply threw the bodies overboard into the harbor. If many slaves died, these "discharges" created a "sanitation problem" that annoyed local residents. *The Courier* reported one of these incidents in 1807. An inquest on the body of an African woman found floating near Craft's Wharf reached a verdict that she

---

[28] James A. McMillin, *The Final Victims: Foreign Slave Trade to North America, 1783–1810* (Columbia: University of South Carolina Press, 2004), 1–5, 52; James A. Rawley, *The Transatlantic Slave Trade: A History* (New York: Norton, 1981); *The Atlantic Slave Trade: Effects on Economies, Societies and Peoples in Africa, Europe, and the Americas*, ed. by Joseph E. Inikori and Stanley L. Engerman (Durham, North Carolina: Duke University Press, 1992); Herbert Klein, *The Atlantic Slave Trade* (Cambridge and New York: Cambridge University Press, 1999).

[29] Philip D. Morgan, *Slave Counterpoint: Black Culture in the Eighteenth-Century Chesapeake and Lowcountry* (Chapel Hill: University of North Carolina Press, 1998), 445.

[30] *The Courier*, Dec. 8, 1806; Elizabeth Donnan, *Documents Illustrative of the Slave Trade to America*, 4 vols. (Washington, DC: Carnegie Institution of Washington, 1930-1935), 4: 343, 358–361, 458–459; Daniel Littlefield, *Rice and Slaves: Ethnicity and the Slave Trade in Colonial South Carolina* (Urbana and Chicago: University of Illinois Press, 1991), 28.

had died "by the visitation of God." They conjectured that she had been on one of the many slave ships then in the harbor and that the crew had thrown her body into the water to save burial expenses. The editor commented that this "nuisance" had become so frequent that the citizens needed to punish those responsible. Not only was the practice "inhumane" – it was also unpleasant to think that the citizens might eat fish "that have fattened on the carcasses of dead negroes."[31]

Such incidents were more frequent – or perhaps more frequently reported in the newspapers – in the years just before the federal ban on the slave trade went into effect in 1808. Traders rushed to profit before the market was permanently closed, and as Adam Smith would have said, supply greatly exceeded effective demand. Many Africans remained on overcrowded and unsanitary ships for months. Almost 16,000 arrived in Charleston during the last four months of 1807. John Lambert, a British traveler who visited the port in January 1808, learned that at Gadsden's Wharf, more than 700 of them (out of some 2,000 on the ships at the time) had died at the wharf in less than three months from dysentery and other contagious diseases. A Charleston merchant told him a "similar mortality" had occurred a few years before.[32] David Ramsay also reported that disease had killed "great numbers of the newly-imported Africans" in 1807. Like Garden earlier, Ramsay blamed conditions aboard the slave ships, "where such crowds of human beings were almost constantly shut up without a supply of fresh air, and frequently with a scanty allowance of unwholesome food and bad water."[33]

THE SUFFERING OF THE SHEPHERDS

In July 1733 the beleaguered Anglican Commissary of South Carolina, Alexander Garden (no relative of the doctor), received some happy news: The Rev. Colladon had arrived to serve the vacant parish of St. James Santee. Unlike some recent ministers, Colladon was acceptable to both the French Huguenots and the English of that parish, because he was fluent in both languages. The relief was short-lived: Soon after his arrival, he contracted a fever that killed him in four days.[34] John Fullerton arrived in South Carolina in May 1735 to minister to Christ Church Parish. One can almost anticipate his

[31] *The Courier*, April 22, 1807.
[32] Donnan, *Slave Trade*, 4: 343; John Lambert, *Travels Through Canada and the United States of America during the Years 1806 and 1807*, 2 vols., 2d ed. (London, 1814), 166–167; James A. McMillin, *The Final Victims: Foreign Slave Trade to North America, 1783–1810* (Columbia: University of South Carolina Press, 2004), 110–114. McMillin estimates that between 1,600 and 2,000 Africans died on the ships in 1807–1808.
[33] David Ramsay, "Remarks on the Yellow Fever and Epidemic Catarrh, as They Appeared in South Carolina During the Summer and Autumn of 1807," *Medical Repository* (1808) 5: 233.
[34] George W. Williams, "Letters to the Bishop of London from the Commissaries in South Carolina," *SCHM* 78 (1977), 214–217.

fate from his first report after his arrival: "the parsonage here is three or four miles from the Church, the house is rotten and situate in a bog." He was dead by September.[35]

The experiences of Colladon and Fullerton were not unusual. During the colonial period, the clergy were highly vulnerable to the local diseases, probably because most came from Britain or the northern colonies. In 1699, yellow fever killed five ministers in Charleston.[36] After 1702, the records of the Society for the Propagation of the Gospel provide abundant documentation of the suffering of the Anglican missionaries and others. Samuel Thomas, the first SPG missionary to arrive in the colony in 1702, was also the first to die there, in the yellow fever epidemic of 1706. Many of his successors experienced a similar fate. In 1717, Francis Le Jau informed the Bishop of London that four SPG missionaries had died within eighteen months. Le Jau joined them that fall.[37] Seventeen out of the fifty Anglican ministers sent to South Carolina between 1701 and 1750 died within ten years of their arrival. Twenty-six died or resigned for health reasons within the same period. After fifteen years, thirty-four had died or resigned. Only four survived in the colony more than twenty years.[38] When Charles Woodmason arrived in the colony in August 1766 to serve as an itinerant Anglican missionary, he found many clergymen dying of fevers. Soon after his arrival, he learned of the deaths of four Anglican and three Presbyterians ministers. In all, seven Anglican ministers died that summer, prompting Woodmason to write the Bishop of London that "as this country ever was the grave of the clergy, it has been bitterly so this summer." In a later letter, he listed twenty-eight ministers, Anglican, Dissenter, and Lutheran, who had recently died.[39]

The frequent deaths, resignations, and extended absences of Anglican ministers left many parishes without incumbents for long periods of time. In 1711, Thomas Hasell reported that half of the parishes had become vacant by death or removal. Reports in the following years often stated that half or more of the parishes were vacant.[40] Getting replacements from England for dead or

---

[35] Frederick Dalcho, *An Historical Account of the Protestant Episcopal Church in South Carolina* (Charleston, 1820), 280–281; John Fullerton, May 5, 1735, SPG Letter Books, A26: 129; George Haddrell, Dec. 17, 1735, SPG Letter Books, A26: 152; Helena Boschi, SPG Letter Books, Nov. 3, 1749, B16: 180.

[36] Extract of a letter from Hugh Adams to Samuel Sewell, Feb. 23, 1700, in Diary of Samuel Sewell, April 22, 1700, Massachusetts Historical Society, *Collections*, 5th series, 6: 11–12.

[37] Klingberg, *Le Jau*, 204–205.

[38] John Duffy, "Eighteenth-Century Carolina Health Conditions," *Journal of Southern History* 18 (1952), 301–302.

[39] Richard J. Hooker, ed. *The Carolina Backcountry on the Eve of the Revolution: The Journal and Other Writings of Charles Woodmason, Anglican Itinerant* (Chapel Hill: University of North Carolina Press, 1953), 4–5, 85 (quotation), 192–193, 200–201; Charles Woodmason to Bishop Terrick, Oct. 19, 1766, Fulham Papers, Lambeth Palace Library, 10: 162–163.

[40] Thomas Hasell, Sept. 4, 1711, SPG Letter Books, A6: 148; William Tredwell Bull, Jan. 3, 1716/17, SPG Letter Books, A12: 129, Thomas Hasell, Dec. 27, 1716, SPG Letter Books, A12: 159; Governor and Council, Charles Town, to the Society, Dec. 20, 1717, SPG Letter Books, A13: 141.

departed missionaries was a slow process that might take many months, and
the new incumbent might himself die, leave, or be removed within a short time.
Missionaries and parish vestries endlessly repeated the same messages: vacant
parishes and clergyman too ill to perform their duties. Anglican Commissary
William Tredwell Bull wrote in 1718 that for more than two months he had
been unable to conduct divine services. He was still very weak from a third
relapse and could not assist the vacant parishes: "[I]n this sickly country we
recover so very slowly after any considerable indisposition that I fear it will
be a long time ere I shall." He requested more ministers, something all the
commissaries had to do regularly. In 1751, the vestry of Prince Frederick
Parish reported that their rector had died. They could not get any help from
three neighboring parishes because they were also vacant. Three years earlier,
Commissary Garden reported that he and his assistant were both sickly and
asked the Society to send someone to assist him, or succeed him, should he
die. The fall fevers even changed the church calendar. They were so common
among the Anglican clergy that in 1733, Commissary Garden changed his
annual visitation of the parishes from the fall to the spring.[41]

The high attrition rate among the SPG missionaries increased the labors
of those who remained able to work. Performing duties for other parishes in
addition to their own – which included visiting the sick, burying the dead,
and teaching the young – often led to exhaustion, illness, death, or resignation for health reasons. The situation was aggravated by the low salaries of
the Anglican clergy and the difficulty they had in getting them paid. Gideon
Johnston spoke for many of his colleagues when he wrote to the bishop of
Salisbury: "I cannot be over fond of staying in such a place and amongst such
a strange sort of people; and especially where the salary is so small." With a
wife and eleven children, his paltry income ensured penury. When Johnston
described his body as a scene of diseases, he added "[and] so is my family
of poverty and misery." The three were intimately connected: "[M]y necessities ... daily increase upon me; for what between poverty, diseases, and debts,
both I and my family ... are in a most miserable and languishing condition."
His continual sickness and that of his wife Harriet, who earned some money
painting portraits of local worthies, reduced their meager income. Johnston
almost immediately and repeatedly asked to return home, even to "the meanest
thing in South Britain." The prospect of riches, real or imagined, may have
helped the merchants or planters bear the onslaught of disorders. The poorly
paid clergy, like most inhabitants, white or black, had no such consolations.[42]

The trials of the ministers undoubtedly weakened Anglican authority and
strengthened Protestant Dissenting sects. Dissenters were numerous from the

[41] William Tredwell Bull, Sept. 25, 1718, SPG Letter Books, A13: 182–183; Manross,
Fulham Papers, 152–153.
[42] Klingberg, *Johnston*, 19–22, 34–35, 60–61, 68. Missionaries complained constantly about the
meagerness of their salaries, which were often eroded by inflation and difficulties in getting
paid.

early days of the colony, because the Proprietors had established religious tolerance to attract Presbyterians, Baptists, Quakers, and French Huguenots. In 1700, Dissenters were a majority in Carolina. SPG missionaries frequently commented on the large number of Dissenters in their parishes and the need to supply more ministers to convert them to Anglicanism. Anglicans made considerable strides in building churches and attracting converts in the early eighteenth century, but the Dissenting sects regained the advantage with the arrival of Swiss, German, Welsh, and Scots-Irish Protestants and the rise of evangelicalism in the 1730s and after. By the time of the Revolution, Anglicanism had lost its bid for dominance. In 1778, the newly independent state of South Carolina disestablished the Church of England. The Episcopal Church, as it was renamed, would soon become the church of a small minority in the state, as it still is.[43]

The frequent illnesses, deaths, absences, and resignations of the Anglican clergy helped bring about this result. The loyalty of many colonists to the Church of England was nominal, and during the often-long periods when Anglican parishes were vacant, some turned readily to their rivals. Johnston and others often noted the ease with which people moved back and forth between the Church and the Dissenting sects: "Many of those that pretend to be Churchmen are strangely crippled in their goings between the Church and Presbytery, and as they are of large and loose principles so they live and act accordingly, sometimes going openly with the Dissenters as they now do." A few years later, when Gilbert Jones arrived to take the post of minister at St. Bartholomew's Parish, Johnston assigned him to Christ Church Parish instead. Christ Church had been without a minister for three years, and Dissenters were making converts among the parishioners. [44]

The Dissenting churches had a major advantage over the Church of England in the contest for souls: They could replace ministers more easily and quickly. Candidates for the Anglican ministry in colonial America had to be ordained by a bishop in Britain, which meant that most of them came from there. The Dissenting sects, in contrast, were more easily able to recruit ministers in America because candidates did not have to go to Britain to get ordained. In the late 1760s, the Anglican Church had one missionary, Charles Woodmason, in the backcountry, which swarmed with clergy of other denominations.[45] Of these, the Baptists were ultimately the most successful, partly

[43] Patricia U. Bonomi, *Under the Cope of Heaven: Religion, Society, and Politics in Colonial America* (New York: Oxford University Press, 2003), 31–32; Thomas J. Little, "The Origins of Southern Evangelicalism: Revivalism in South Carolina, 1700–1740," *Church History*, Dec. 2006, 1–36; Ebenezer Taylor, July 28, 1713, SPG Letter Books A8: 14; William Guy, Jan. 10, 1714/15, SPG Letter Books, A10: 13.

[44] Klingberg, *Johnston*, 20–50; Gideon Johnston, Report on the Gilbert Jones-Christ Church Controversy, 1712, SPG Letter Books, A:8, unnumbered.

[45] Manross, *Fulham Papers*, 144; Woodmason, *Carolina Backcountry*; Bradford J. Wood, "'A Constant Attendance on God's Alter': Death, Disease, and the Anglican Church in Colonial South Carolina, 1706–1750," *SCHM* 100 (1999), 204–220; "Documents

because they proselytized strenuously, but also because they did not demand a highly educated clergy. Baptist ministers were readily replaceable and they were more likely to come from the ranks of the people they served. They were often recruited locally and thus may have enjoyed greater immunity to local diseases than ministers coming from Europe. In contrast, Presbyterians and Congregationalists, like Anglicans, demanded a highly trained pastorate. They secured most of their ministers during the colonial period from New England, and the rest from Britain. These men were often as susceptible to fevers as the Anglicans. Several ministers of the Charleston Congregational Church died or left after short tenures. Benjamin Pierpont, who arrived in 1691, did better than most. He died, probably of smallpox, in 1698. His successor, Hugh Adams, suffered from a myriad of disorders, which he listed as putrid fever, tertian ague and fever, dropsy, scurvy, pestilence, gout, and – perhaps unsurprisingly – hypochondriac melancholy. Adams soon resigned and returned to New England. His replacement, John Cotton, died within months of his arrival in the yellow fever epidemic of 1699. Nathan Bassett survived fourteen years, only to die of smallpox in 1738. Four other colonial ministers died after two to five years in the post. One of them, William Hutson, also lost two wives during his brief tenure. The last colonial Congregational pastor, William Tennent, died of fever at age thirty-seven in 1777.[46]

After independence, mortality among the clergy was lower, probably because more were born locally. But those who came from other places were still at high risk. In 1817, yellow fever claimed the lives of several Charleston ministers, including Theodore Dehon, the Episcopal bishop of South Carolina. Dehon had been born and lived in New England most of his life, coming to Charleston only in 1810.[47] Yellow fever also took a heavy toll on the men who served on the faculty of the College of Charleston, which opened in the late 1780s. Most were newcomers from northern seminaries or Britain and thus susceptible to local fevers. Three headmasters died from disease between 1800 and 1810, a period of frequent yellow fever epidemics. Two of their deaths were attributed to yellow fever; the third probably died of it. After recording the death of headmaster Elijah Ratoone in 1810, a historian of the college comments: "Thus for the third time within the space of ten years, the College was deprived by death of a man who might have found a solution of its many problems." Several faculty also left the college during this period to avoid the

Concerning Rev. Samuel Thomas," *SCHM* 5 (1904), 39; Walter Edgar, *South Carolina: A History* (Columbia: University of South Carolina Press, 1998), 181–183, 293.

[46] George N. Edwards, *A History of the Independent or Congregational Church of Charleston, South Carolina* (Boston: The Pilgrim Press, 1947), 8–13, 21–29, 152, 157; George Howe, *History of the Presbyterian Church in South Carolina* (Columbia, 1870), 372–373; "A Faithful Ambassador: The Diary of William Hutson, Pastor of the Independent Meeting in Charleston, 1757–1761," ed. by Daniel J. Tortora, *SCHM* 107 (2006), 273–306, 108 (2007), 32–100.

[47] *The Courier*, Aug. 8, 1817; Joshua B. Whitridge to Dr. William Whitridge, Sept.19–21, 1817, Whitridge Papers, SCHS.

local fevers, or failed to show up after being hired citing the fear of fever as their reason. Yellow fever increased the difficulties that the college's trustees faced in trying to establish a stable and effective academic environment. In 1836, the college closed down due to lack of students and income. It reopened in 1838 as the first municipally funded college in America. Coincidently or not, 1838 was also the year of a virulent yellow fever epidemic. The college's new identity partly reflected the difficulty of attracting faculty and students from healthier regions.[48]

THE DANGEROUS ACADIANS

Another identifiable group that suffered heavily from disease was French Acadians. More than 1,000 of them were interned in South Carolina in the winter of 1755–1756 following the outbreak of war between the French and British in North America. In an early example of ethnic cleansing, the British governor of Nova Scotia (formerly the French colony of Acadia) had ordered that the Acadian population be dispersed among the colonies to the south for fear they would aid the French war effort. An influx of white people would normally have been welcome, as fear of the black majority was ever present. Not in this case. The Acadians' arrival in Charleston aroused a host of fears in the town, partly because they were French Catholics injected into a rabidly anti-papist community fearing imminent attack by Catholic France. They also raised fears of epidemic disease.[49]

After the first ships arrived from Nova Scotia in late November, the port physician had inspected the first transports and reported them free of any contagious or malignant disorder. Nevertheless, the colonial assembly ordered them to be quarantined at the pest-house on Sullivan's Island for five days to "purify and cleanse themselves." After that, the "turbulent and seditious" were to be sent to the workhouse and the rest to be lodged under guard and given a sunset curfew. Able-bodied men were put to work on the city's fortifications, then being readied for a possible French attack. By late January, many of the Acadians were ill. A committee of the Assembly claimed that their disorders were due to overcrowding and poor accommodation.[50] Concern heightened when another transport arrived in January 1756 with 340 more Acadians, bringing their number to more than 1,000 in a town that numbered perhaps 9,000. After lengthy debates centered on fears that the new arrivals would bring an epidemic into the town, they were landed on Sullivan's Island in mid-February. Many of them quickly became ill there, probably

---

[48] J. H. Easterby, *A History of the College of Charleston* (Charleston, S.C., 1935), 46–47, 55, 60.

[49] Ruth Allison Hudnut and Hayes Baker-Crothers, "Acadian Transients in South Carolina," *American Historical Review* 43 (1938) 500–513; Marguerite B. Hamer, "The Fate of the Exiled Acadians in South Carolina," *Journal of Southern History* 4 (1938), 199–208; Chapman J. Milling, *Exile Without an End* (Columbia, SC: Bostick and Thornley, Inc., 1943).

[50] *JCHA*, 14: 20–23, 64–65, 87–88; *SCG*, Jan. 1, May 1, Dec. 23, 1756.

from dysentery. They were allowed to move into town in late March, after the Assembly reported that many had died due to bad water and poor care and that many more would die if they remained on the island. In early April, a new complication arose: A British naval squadron landed more than 100 French prisoners of war in the city. Their arrival heightened concerns that the French would stir up rebellion among the black majority.[51]

Fear that the new arrivals might set off an epidemic also increased. Members of the assembly urged that they be dispersed throughout the province to remove a potential source of pestilence: "[A]s the hot season is coming on, your committee is apprehensive that some contagious distemper may break out amongst them, which will prove of fatal consequence to the inhabitants of the Town." The assemblymen had apparently learned that the arrival of large numbers of newcomers in Charleston could trigger yellow fever in the warm months. In July 1756, the assembly passed an act for "Disposing of the Acadians." By then, more than 100 had already died. Another 273 had been sent to other colonies or had escaped. Four-fifths of the 645 who remained were to be sent to other parishes and one-fifth to remain in town.[52] Dispersal did not improve the Acadians' situation or resolve concerns about them. Many of them died and others gradually drifted back to Charleston. In November 1757, the vestry and church wardens of St. Philip's Parish complained to the assembly about the "intolerable" burden of caring for the large numbers of sick and infirm Acadians who had returned to the town. The parish was already in straitened circumstances from caring for large numbers of sick soldiers and their dependents. The church wardens declared that most of the Acadians would have died had they not received medical care and food. The wardens repeated the same complaint in July 1759 and threatened no longer to care for the Acadians unless the Assembly voted funds.[53] In January 1760, about 320 Acadians remained in Charleston. Smallpox killed about one-third of them in the next few months. After the Seven Years' War ended in 1763, most of the survivors went to the French West Indies and then to Louisiana, where they and other Acadians became the "Cajuns."[54]

CALCULATING DEATH

Much of the evidence for the deadliness of the lowcountry disease environment is impressionistic, but some statistical data exist. Calculating accurate mortality rates from the fragmentary vital statistics is a hazardous business,

---

[51] *JCHA*, 14: 123, 139, 151, 158, 200; BPRO/SC 27: April 14, June 16, 19, 1756.
[52] *Stats.* 4: 31, July 6, 1756; BPRO/SC 27: June 16, 19, 1756.
[53] *JCHA*, 14: 278, 311; JCHA, 1757–1761, computer file, 31–32, 413.
[54] Milling, *Exile*, 46–54. Milling says the Acadians died of stranger's fever, a nineteenth-century term for yellow fever. Some of them may well have died of that disease, but smallpox was severely epidemic in the winter and spring of 1760.

but it is clear that people died at rates higher – in some cases much higher – than in other parts of North America and Europe. Among British American colonies, only Jamaica was deadlier. On balance, blacks suffered as much as whites from disease, possibly more. Blacks, like whites, had difficulty sustaining their population through natural increase, at least before the 1770s, and disease played a large role in limiting their population growth, especially in the case of those who worked on rice plantations.[55]

From an analysis of the death records of St. Philip's Parish in Charleston between 1722 and 1732, Peter Coclanis estimated that the crude death rate was between about 52 and 60 per 1,000. As he points out, mortality rates of this sort were extremely high, "even by pre-industrial standards." Between 1721 and 1770, deaths outnumbered births in St. Philip's Parish by almost 4 to 1: 5,398 to 1,540. The great excess of deaths over births in the town is somewhat misleading because deaths were more likely to be recorded than births, and many of the dead were transients: sailors, soldiers, the poor, and people who came from the country to get medical attention. On average, several hundred transients lived in the town at any time. Nevertheless, early-eighteenth-century Charleston was a deadly place, roughly twice as deadly as the average town or parish in England or New England at the time.[56]

Mortality rates, especially for infants and children, were often appalling. They constituted a large majority of burials in many years. In Christ Church Parish, 86 percent of the white children whose births and deaths were recorded during the early eighteenth century died before the age of twenty. In St. John's Berkeley Parish, only 21 percent of white males born between 1680 and 1720 reached age twenty. This figure rose slightly, to 26 percent, between 1720 and 1760, and then more significantly, to 45 percent, between 1760 and 1800. The white population of St. John's grew almost totally by immigration from Europe and the West Indies until just before the Revolution. Few families managed to establish a second generation, or if they did, lived to see the beginning of a third. Between 1680 and 1720, more than 55 percent of whites reaching twenty years of age did not live to be fifty. Between 1721 and 1760, 45 percent did not reach fifty. General mortality improved in St. John's after mid-century. Between 1760 and 1800, 45 percent of those reaching twenty survived past seventy, and only 18 percent did not reach fifty. Women's mortality rates in St. John's were even worse than men's during the first decades of

---

[55] Peter Coclanis, *The Shadow of a Dream: Economic Life and Death in the South Carolina Low Country* (New York: Oxford University Press, 1989), 43–45.

[56] Coclanis, "Death in Early Charleston: an estimate of the crude death rate for the white population of Charleston, 1722–1732," *SCHM* 85 (1984), 280–291; Coclanis, *Shadow of a Dream*, 290; Richard Waterhouse, *A New World Gentry: The Making of a Merchant and Planter Class in South Carolina, 1670–1770* (New York and London: Garland Publishing, Inc., 1989), 105–106. On Jamaican mortality, see Trevor Burnard, "'The Country Continues Sicklie': White Mortality in Jamaica, 1655–1780," *Social History of Medicine* 12 (1999), 45–72.

settlement. They were particularly vulnerable to malaria during pregnancy.[57] Elite families sometimes suffered appalling losses. Between 1750 and 1779, planter Henry Ravenel and his wife had sixteen children. Only six survived past the age of twenty-one. Eight died before the age of five. Of their seven daughters, none lived to be twenty. Elias Ball and Mary Delamere, who married in 1721, had six children, and all of them died before age twenty. Peter Gaillard and his wife Elizabeth had twelve children, of whom only three lived until twenty; one of those died at twenty-three. The reports of the Anglican clergy often mentioned that disease and flight had "thinned" their congregations.[58] The deaths of children were a tragedy. The deaths of breadwinners were often disastrous, leaving their families destitute.[59]

TALK ABOUT SUFFERING

The lowcountry's cornucopia of diseases produced enormous agony. The most compelling evidence of the suffering from disease comes from the testimony of the victims themselves, or those close to them. Affra Coming wrote of the death of her husband from a fever in 1694 that she had never seen someone experience such "extreme burning" before. He suffered so much that he prayed for death and "welcomed it when it came."[60] Mary Stafford wrote in 1711 that the flux had killed "abundance of newcomers" and that many others had suffered the crippling agony of the dry belly ache, "a sad distemper in this country." The belly ache, also known as the dry gripes or the colic, probably resulted from lead poisoning. Many people consumed large quantities of rum distilled through lead pipes and used pewter pots and drinking vessels. Consumption of rum punches was particularly high during the fever season, and the belly ache added one more agony to those months. Francis Le Jau frequently mentioned this "strange distemper" that paralyzed people's limbs and produced "intolerable pains."[61] West Indian doctor Richard Towne described it as an "unmerciful torture: The belly is seized with an

57 Terry, "'Champaign Country,'" 90–97; Merrens and Terry, "Dying in Paradise." See also, Anne B. L. Bridges and Roy Williams III, *St. James Santee, Plantation Parish: History and Records, 1685–1925* (Spartanburg, SC: Reprint Co. Publishers, 1997), 417–431.
58 Diary and Account Book of Rene and Henry Ravenel of Hanover, 1731–1860, Thomas Porcher Ravenel Collection, SCHS, 12/313/1; Anne Simons Deas, *Recollections of the Ball Family of South Carolina and the Comingtee Plantation* (Charleston, South Carolina Historical Society, 1978, c.1909), 43; Terry, "'Champaign Country,'" 90–97; Merrens and Terry, "Dying in Paradise"; William Guy, January 10, 1738/9, SPG Letter Books, B7: 221; John Fordyce, Oct. 3, 1744, April 2, 1746, SPG Letter Books, B12: 90, 93.
59 Petition of Martha Osborne, [Feb. 1715/16], SPG Letter Books, A11: 25–26; Frederick Dalcho, *An Historical Account of the Protestant Episcopal Church in South Carolina* (Charleston, 1820), 280–281; John Fullerton, May 5, 1735, SPG Letter Books, A26: 129; George Haddrell, Dec. 17, 1735, SPG Letter Books, A26: 152; Helena Boschi, Nov. 3, 1749, SPG Letter Books, B16: 180; SPG Letter Books, B5: 250.
60 Deas, *Recollections of the Ball Family*, 27.
61 Klingberg, *Le Jau*, 53–54.

intolerable piercing pain" that might last for weeks. Nathaniel Johnson refused the governorship of Carolina for a time because of its effects (he later took the job). Gideon Johnston's hands were so badly affected by the dry gripes that he was often unable to write. A Swiss immigrant who probably suffered from the gripes recalled that his "whole belly was so swollen so that I might have burst."[62]

New arrivals usually believed that they could withstand lowcountry diseases. Francis Le Jau was sure that he and his family would enjoy good health once they had become "seasoned" to the climate. They never enjoyed good health for long. In September 1708, he stated that he had been in poor health for sixteen months and that his entire family of nine persons had been taken ill simultaneously. In 1715, he calculated that he had been ill six full years of the ten he had spent in the province. Two years later, he died after yet another lingering illness.[63] His colleague Robert Maule recalled that when he had first come to Carolina, he believed that he could withstand any disease. Experience taught him "that the climate can break even the strongest constitution." He preceded Le Jau to the grave by a few months, having suffered almost constant illness for three years.[64]

Some sufferers quickly became skeptical about their chances for survival. In December 1738, Stephen Roe of St. George's Parish reported that since the previous summer he had been afflicted with intermittent fever, dysentery, a cough, and spitting of blood. During the next two years, he was "perpetually harassed with fevers" and declared that he did not expect to survive, "a fever either continued or intermitting perpetually pursuing me with all its roasting consequences." The callousness of his parishioners added to his agonies. Suffering from fever and flux, with his cellars flooded, he applied to the vestry to drain off the water, but "they had not the humanity or compassion to regard it: may God forgive them and turn their hearts." He confessed himself "almost wearied out with the perverseness of the people added to the unhealthfulness of the country."[65]

Natives and long-term inhabitants were less likely to make sweeping or anguished statements about the local disease environment than visitors or newcomers. This was probably because they had developed some immunities to the local maladies or because they did not feel the need to emphasize something

---

[62] Mary Stafford to Mrs. Randall, Aug. 23, 1711, Sloane Mss. 3338.f.33, British Library, photocopy, WHL; Edward Marston to Rev. Dr. Thomas Bray, Feb. 2, 1702/3, SPG Letter Book, A1: 60; Richard Towne, *A Treatise on the Diseases Most Frequent in the West Indies* (London, 1726), 87–88; Thomas Hasell, April 25, 1710, SPG Letter Books, A5: 296; see also, *The Journal of William Stephens, 1743–1745* ed. by E. Merton Coulter (Athens: University of Georgia Press, 1959), 175; R. W. Kelsey, "Swiss Settlers in South Carolina," *SCHM* 23 (1922), 89.
[63] Klingberg, *Le Jau*, 18, 26, 32, 34, 42, 60, 188, 204.
[64] Robert Maule, March 6, 1708/9, SPG, Letter Books, A4: 472; Klingberg, *Le Jau*, 191.
[65] Stephen Roe, July 17, 1739, Dec. 22, 1741, SPG Letter Books, B7: 223, B10: 171; Andrew Leslie, April 28, 1739, SPG Letter Books, B7: 227.

everybody around them knew. But the surviving letters, journals, and diaries of the elite contain constant references to sickness, especially fevers, in the summer and autumn months. Ann Manigault's journal and Eliza Pinckney's letter book read like hospital morbidity and mortality reports.[66] Dr. Alexander Garden's letters contain constant laments about his inability to pursue his beloved natural history due to fevers and other diseases – his own and those of his patients.[67] The huge business correspondence of Henry Laurens often mentions illness.[68] Planter John Ball's letters are filled with laments of his constant suffering from the "country fevers" he contracted on visits to his plantations. On one occasion, he wrote his son, away at Harvard: "The dangers to which I am exposed in this sickly climate by going [from town to country and back] in order to attend my business, and see my family, will probably shorten my life, or even cut me off 'ere you return."[69]

During the fall of 1817, when yellow fever produced numerous fatalities all across the region, Hetty Heyward wrote her mother that "it will be a long time before any of us can enjoy the happiness that we once felt, for even if all of us have not to mourn the loss of a beloved husband or child, still our hearts must bleed at the idea of what some of our nearest and dearest connections are suffering."[70] All this "talk about suffering" makes it abundantly clear that disease took a massive physical toll on the population. The lowcountry's virulent disease environment also helped shape its economic, political, racial, and cultural destiny. Disease even helped transform the British colonies into the United States.

[66] "Extracts from the Journal of Mrs. Ann Manigault, 1754–1781," *SCHM* 20 (1919), 57–63, 128–141, 204–212, 256–259, 21 (1920), 10–23, 59–72, 112–120. See also, Manigault FP, SCL; "Letters of Eliza Lucas Pinckney, 1768–1782," *SCHM* 76 (1975), 143–167; Elise Pinckney, ed., *The Letterbook of Eliza Lucas Pinckney, 1739–1762* (Chapel Hill: University of North Carolina Press, 1972).
[67] James E. Smith, *A Selection of the Correspondence of Linnaeus and Other Naturalists* 2 vols. (New York, Arno Press, 1978) 1: 316–582.
[68] *HLP*, esp. volumes 4–7; "Letters from Henry Laurens," *SCHM* 24 (1923): 11. See also, the Oliver Hart Papers and Oliver Hart Diary, SCL.
[69] John Ball, Sr., to John Ball, Jr., Aug. 15, 1799, Ball FP, SCHS, 11/516/11B; see also, John Ball, Sr. to John Ball, Jr., Sept. 11, Sept. 30, 1798, Aug. 8, 1799, SCHS, 11/516/10, 11/516/11B.
[70] Hetty Heyward to Mother, Nov. 8, 1817, Heyward and Ferguson FP, COCSC.

4

Wooden Horse

> The slave trade in the American republic ... is to the body politic what yellow fever is to an individual. Every ship that arrives in Charleston is to our nation what the Grecian wooden horse was to Troy.
>
> Thomas Branagan, preface to *The Penitential Tyrant*, 1805

> For the last sixteen years the yellow fever has recurred much oftener than in any preceding period. This has not been satisfactorily accounted for.... No visible cause can be designated why it should have recurred almost every year of the last fifteen, and not once as an epidemic disease for the forty years which immediately preceded the year 1792.
>
> David Ramsay, *History of South Carolina*, 1809

"THE PREVAILING DISORDER"

"Its appearance being sudden, the inhabitants were seized with a panic, which caused an immediate *sauve qui peut* seldom witnessed before. I left, or rather fled, for the sake of my daughters.... They were dreadfully frightened.... Of a population of fifteen thousand, six thousand who could not get away remained, nearly all of whom were more or less seized with the prevailing disorder."[1] This reaction to a yellow fever epidemic in Savannah in the 1850s conveys the panic the disease could inspire, akin to that aroused by the arrival of plague in the Old World. Like plague, yellow fever could spark a mass exodus from cities, in part because people recognized early on that, unlike malaria or smallpox, it was preeminently an urban disease, in North America at least. Like *falciparum* malaria, yellow fever's prominence in the lowcountry was partly due to the warm and humid climate. But it was also due to the lowcountry's economic dependence on slaves from Africa and trade with the Caribbean, both places where the disease was common, if not endemic.

---

[1] Quoted in Frederick Law Olmsted, *The Cotton Kingdom* 2 vols. (New York, 1861) 1: 258–259.

In colonial South Carolina, epidemics of yellow fever seem to have been largely restricted to Charleston. In a report to the British Board of Trade in 1751, Governor James Glen remarked that "this dreadful distemper has never spread its fatal influence in the country. Numbers of country people have been infected by it here, and have carried it home, where they have died of it, but hitherto, there is no instance of its having been communicated to any person in the country."[2] Charlestonian John Moultrie, Jr., who wrote a medical dissertation on yellow fever at Edinburgh University in 1749, claimed that it was an urban disease. David Ramsay called it "eminently the disease of cities," and his colleague Tucker Harris claimed that at certain periods it had "been nearly coeval with this town."[3] Yellow fever also struck northern cities, but it was more frequent in Charleston. In the 1950s, John Duffy declared that Charleston had suffered seven major yellow fever epidemics in the colonial period whereas New York and Philadelphia had four each. Duffy undoubtedly underestimated the number of epidemics in Charleston. Moreover, whereas yellow fever retreated from the North after the early 1800s, it struck Charleston frequently until the 1870s.[4]

The name "yellow fever" may even have originated in South Carolina. Some histories claim that the term was first used in Barbados in 1750. But nine years earlier, in 1741, the journal of the South Carolina colonial assembly referred to an epidemic in 1739 as "yellow fever."[5] In the 1750s, John Lining applied the name retrospectively to an epidemic of 1732. Prior to the 1740s and for decades after, contemporary sources refer to yellow fever by a bewildering variety of names, including malignant fever, pestilential fever, putrid bilious fever, Siam distemper, black vomit, or simply plague, pestilence, or sickness. In the late eighteenth and early nineteenth centuries, new names were coined. Into the nineteenth century, people often referred to "a yellow fever" rather than "the yellow fever," indicating the widespread view that it was a type of a generic fever rather than a specific disease. Adding to the

[2] Roy H. Merrens, ed., *The Colonial South Carolina Scene: Contemporary Views, 1697–1774* (Columbia: University of South Carolina Press, 1970), 185; BPRO/SC, 24: 303–330; *The Wellcome Trust Illustrated History of Tropical Diseases* (London: The Wellcome Trust, 1996), 143; Kenneth Kiple, ed., *The Cambridge World History of Human Disease* (Cambridge: Cambridge University Press, 1993), 1102–1103.

[3] David Ramsay, "Extracts from an address delivered before the Medical Society of South Carolina, on the 24th of September 1799," *Medical Repository* 4 (1801): 100–102; Joseph I. Waring, "John Moultrie, Jr., M.D., Lieutenant Governor of East Florida, His Thesis on Yellow Fever," *The Journal of the Florida Medical Association* 54 (Aug. 1967), 775. Moultrie's Latin thesis was entitled *De Febre Maligna Biliosa Americae* (Edinburgh 1749); Tucker Harris, "On the Yellow Fever of Charleston," *Philadelphia Medical and Physical Journal* 2 (1805): 25.

[4] John Duffy, *Epidemics in Colonial America* (Baton Rouge: Louisiana State University Press, 1953), 142–162.

[5] *JCHA*, 3:85; Henry Rose Carter, *Yellow Fever: An Epidemiological and Historical Study of Its Place of Origin* (Baltimore: The Williams and Wilkins Co.: 1931), 197; Kiple, *Cambridge World History of Human Disease*, 1100.

confusion, some observers also used "yellow fever" to describe any disease that produced jaundice.

Yellow fever was perhaps the most dreaded disease to strike the lowcountry during the colonial and early national periods. Smallpox could arouse similar terror, especially in the eighteenth century, but it was less mysterious and no more common in the region than in other parts of America. Together with malaria, yellow fever helped establish the lowcountry's reputation as a dangerously unhealthy place. Like malaria, yellow fever is transmitted by mosquitoes and strikes in warm weather. Epidemics usually began in mid-to-late summer, peaked in September, and ended with the onset of cold weather, usually sometime between late October and early December. People sometimes noticed the coincidence of the mosquito season and the yellow fever season, as they did with malaria. But as with malaria, the role of mosquitoes in its transmission was not established until the end of the nineteenth century. Although no one knew it before then, yellow fever was largely confined to urban locations because of the habits of its local vector. *Aedes aegypti* is a domestic mosquito well adapted to dense human settlements and urban conditions. It relishes human blood above all and prefers to lay its eggs in man-made containers such as barrels, pots, jugs, and cisterns. It flourished where people purposely or inadvertently collected rainwater. In Charleston, surrounded by salt water, the ground water is brackish, and spring and early summer are often dry. Before the advent of piped water systems, people collected rainwater in barrels and cisterns, providing ideal breeding places for the mosquito vector. Ships anchored in the harbor and on the city's wharves also carried water barrels and other containers suitable for mosquito breeding. Late summer and early fall rains often filled these containers and helped lay the foundations for epidemics. In the 1820s, Dr. Samuel Henry Dickson repeated an observation of an "old inhabitant" that he could "foretell an unhealthy fall by the permanent fullness of his well, and the remark is a common one."[6]

The flight range of the vector is only a few hundred yards, but as it resides close to human habitations, this is no obstacle to its spreading yellow fever where populations are dense, as in towns. *Aedes aegypti* is also adept at hitching rides aboard ships, which is why the disease was prevalent in ports and along navigable rivers. Ports favored yellow fever for another reason: They attracted the nonimmune individuals needed to provide the virus with new sources of infection. Charleston was the only city in South Carolina in the colonial and early national eras, and parts of it – especially near the wharves – were often densely packed with new immigrants, transients, sailors, and in time of war, soldiers. The subtropical climate, in which frosts seldom came before the late fall or early winter, if at all, was friendly to the vector. *Aedes aegypti* requires temperatures above 62 degrees Fahrenheit (17 degrees Celsius)

---

[6] Samuel Henry Dickson, "Account of the epidemic which prevailed in Charleston, S. C. during the summer of 1827," *The American Journal of the Medical Sciences* (1828), 2: 2; McNeill, *Mosquito Empires*, 59.

to bite and generally above 50 degrees Fahrenheit (10 degrees Celsius) to survive. Temperatures in the city rarely fall outside those parameters between April and November. Warm autumns sometimes allowed the mosquitoes to spread the virus into December. Epidemics that ended earlier may have done so from a lack of nonimmunes rather than cold weather. During epidemics, many people fled the city while others avoided it, depriving the virus of its fuel.[7]

As a source of morbidity and mortality, yellow fever was less important than malaria and dysentery. But it was feared more than either and in Charleston it was often a major killer. Moreover, it had a powerful effect on the development and outlook of the city and its region.[8] People in the region dreaded it not only for the mortality and agony it produced, but also because it could have a devastating impact on public business, commerce, and immigration. Much of the population would flee in panic to the countryside, to the sea islands such as nearby Sullivan's Island, and to cooler points farther north and higher in altitude. Country people avoided the city. Meetings of the legislature and the courts might be suspended, and trade brought to a virtual standstill for months. Yellow fever was also a major deterrent to white immigration. The numerous epidemics that struck the city, especially after the 1790s, partly explain why Charleston – the fourth-largest city in the United States in 1790 – never attracted the hordes of European immigrants who flocked to cities further north. After the epidemic of 1817, Roger Pinckney predicted that yellow fever would "injure the prosperity of Charleston considerably as persons will not settle where they are obliged every summer to fly; every stranger that has not left the place has died."[9]

Because of yellow fever's economic impact and the need to establish an effective public policy to deal with it, theories about its origins and transmission aroused enormous controversy everywhere until 1900, when U.S. Army physicians, led by Walter Reed, confirmed the role of the mosquito vector. On one side were those who believed yellow fever was an imported and probably contagious disease. On the other were people who argued that the disease was not contagious and originated locally. The first group demanded strict enforcement of quarantine regulations. The second group generally urged relaxation or elimination of quarantine laws and a focus on sanitary measures. In between were some people who hedged their bets and advocated

---

[7] Daniel Horlbeck to Judge Glover, Oct. 29, 1858, MSS 945, WHL; Joseph I. Waring, *Medicine in South Carolina, 1825–1900* (Charleston: South Carolina Medical Association, 1967), 130–135; McNeill, *Mosquito Empires*, 40–44; Kenneth Kiple, *The Caribbean Slave* (1984), 18; Margaret Humphreys, *Yellow Fever and the South* (Baltimore and London: Johns Hopkins University Press, 1992); Thomas P. Monath, "Yellow Fever: An Update," *Lancet Infectious Diseases* (2001) 1: 11–20; *Cambridge World History of Human Disease*, 1100–1101.

[8] John Duffy, "Yellow Fever in Colonial Charleston," *SCHM*, 52 (1951), 197; Waring, *Medicine in South Carolina, 1825–1900*, 30.

[9] Roger Pinckney to his aunt, Oct. 2, 1817, Roger Pinckney Correspondence, 1783–1823, SCHS; William Hume, "The Yellow Fever of Charleston, considered in its relation to the West Indian commerce," *Charleston Medical Journal and Review* 15 (Jan. 1860), 1–3, 11, 22–25, 28–31.

both approaches. Both methods of preventing yellow fever aroused opposition. Strict quarantine disrupted trade; sanitary improvements were expensive and interfered with property rights.[10] Not surprisingly, public officials were reluctant to admit the presence of a disease whose loathsome reputation could bring commerce to a virtual halt. In these circumstances, physicians might be reluctant to diagnose yellow fever, especially in the early stages of an epidemic, when it could be easily mistaken for another disease. Later chapters will address these issues in detail.

INTRODUCING YELLOW FEVER

To better understand pre-1900 reactions and responses to yellow fever, we need to consider the modern picture of the disease. Yellow fever probably originated in Central or East Africa. Its transmission to the Americas resulted from the slave trade. It is caused by a flavivirus, a genus that includes the dengue and West Nile viruses among many others. The name "yellow fever" derives from one of its common symptoms, a jaundice produced by the virus's attacks on the liver. Other symptoms include high fever, vomiting, exhaustion, convulsions, delirium, severe bodily aches, and internal and external bleeding. Severely ill patients often vomit dried and blackened blood that has the appearance of coffee grounds, hence the Spanish names *vomito negro* or *vomito prieto* – "the black vomit." The disease has an incubation period of three-to-six days from infection. It generally runs its course within two weeks, but it can kill in two or three days from onset of symptoms. Like many viral diseases, it has no known cure. Historically, estimated case mortality rates (the percentage of the infected who die) for yellow fever have varied considerably, from less than 10 percent to more than 80 percent. In August 1819, doctors of the Medical Society of South Carolina reported a case mortality rate of 50 percent. In the 1840s, Dr. Samuel Henry Dickson estimated that the average case mortality of epidemics was about one in five or six, but that it occasionally reached levels as high as three out of four.

A major problem in establishing case mortality rates for yellow fever is determining how many people have been infected. Infections often result in mild or even subclinical cases that go unreported. If there are a large number of such cases, the reported mortality rate will be inaccurately high, because those with the most prominent symptoms are also the most likely to die. Patients who survive the disease are henceforth immune, but may not know they have ever had it. In places where the disease is endemic or frequently epidemic, most victims are young children and newcomers because nearly

[10] Humphreys, *Yellow Fever and the South*; Blake, "Yellow Fever," 680–683; Jo Ann Carrigan, "Yellow Fever: Scourge of the South," in *Disease and Distinctiveness in the American South*, ed. by Todd L. Savitt and James Harvey Young (Knoxville: University of Tennessee Press, 1988), 57–58; Margaret Humphreys, "Dengue Fever: Breakbone Fever," in Kenneth F. Kiple, ed., *Plague, Pox and Pestilence: Disease in History* (London: Weidenfeld and Nicholson, 1997), 96.

everyone else will be immune from having survived an attack. If the number
of nonimmunes is small, yellow fever may appear as a sporadic disease or not
at all due to "herd immunity." People who are immune are virus killers. If
their percentage among the population is sufficiently large – around 80 percent – they will protect the immunes within the population by stopping the
circulation of the virus. An influx of susceptible newcomers, especially young
adults, however, can set off an epidemic if the right conditions exist for the
breeding and biting of the mosquito vector. Young adults also tend to have the
highest mortality rates from yellow fever, perhaps the result of an over-reaction
of the immune system. In places where yellow fever was endemic or common,
most victims were newly arrived immigrants, merchants, sailors, and soldiers.
Many Africans were immune from having survived the disease or perhaps from
a genetic resistance, an issue that will be fully discussed in a later chapter.[11]

Drawing an accurate epidemiological picture of yellow fever is extremely
difficult. No one doubts that yellow fever was frequently epidemic in South
Carolina in the eighteenth and nineteenth centuries, but its presence or absence
at a specific time may be open to dispute. Unlike smallpox, which was seldom
mistaken for anything else, yellow fever has historically been confused with
several other diseases that present similar symptoms, notably the jaundice,
that led to it being called yellow fever. Confusion was particularly likely in
mild cases of the disease, which were common, especially among children.
Diseases sometimes confused with yellow fever include malaria, dengue, hep-
atitis and other liver diseases, relapsing fever, spirochetal diseases, typhus,
typhoid, and scurvy. Confusion in the past was increased by the numerous
and not terribly descriptive names used to denote the fever at various times
and places. An example is the French name *mal de Siam*, born of the mistaken
notion that the disease had originated in that country. Another French name,
fievre de matelotte, or sailor's fever, was accurate in that seamen were one of
the groups most prone to getting it. But it did not do much to distinguish it
from other diseases, for the same was true of scurvy and typhus, both often
called "ship fever." The "black vomit" is not uniformly descriptive, because
that dramatic symptom did not appear in many cases of the disease. The name
"yellow fever" is not particularly helpful, either. As early as 1768, British
naval surgeon James Lind pointed out that jaundice was found in many other
diseases "so cannot properly be a distinguishing mark." Others observed that
jaundice was a not a universal symptom in yellow fever.[12]

[11] J. R. McNeill provides the best recent discussion of the ecology of yellow fever and its effects
in the Caribbean region from the seventeenth to the early twentieth century. See his *Mosquito
Empires: Ecology and War in the Greater Caribbean, 1640–1914* (Cambridge: Cambridge
University Press, 2010), esp. chapter 2; Kiple, *Cambridge World History of Human Disease*,
1101; Margaret Humphreys, "Yellow Fever: the Yellow Jack," in Kiple, *Plague, Pox and
Pestilence*, 86–91; MSM, Aug. 20, 1819, 142; Samuel Henry Dickson, *Essays on Pathology
and Therapeutics* 2 vols. (Charleston, 1845), 1: 342–343.
[12] James Lind, *An Essay on Diseases Incident to Europeans in Hot Climates* (London, 1768),
118; Benjamin Moseley, *A Treatise on Tropical Diseases* (London, 1792), 413.

Malaria was often mistaken for yellow fever (and vice versa). Malaria is generally less deadly than yellow fever, although the former can produce high mortality in children. People could have contracted both malaria and yellow fever at the same time or in succession, thus complicating diagnosis. Another complication is that dengue or break-bone fever can easily coexist with yellow fever and may even provide some protection against it. Dengue, like yellow fever, is a viral disease transmitted by the same species of mosquitoes, *Aedes aegypti*. Charleston doctors noted the presence of dengue in the city on numerous occasions and some argued that it could be confused with yellow fever.[13] In addition, as previously noted, yellow fever often produces mild symptoms or is even asymptomatic, especially in infants. As a result, its presence in a community where most adults are immune from previous attacks can easily pass unnoticed or be mistaken for a less virulent disease.[14] Depending on the circumstances, yellow fever may be overdiagnosed or underdiagnosed. These problems were compounded by the desire of local officials not to admit its presence because it caused panic and scared off nonresidents, with potentially devastating economic effects.

It should be clear from the foregoing that historical pronouncements about the presence or absence of yellow fever may be highly tentative. This is especially true in the many cases when no observer provided a detailed clinical description of the disease. Throughout the eighteenth and most of the nineteenth centuries, doctors debated the proper name, nature, identity, and specificity of the disease. Some of them viewed yellow fever as a virulent form of what we would call malaria, aggravated by peculiar circumstances of the atmosphere and the individual victim. Others considered it a separate pestilential disease, similar to or perhaps related to typhus or plague. In the 1740s, British doctor Henry Warren argued that the disease was "commonly mistaken for a bilious fever [but was] truly of the pestilential kind." By this, he apparently meant it was more like plague, smallpox, or typhus than malaria, which was often called a bilious fever. In contrast, Benjamin Rush, mentor of many American doctors, argued in the 1790s that yellow fever was simply "a higher grade of the common bilious fever of warm climates and seasons." In his view, changes in atmospheric conditions, personal habits, and improper medical treatment could transform an intermittent fever into a bilious fever, which could, given the right circumstances, turn into a yellow fever. Many South Carolina doctors agreed. Rush's protégé, David Ramsay, followed him closely. He declared that fevers were "the proper endemics of Carolina.... In their mildest season they assume the type of intermittents; in their next

[13] Benjamin B. Strobel, *An Essay on the Subject of Yellow Fever Intended to Prove its Transmissibility* (Charleston, 1840), 170–171; MSM, July 28, 1827, 337, May 1831, 433, Sept. 1, 1858, 407; Humphreys, "Dengue Fever"; McNeill, *Mosquito Empires*, 39; Carter, *Yellow Fever*, 49–81.

[14] Humphreys, "Dengue Fever,"; Humphreys, "Yellow Fever"; Carter, *Yellow Fever*, 49–81; K. D. Patterson, "Yellow Fever Epidemics and Mortality in the United States, 1693–1905," *Social Science Medicine* 34 (1992), 857, Table 1.

grade they are bilious remittents, and under particular circumstances in their highest grade constitute yellow fever."[15] In the 1750s, British doctor William Hilary claimed that "the propriety or impropriety of calling yellow fever a putrid bilious fever" was "only a dispute about words," and used the terms "yellow," "putrid," and "bilious" synonymously. Other doctors did the same, and the result was confusion for contemporaries and historians, often with deadly results for the contemporaries.[16]

DISCOVERING YELLOW FEVER

The first known epidemic of yellow fever in South Carolina occurred in 1699. Several historians have claimed that yellow fever struck Charleston in the early 1690s, but none provided evidence. Yellow fever could have been among the malignant fevers that produced heavy mortality among new arrivals – especially Scots and Huguenots – in the mid-1680s, but no one left a description of the disease or diseases responsible.[17] In 1699, the evidence points much more clearly to yellow fever. The disease was raging in the Caribbean in the 1690s following the arrival of European military expeditions fighting in the Nine Years' War, and Carolinians plied a regular trade with Barbados and other West Indian islands. Yellow fever was one of the diseases that destroyed the Scots colony at Darien in Panama between 1698 and 1700.[18] Carolina officials stated that the epidemic of 1699 was the same disease that had recently attacked several other English colonies and believed that it had come from Barbados or Providence in the Bahamas. The epidemic killed almost 200 people, including one-third of the colonial assembly and several high-ranking officials, and paralyzed trade and public business for weeks. Yellow fever returned in 1706 and became a frequent visitor during the next forty years.[19] Anglican

---

[15] Ramsay, *History of South Carolina*, 2: 54; Benjamin Rush, *An Account of the Bilious Remitting Yellow Fever, as it Appeared in the City of Philadelphia, in the Year 1793* (Philadelphia, 1794), 178–179.

[16] William Hillary, *Observations on the Changes of the Air and the Consequent Epidemical Diseases, on the Island of Barbados, to Which is Added, a Treatise on the Putrid Bilious Fever, Commonly Called the Yellow Fever* (London, 1759), 143–144; *Letters of Benjamin Rush* ed. by L.H. Butterfield 2 vols. (Princeton, NJ: Princeton University Press, 1951), 2: 881; Henry Warren, *A Treatise Concerning the Malignant Fever in Barbados and the Neighboring Islands* (London, 1741); Richard B. Sheridan, *Doctors and Slaves: A Medical and Demographic History of Slavery in the British West Indies, 1680–1834* (Cambridge: Cambridge University Press, 1985), 23, 68.

[17] Noble David Cook, *Born to Die: Disease and New World Conquest, 1492–1650* (Cambridge and New York: Cambridge University Press, 1998), 181; Kiple, *Cambridge World History of Human Disease*, 1103; K. D. Patterson, "Yellow Fever Epidemics and Mortality in the United States, 1693–1905," *Social Science Medicine* 34 (1992): 857, Table 1; Julien St. Ravenel Childs, *Malaria and Colonization in the Carolina Low Country, 1526–1696* (Baltimore: The Johns Hopkins University Press, 1940), 207; "Arrival of the Cardross Settlers" *SCHM* 30 (1929), 72.

[18] Kiple, *Caribbean Slave*; Blake, "Yellow Fever," 673–674; Humphreys, "Yellow Fever," 86. On the Darien colony, see McNeill, *Mosquito Empires*, 105–123, 144–149.

[19] *Commissions and Instructions from the Lords Proprietors of Carolina to the Public Officials of South Carolina, 1685–1715*, ed. by A. S. Salley, Jr. (Columbia, 1916), 129; Hugh

missionaries often referred to pestilential and malignant fevers in the summers and autumns in the 1710s. The assembly was prorogued several times in this period during the autumn months, a pattern consistent with later yellow fever epidemics.[20] In the fall of 1728, an epidemic killed "multitudes," according to Alexander Hewatt. The disease was "suddenly caught" and "quickly fatal." So many people were sick and dying that it was impossible to bury the dead properly. Although they were often buried the day they died, "so quick was the putrefaction, so offensive and infectious were the corpses, that even the nearest relations seemed averse from the necessary duty." Country people avoided Charleston, business came to a halt, food prices soared, and many people went hungry. The assembly, scheduled to meet in September, could not achieve a quorum all autumn and did not convene until January.[21]

Such scenes occurred repeatedly during the 1730s and 1740s.[22] An epidemic of 1732 was the first to be reported in the recently established *South Carolina Gazette*. On July 15, the paper announced that a number of people had "died suddenly" of fevers in town. By early August, an "uncommon mortality" raged. The dead included the son of Governor Robert Johnson. The assembly was prorogued several times until December.[23] Anglican Commissary Alexander Garden wrote to the Bishop of London in November that "a plague" had been raging since July, with as many as "ten funerals a day." Garden was not exaggerating, at least not much. On July 23, the St. Philip's Parish register records ten people buried, and on July 26, nine. In July and August, the parish alone buried ninety-three people, and there were several other churches (or meeting houses) in the town. The number of deaths in the city in 1732 was the highest of the decade 1722–1732. The second highest was 1728, another yellow fever year.[24]

Adams to Samuel Sewell, Feb. 23, 1700, Massachusetts Historical Society, *Collections*, 5th ser., 6: 11–12; Thomas Hasell, Sept. 6, 1707, SPG Letter Books, A3: 281–284; BPRO/SC, 5: 161–162, 171–174; Salley, *Narratives*, 304, 308; *JCHA*, Nov. 20, 1706-Feb. 8, 1707, 3, 5; Klingberg, *Le Jau*, 16–21, 85–87, 104.

[20] Thomas Hasell, Aug. 18, 1712, SPG Letter Books, A7: 435; *Commissions and Instructions*, 273; JCHA, Aug. 4, 1716, Oct. 10, 1717, SCDAH; Thomas Hasell, Oct. 11, 22, 1718, SPG Letter Books, A13: 190; William Treadwell Bull, Nov. 24, 1718, SPG Letter Books, A13: 236; Waring, *Medicine in South Carolina, 1670–1825*, 27; John Duffy, "Yellow Fever in Colonial Charleston," *SCHM* 52 (1951), 196; Duffy, "Carolina Health Conditions," 299–302.

[21] Alexander Hewatt, *An Historical Account of the Rise and Progress of the Colonies of South Carolina and Georgia*, 2 vols. (London, 1779) 1: 316–318; Journals of His Majesty's Council of South Carolina, Sept. 21, Oct. 31, Nov. 21–23, 1728, SCDAH; JCHA, Jan. 18, 1728/29, SCDAH; Walter Fraser, *Charleston! Charleston! The History of a Southern City* (Columbia: University of South Carolina Press, 1989), 7–44.

[22] John Lining, "A Description of the American Yellow Fever," *Essays and Observations, Physical and Literary* 2 (1756): 370–395; Ramsay, *History of South Carolina*, 2: 47.

[23] *SCG*, July 15, Aug. 5, 12, 19, Sept. 2, 15, 23, Oct. 20, Dec. 16, 1732; Council Journals, August 30, Nov. 9–10, Dec. 5, 1732, SCDAH; *Collections of the South Carolina Historical Society* 5 vols. (Charleston, 1897), 3: 316–317; Robert Johnson to Board of Trade, Dec. 15, 1732, BPRO/SC 16: 4.

[24] Alexander Garden to Bishop of London, Nov 8, 1732, Fulham Palace Mss., Library of Congress, transcript summary of letters from Garden to Bishop of London, copies in SCHS; Coclanis, *Shadow of a Dream*, 164, Table B1, 169–170, Tables D1-D3.

Yellow fever returned several more times during the 1730s and 1740s. St. Philip's Parish register shows substantial jumps in the number of burials in the late summer and fall in many of these years. Obituaries in the *Gazette* often reported warm weather deaths as "sudden" or occurring after a short illness, a pattern more characteristic of yellow fever than malaria. A virulent epidemic of yellow fever struck the town in 1739, on the heels of a major smallpox epidemic the previous year. Trade and public business were paralyzed. Ships coming into the port could not get needed supplies or had to wait weeks to get the goods they had come for.[25] The number of burials at St. Philips parish in 1739 –198 – was the second highest of the period 1720–1758. (The highest was the previous year, one of smallpox.) The deaths, illnesses, and panic in 1739 may have encouraged and certainly aided the Stono Rebellion that September, the most serious slave uprising of the colonial period. The disease returned the following year. A "malignant distemper" in town convinced the colonial assembly to disband. Burials surged in September and October, though not as much as in 1739.[26]

Yellow fever made its way to Savannah, capital of the new colony of Georgia, in the early 1740s. War or Carolinians probably brought it there, as slavery was not yet legal. Between 1740 and 1742, British forces lost thousands of men to the disease on expeditions against Spanish possessions in the Caribbean. In the latter year, Georgia official William Stephens described an epidemic that struck Savannah as "a malignant fever of the worst sort." In its wake, the town had "grown thin."[27] In contrast, epidemic yellow fever spared Charleston during the early 1740s. Recent epidemics had probably immunized most of the survivors. The Stono Rebellion of 1739 also led to the imposition of a prohibitive duty on slave imports. But the slave trade surged after 1745, and epidemic yellow fever returned immediately. An Anglican missionary reported

[25] James Kilpatrick, *An Essay on Inoculation* (London, 1743), 56–57; Walter Edgar, *Letterbook of Robert Pringle* 2 vols. (Columbia: University of South Carolina Press, 1972), 1: 140, 143; William Bull to Duke of Newcastle, Nov. 20, 1739, *Collections of South Carolina Historical Society*, 2: 273; BPRO/SC, 20: 192–193, 300–331; Duffy, "Yellow Fever," 194; Wood, *Black Majority*, 312–313; Alexander Garden to the Bishop of London, April 24, 1740; "Letters to the Bishop of London from the Commissaries in South Carolina" ed. by George W. Williams, *SCHM* 78 (1977), letter 43; James Kirkpatrick, *The Analysis of Inoculation* (London, 2d ed., 1761), 64.

[26] *Death Notices in the South Carolina Gazette*, 8, 11–14, 20–22; Frank J. Klingberg, *An Appraisal of the Negro in Colonial South Carolina: a Study in Americanization* (Washington, DC: Associated Publishers, 1941), 61; *Register of St. Philip's Parish*, 244–266; *JCHA*, 2: 398, 400; Waring, *Medicine in South Carolina, 1670–1825*, 372, 412; Andrew Leslie, Jan. 7, 1739/40, SPG, B7, 2: 243–244;. Historians have provided several explanations for the timing of the Stono Rebellion. See Mark M. Smith, ed. *Stono: Documenting and Interpreting a Southern Slave Revolt* (Columbia: University of South Carolina Press, 2005); Matthew Mulcahy, "Melancholy and Fatal Calamities," in Jack P. Greene, Rosemary Brana-Shute, and Randy Sparks, eds., *Money, Trade, and Power: The Evolution of South Carolina's Plantation Economy* (Columbia: University of South Carolina Press, 2001), 281; Wood, *Black Majority*.

[27] *Journal of William Stephens*, 116–126; McNeill, *Mosquito Empires*, 149–169.

that fall that Charleston was "very much afflicted with a great and malignant sickness called the yellow fever, in which they die suddenly." Burials soared during September and October. The number of St. Philip's burials for the year was the third highest of the period 1720 to 1758.[28]

Yellow fever was probably active in Charleston nearly every year in the later 1740s. A petition to the colonial government in 1749 lamented that the town had "divers times of late years been greatly afflicted with an epidemical sickness, commonly called the yellow fever, attended with great mortality." St. Philip's Parish records show a sharp spike in burials during the warm months of the late 1740s. Meetings of the assembly were generally delayed until late fall or winter. Large numbers of Indians, including the friendly king of the Catawba, perished of pestilence in 1749 while on a diplomatic visit to Charleston. This happened in spite of the fact that Governor Glen met them a few miles outside the town, where the air and water were allegedly more pure.[29]

STEALTH YELLOW FEVER: 1750–1792

Around 1750, the perception – if not the reality – of yellow fever changed. Most accounts claim that epidemic yellow fever retreated from Charleston after 1748 – except for sporadic cases in the early 1750s – and did not reappear until the early 1790s. Some historians have argued that epidemic yellow fever seemingly disappeared entirely from British North America between the 1760s and early 1790s. In 1968, John Blake stated that Philadelphia's yellow fever epidemic of 1762 was apparently the last one to ravage the British North American mainland until the famous epidemic in that city in 1793. He noted, however, that some historians had listed an epidemic in Charleston in 1792, and declared: "[T]he origin of this outbreak, if indeed it was yellow fever, deserves further investigation."[30] Blake was correct. The Charleston epidemic of 1792 – and others that soon followed it – deserve further investigation because they shed light on the alleged disappearance of yellow fever between the 1750s and the 1790s.

David Ramsay claimed that no epidemic of yellow fever had occurred in Charleston between 1748 and 1792. The disease had become epidemic in the latter year and returned almost every year since. Ramsay was justifiably mystified by both the apparent absence of epidemics for more than forty years

---

[28] John Fordyce, Nov. 4, 1745, SPG Letter Books, B12: 92; *SCG*, Sept. 15, Oct. 7, Nov. 11, 1745; *JCHA*, 6: 12; *Journal of William Stephens*, 243, 250; Charles Boschi, Oct. 30, 1745, SPG Letter Books, B12: 112; Council Journals, Oct. 5, Nov. 6, Dec. 5, 7, 1745, SCDAH; *Register of St. Philip's Parish*, 198–204.

[29] *JCHA*, 9: 168, 200; Journal of the Upper House of Assembly of South Carolina, 1748–1749, SCDAH; Levi Durand, April 23, 1747, SPG Journals, 10: 287; *SCG*, Sept. 6, 1747; *Register of St. Philip's Parish*, 206–213, 264–265; *HLP*, 1:171; *SCG*, Sept. 6, 1748; Charles Boschi, Feb. 10, 1749, SPG Letter Books, B16–17: 345–346, quoted in Duffy, "Yellow Fever," 196; Jonathan Mercantini, *Who Shall Rule at Home? The Evolution of South Carolina Political Culture* (Columbia: University of South Carolina Press, 2007), 72–73.

[30] Blake, "Yellow Fever," 674–675; Duffy, "Yellow Fever," 196.

and the sudden return of epidemics nearly every year for the next sixteen years after that.[31] Later writers repeated Ramsay's account and shared his puzzlement. Some of them argued that the absence of epidemic yellow fever was related to a decline of the disease in the British West Indies.[32] In fact, the evidence indicates that yellow fever did not disappear from Charleston after 1748, but was often present without being explicitly acknowledged or perhaps recognized as such. The latter scenario makes sense given what happened when the disease "returned" in the 1790s and early 1800s. The epidemics of that period spared most natives and long-term residents, whereas nearly all the victims were newcomers and young children. This could not have been the case if yellow fever had disappeared for more than forty years.

Indeed, in 1805, Ramsay's colleague Tucker Harris claimed that yellow fever epidemics had struck the city frequently since 1748. Harris concluded that the disease was practically endemic to Charleston, as did James Kilpatrick in the 1740s.[33] Retrospectively, it is possible to identify several epidemics from the late eighteenth century that may have been yellow fever but are not called yellow fever in official documents. Because investigators from the later eighteenth century on have not found the term "yellow fever" in the sources of this period, they have generally assumed that it had disappeared. It did undoubtedly become less of a problem as the proportion of immunes in the population increased. It is also highly likely that locals had chosen to avoid a name that conveyed such terror and had such adverse economic consequences. A straw in the wind came during the epidemic of 1748, when the *South Carolina Gazette* hesitated to declare the disease the same as "the yellow fever of the West Indies" but noted that it killed "very healthy and strong men" in a few days, a pattern typical of yellow fever. A few years later, John Lining declared in his essay on the disease that the epidemic of 1748 had indeed been yellow fever.[34] But then something very odd happened. Even before Lining's essay was published, the frightful name "yellow fever" disappeared from public discussion in Charleston. In 1755, the *Gazette* reported that adult mortality had been above average for the past two years but did not even mention yellow fever as a possible cause of the increase.[35] Two years later, high mortality occurred among soldiers posted to

[31] Ramsay, *History of South Carolina*, 2: 45–47; *South Carolina, Resources and Population, Institutions and Industries* (Charleston, 1883), 22.

[32] Thomas Y. Simons, "Observations on the Yellow Fever, as it occurs in Charleston, South Carolina," *Carolina Journal of Medicine, Science, and Agriculture* 1 (1825), 2; Blake, "Yellow Fever," 675. Joseph I. Waring claimed that yellow fever struck Charleston in 1758, 1759, and 1762 but provided no evidence. See Waring, *Medicine in South Carolina, 1670–1825*, 372, 412.

[33] Harris, "Yellow Fever of Charleston," 24–25; Kilpatrick, *Essay on Inoculation*, 56.

[34] Levi Durand, April 23, 1747, SPG Journals, 10: 287; Duffy, "Yellow Fever in Colonial Charleston," 195; *SCG*, Sept. 6, 1747; *Register of St. Philip's Parish*, 206–210, 264–265; *HLP*, 1: 171; *SCG*, Sept. 6, 1748; Journal of the Upper House of Assembly of South Carolina, 1748, SCDAH; Charles Boschi, Feb. 10, 1749, B16–17: 345–346, cited in Duffy, "Yellow Fever," 196.

[35] Robert Stone, March 6, 1749/50, March 22, 1750/51, SPG, B17: 182, B18: 186; William Langhorne, March 8, 1750/51, SPG, B18: 190; *SCG*, June 13, 1755, cited in Duffy, "Yellow Fever," 196.

Charleston to guard against a possible French attack, and again no one even mentioned yellow fever. This episode deserves a closer look.

In June 1757, Lieutenant-Colonel Henry Bouquet arrived in Charleston with about 700 colonial soldiers. Many of his men soon became sick at their camp at the race course, about two miles north of town. By late August, with heavy rains and "the number of sick increasing every day," Bouquet moved his men into town to get them "under cover." At the end of the month, he was reinforced with the arrival of about 1,000 Scots Highlanders. By now, a town of perhaps 8,000 residents was inundated with about 1,700 soldiers, in addition to several hundred French Acadians and more than 100 French prisoners of war. The provincial government had not prepared adequate quarters for the soldiers, pleading lack of time. Bouquet blamed stinginess, noting that the local elite had begged for soldiers to protect them and then refused to provide them decent accommodation. The result was a political crisis over housing soldiers in private homes without consent, one of the issues that later led to the American Revolution. In 1757, the lack of adequate quarters contributed to illness and death among the soldiers. The causes of death may well have included yellow fever.

Lord Loudoun, the British commander in chief, had feared such an outcome. In early September 1757, he wrote Governor William Lyttleton that if the soldiers he was sending were not properly housed and cared for, they "will be very sickly in your climate." When the Highlanders landed on September 3, both Lyttleton and Bouquet proclaimed them to be in good health. Within a week, Bouquet was reporting that they "grow very sickly." Some of the Highlanders were initially quartered in warehouses along the wharves, where yellow fever generally lurked. Others were housed in the half-finished St. Michael's Church nearby and in empty houses. Most had to lie outside upon the ground, easy prey for mosquitoes. By the end of September, more than 500 were ill, more than half their number. Among the colonial troops, only 300 men were fit for duty. A delegation of the Creek Nation whom Lyttleton invited to Charleston that September decided not to come when they heard about the sickness there. On October 22, Bouquet wrote that the heat had moderated but "the whole country is sick; our men die very fast, and we have lost more in one month, than in the whole winter at Philadelphia." At the time, Lyttleton informed Loudoun that the autumn had been the unhealthiest in Carolina for many years and that sickness was "universal." Yet in a letter to Gen. Jeffery Amherst three years later, Lyttleton declared that the Highlanders had suffered "little sickness" and few deaths in the fall of 1757. He also claimed that the soldiers' housing was adequate.

Bouquet told a radically different story. In early December, he reported that 60 Highlanders had died since they landed, and claimed that many more would have died had not compassionate locals taken more than 200 of them into their own houses. Bouquet did not report the number of deaths among the colonial soldiers or the final tally for the Scots. But between August 3 and December 24, St. Philip's register lists the burials of sixty-five soldiers, along with several of their wives and children, and a number of sailors. Soldiers and sailors continued to be buried there in large numbers in the following months. Between June 1757 and September 1759, soldiers made up by far the largest category in the parish burial list. In contrast, just before and after those dates, most of the deaths were among children. The register does not distinguish how many of the dead were Highlanders and how many were colonial soldiers. Some deaths in both groups may not have been recorded because they were buried in the city's Dissenting churches.

No one left a description of the disease or diseases that scourged the army (or the Acadians also present in the town), but yellow fever is a highly likely culprit in the case of the Highlanders who became ill within a week after their arrival in town. Malaria has an incubation period of about two weeks after infection, whereas symptoms of yellow fever appear three to six days after the virus enters the bloodstream. In Charleston, yellow fever epidemics usually began near the wharves along the Cooper River, where some of the Scots were camped in exposed conditions. It is probable that yellow fever, if it was responsible for their illnesses, was confined to the area near the wharves. The soldiers scattered about town in private houses may have been protected by distance from the wharves and/or herd immunity among the locals. The total number and percentage of deaths, while significant, was small compared to the huge losses to yellow fever sustained by European forces in the Caribbean campaigns of the eighteenth century. Other diseases probably accounted for some or most of the illnesses among the soldiers.[36]

Epidemic yellow fever almost certainly struck Charleston in 1761. The disease was epidemic in Havana that summer. St Philip's Parish register shows a surge of burials from August to December 1761, and soldiers once again fell in large numbers.[37] Dr. Alexander Garden reported that a "violent epidemic" of "putrid bilious fever" – a name some doctors used to describe what we would now call yellow fever – had attacked him and subsequently kept him busy in town with patients for months.[38] Some people called the disease

---

[36] *The Papers of Henry Bouquet* 2 vols. (Harrisburg: The Pennsylvania Historical and Museum Commission, 1972), 1: 150–151, 172, 196, 203, 211–212, 216–217, 226, 248–249; *Register of St. Philip's Parish*, 284–296; Council Journals, Sept. 1, 2, 29, 1757, SCDAH; William Henry Lyttleton to William Pitt, Sept. 3, 1757, Lyttleton to the Board of Trade, Sept. 15, 1757, BPRO/SC: 27; Lyttleton to Lord Loudoun, Oct. 20, 1757, WO34/35; Lyttleton to Amherst, March 31, 1760, WO34/35, PRO; Mercantini, *Who Shall Rule?*, 131–132; Peter Coclanis, "Death in Early Charleston: an estimate of the crude death rate for the white population of Charleston, 1722–1732," *SCHM* 85 (1984), 285–286; Leonard Jan Bruce-Chwatt, *Essential Malariology*, 2d edition (New York: John Wiley and Sons), 32; Kiple, *Cambridge History of Disease*, 1102.

[37] McNeill, *Mosquito Empires*, 175–187; "Extracts from the Journal of Mrs. Ann Manigault," *SCHM* 20 (1919), 139; Robert Raper Letterbook, SCHS, [September?], 1761, Feb. 27, 1762; J[oh]n Drayton to James Glen, Oct. 11, 1761, ALS, James Glen Papers, SCL; *Register of St. Philip's Parish*, 298–299. Twenty-six soldiers were recorded as buried in St. Philip's Cemetery between August 11 and December 28, 1761.

[38] Alexander Garden to John Ellis, Feb. 26, 1762, James E. Smith, *A Selection of the Correspondence of Linnaeus and Other Naturalists* 2 vols. (New York, Arno Press, 1978), 1: 513–515.

"yellow fever" – in private correspondence. On August 6, Ann Manigault recorded in her diary that a young man was reported to have died of yellow fever. In October, planter John Drayton reported in a letter that yellow fever was in Charleston. Factor Robert Raper also noted in letters that "a yellow fever epidemic" afflicted many families in the fall and that most of the wealthy retreated to the country. Decades later, Tucker Harris, then studying medicine with Lionel Chalmers, declared that the epidemic of 1761 was yellow fever. Most of the fatalities, he recalled, had been among strangers, and only one long-time resident died, a picture consistent with yellow fever attacking a community with a high percentage of immunes. Harris stated that Chalmers was so alarmed at the outbreak that he sent his family to the country, a common strategy for avoiding the fever.[39]

Although no one *declared* publicly in 1761 that the epidemic was yellow fever, one group *denied* publicly that it was: the slave merchants. In early September, Henry Laurens and his partners took out an advertisement in the *Gazette* stating that they had "good reason to believe that Charleston is not infected with yellow fever." Perhaps they believed it. But they added, less sincerely, "or any other epidemic distress." The Laurens group had two cargoes of Africans for sale. They knew from experience that an announcement of yellow fever or any malignant disease in town would scare off potential buyers from the surrounding countryside. They also knew that newly arrived slaves had a high morbidity and mortality rate. Before sale they had to be fed and doctored, a deduction from the merchants' profits. The smallpox epidemic the previous year had been financially devastating for local merchants. The slave traders' advertisement indicates that potential buyers were avoiding the town because they had heard that yellow fever or some other pestilential fever was there. Despite the sellers' assurance that there was no danger in Charleston, they added that they would bring the slaves to the country "in order to remove all cause of apprehension."[40] The advertisement is eerily similar to assurances nineteenth-century officials, doctors, and newspapers often made to outsiders thinking of coming to the city.

When Anglican missionary Charles Woodmason arrived in Charleston in August 1766, a virulent fever was killing large numbers of people. Woodmason never used the name yellow fever, but a planter quickly took him to his country home – a common strategy to avoid the fever in town. Woodmason later complained that some members of the local elite had persecuted him for "branding the province a sickly clime." Woodmason was not exaggerating the mortality. In a private letter, Henry Laurens confirmed that the summer of 1766 had brought an "abundance of mosquitoes" and many deaths to South Carolina and Georgia. The *Gazette* and the St. Philip's Parish register reported a larger than usual number of burials during the fever season. The dead included many recent immigrants – mostly Scots-Irish – drawn to the colony by a bounty the South Carolina colonial assembly established in 1761 to attract white

[39] *Columbian Herald*, March 10, 1794; Harris, "Yellow Fever of Charleston," 24–25.
[40] HLP, 3: 79.

Protestant settlers. The parish buried many more immigrants in the following summer. Between May 29 and November 18, 1767, St. Philip's Parish register lists sixty-seven burials of people from Ireland, sixty-one of them between June and September. Several others from England were buried during this period. Given the timing of their arrival, their status as newcomers, and the fact that many died weeks after they arrived, yellow fever was likely at work.[41]

Tucker Harris claimed that yellow fever had been epidemic in 1770, although he cited no evidence. His preceptor Lionel Chalmers inadvertently provided some, however. Chalmers wrote little about yellow fever in his book on weather and diseases in South Carolina, published in London in 1776. The omission is odd because he had been in Charleston since 1737 and had observed several epidemics. He had also been a partner of John Lining, who authored one of the first accurate clinical descriptions of the disease in the 1750s. Chalmers did mention, however, that a "putrid bilious fever" had attacked Charleston in the warm months of 1770. The fever had produced "such symptoms of a confirmed putrefaction, as to differ but little sometimes from the pestilential yellow fever." In fact, his description fits yellow fever remarkably well. Victims experienced a "prostration of strength" that was "sudden and great." Hemorrhages often occurred, blood being "constantly spurted out" from the mouth, "so that were the tongue, gums, and insides of the cheek to be wiped clean, the blood would immediately ooze out." Blood often poured from the nostrils as well. The blood had "such a cadaverous smell, as carcasses emit when in the first stage of putrefaction." Few patients, he added, "will recover from such a state."[42] An example of the fever's lethality is contained in a note in a family bible. It states that "Mary Gillon died in November 1770 within twenty-four hours illness of the putrid fever."[43] Yellow fever can kill within a day or two of the onset of symptoms. Perhaps Chalmers believed that the epidemic was yellow fever but feared to call it that lest he too be accused of "branding the province a sickly clime."

Chalmers' description of the epidemic of 1770 as resembling but not identical to yellow fever was significant. In 1792, Dr. William Currie of Philadelphia, who drew heavily from Chalmers' book, claimed that the excessive heat of late summer "during the growth of the rice ... has sometimes produced a remitting fever with malignant symptoms, similar to that which in the West Indies goes by the name yellow fever." But it was only similar, he insisted, not

[41] Richard J. Hooker, ed., *The Carolina Backcountry on the Eve of the Revolution: The Journal and Other Writings of Charles Woodmason, Anglican Itinerant* (Chapel Hill: University of North Carolina Press, 1953), 4–9, 84–87, 191–192, 200–201; *HLP*, 5: 198, 165; *Death Notices in the South Carolina Gazette*, 34–35; *Register of St. Philip's Parish*, 13–322; Council Journals, July 7, Sept. 8, 1767, SCDAH; *A Compilation of the Original Lists of Protestant Immigrants to South Carolina, 1763–1773*, comp. by Janie Revell, (Baltimore: Genealogical Publishing Co., 1968).

[42] Lionel Chalmers, *An Account of the Weather and Diseases of South Carolina* 2 vols. (London, 1776), 1: 163–164.

[43] "Records from the Bible belonging to Alexander Gillon," *SCHM* 19 (1918), 146.

the same. Whatever was true in the West Indies, Currie concluded, the South Carolina fever was not a specific disorder, only an aggravated form of the "bilious remittent fevers of hot climates or hot seasons of any climate." Currie cited Chalmers' description of the disease as evidence, and stated that John Lining had made "a very great error" in describing yellow fever as a distinct disorder.[44] Many Charleston doctors agreed. In the 1790s, they concluded that the fever that struck Charleston several times that decade was similar to but not the same as the yellow fever of the Caribbean.

Chalmers published his book on the weather and diseases of South Carolina in 1776. Between then and the epidemics of the 1790s came the American War for Independence. The Revolutionary Era was not a healthy one in the Lower South. Yet in 1796, David Ramsay inexplicably claimed there had been no serious epidemics of any kind in South Carolina in the past twenty years, except for "camp" fevers among the soldiers.[45] How Ramsay came to this astonishing conclusion is mystifying. He was not the best witness, because he was absent from the state from the summer of 1780 until well into the following year, when health conditions were at their worst. Smallpox and fevers killed many people, especially soldiers and large numbers of blacks, in 1780 and 1781. Despite his absence, Ramsay could not have been totally unaware of these events. He was also not being entirely truthful in public. In January 1780, he wrote to Benjamin Rush that the fevers of the previous summer and fall had been the most "speedily mortal" he had experienced since coming to South Carolina. In his *History of South Carolina*, published in 1809, he admitted that smallpox had circulated around the state in 1780 but had not caused "any considerable loss or inconvenience." In fact, thousands had died. Most of the dead were blacks, but many whites died as well. Even those who survived presumably experienced some "inconvenience."[46]

In his memoirs of the Revolution, General William Moultrie claimed that yellow fever had broken out among American prisoners of war after Charleston surrendered to the British in May 1780. Many of the American POWs were interned at a camp across the harbor in Christ Church Parish. Moultrie provided no description of the disease but he was surely familiar with yellow fever, and not only from living in Charleston. His father, John Moultrie, and his brother, John Moultrie, Jr., were both physicians. The latter, as we have seen, wrote one of the first clinical descriptions of yellow fever in 1749. General Moultrie's claim may be supported by a letter from Peter Fayssoux, surgeon to the Continental Army, to Ramsay. Fayssoux described

[44] William Currie, *An Historical Account of the Climates and Diseases of the United States of America* (Philadelphia, 1792), 380n, 390.

[45] David Ramsay, *A Sketch of the Soil, Climate, Weather, and Diseases of South Carolina* (Charleston, 1796), 25.

[46] Harris, "Yellow Fever of Charleston," 25–26; Ramsay, *History of South Carolina*, 2: 44–45; Fenn, *Pox Americana*; Robert L. Brunhouse, ed. *David Ramsay, 1749–1815: Selections from his Writings*, Transactions of the American Philosophical Society, N.S. 55: Part 4, (Philadelphia: American Philosophical Society,1965), 64.

a malignant fever that killed many American POWs on British prison ships in Charleston harbor in the fall of 1780. The description fits yellow fever, although it also fits typhus or typhoid. It produced a high mortality and a yellow suffusion over the victims' bodies. It was also marked by red and purplish spots on the torso.[47] British Major George Hanger claimed that he and other British soldiers had suffered from yellow fever in September 1780. The disease he described was highly malignant. Five fellow officers who became ill at the same time died of it. They contracted it in the upper part of the state, however, presumably out of the normal range of yellow fever in that period. It seems unlikely that infected mosquitoes could have made the journey, but it is not impossible. The yellow fever mosquito can remain infected for up to 180 days and it travels well on boats. The eggs of infected mosquitoes can also carry the virus. The disease often moved far inland in the nineteenth century. Armies, like towns, are highly dense communities, but also mobile, and the British were supplied and reinforced via river transport from Charleston and Georgetown.[48]

Further complicating the picture is the fact that dengue fever was also epidemic during the revolutionary years. Henry Laurens reported that "a vile fever called break-bone" had been prevalent in the Charleston area in 1778. Historians generally date the first recognition of dengue by American physicians to 1780, but some think it has been present in America much longer. Benjamin Rush described an outbreak in Philadelphia in 1780, calling it bilious remitting fever; others called it break-bone. Laurens' use of the term "break-bone" in 1778 indicates that recognition of the disease and the name predates that outbreak by at least a few years. Tucker Harris claimed that break-bone was common in Charleston during the later stages of the war, but that he never saw any cases of yellow fever during that time.[49] Classic dengue fever is rarely fatal, but it is easily mistaken for yellow fever. Conversely, dengue could also have masked the presence of yellow fever, especially in the chaotic conditions of war and occupation, which allowed little time for careful observation and reflection. Conditions in the region continued to be chaotic for several years after independence. The state's economy remained depressed for much of the 1780s, and large numbers of unemployed, transient, and immigrant whites crammed into Charleston's poorer and more unsanitary

[47] William Moultrie, *Memoirs of the American Revolution* 2 vols. (New York, 1802), 2: 112; George Hanger, *The Life, Adventures, and Opinions of George Hanger* (London, 1801), 172, 179–181; George Hanger, *An Address to the Army; in Reply to Strictures, by Roderick Mackenzie on Tarleton's History of the Campaigns of 1780 and 1781* (London, 1789), 68–70; Peter Fayssoux to David Ramsay, March 26, 1785, in Robert Gibbes, *Documentary History of the American Revolution*, 3 vols. (New York, 1853), 119.

[48] Hanger, *Life, Adventures, and Opinions*, 172, 179–181; Hanger, *Address to the Army*, 68–70.

[49] *HLP*, 14: 414; Humphreys, "Dengue Fever: Breakbone Fever," 93–94; *Cambridge World History of Human Disease*, 663; *The Wellcome Trust Illustrated History of Tropical Diseases* (London: The Wellcome Trust, 1996), 149–150; Harris, "Yellow Fever of Charleston," 25–26.

districts, many of them close to the wharves on the Cooper River. The population increased from about 11,500 in 1770 to more than 16,000 in 1790 and more than 20,000 in 1800. The influx of newcomers paved the way for the resurgence of yellow fever in a form that ultimately could not be denied.[50]

YELLOW FEVER RESURGENT

If yellow fever was not a major problem during the Revolutionary War, it may have been because the disease also declined in importance throughout the Caribbean region from the 1760s to the 1790s. The major reason for this was probably the emergence of a largely immune population. Another contributing factor was that the war disrupted trade and reduced the number of European and African newcomers for several years, with the exception of the British army that arrived in May 1780.[51] Commerce with the West Indies and Africa was the main source of infected people and mosquitoes. European immigration provided nonimmunes who could sustain an epidemic. Immigrants began to flow into the city soon after the Revolution. Planters once again began to import large numbers of slaves. The state banned the slave trade between 1787 and 1803, but a clandestine trade continued; thousands were bought from Georgia traders. The South Carolina General Assembly reopened the trade in December 1803 and between then and January 1808, when a federal prohibition began, about 40,000 slaves were imported.[52]

Regular trade with the Caribbean region resumed after the Revolution. In 1799, Charles Caleb Cotton noted that Charleston was involved in "a vast trade to the Havannah" and a highly profitable "clandestine trade to the Spanish Main, La Vera Cruz, New Orleans, etc."[53] Coincidentally or not, yellow fever was epidemic in Charleston frequently in the 1790s and early 1800s. In the antebellum period, several observers linked the revival of the disease to the Caribbean trade. One of them, William Hume, argued that the fever's resurgence was related to the passage of the American Navigation Acts of 1789 and 1792. These acts, he argued, increased the volume of trade with the West Indies and changed the nature of the ships' crews involved in it. Prior to the acts, the trade, Hume claimed, had been carried out largely by West Indian and Charleston crews "habituated" to yellow fever. The acts

[50] Peter Coclanis, *The Shadow of a Dream* (Oxford and New York: Oxford University Press, 1989), 115, Table 4–4.

[51] Sylvia R. Frey, *The British Soldier in America* (Austin: University of Texas Press, 1981), 42–43; John Blake, "Yellow fever in eighteenth century America," *Bulletin of the New York Academy of Sciences* 44 (1968), 675; J. R. McNeill, "Ecology, Epidemics, and Empires: Environmental Change and the Geopolitics of Tropical America, 1600–1825," *Environment and History* 5 (1999), 175–184.

[52] Fraser, *Charleston! Charleston!*, 176, 185, 188; Philip D. Morgan, *Slave Counterpoint: Black Culture in the Eighteenth-Century Chesapeake and Lowcountry* (Chapel Hill, University of North Carolina Press, 1998), 62.

[53] "The Letters of Charles Caleb Cotton, 1798–1802," *SCHM* 51 (1950), 142, 222.

increased the number of ships with northern and European crews more likely to be susceptible to yellow fever, and hence capable of carrying it from one port to another.[54]

A common explanation for the resurgence of yellow fever in the Americas more generally is the Haitian Revolution that began in the early 1790s, combined with the beginning of war between Revolutionary France and Britain in 1793. These events brought large numbers of susceptible soldiers and sailors to the Caribbean and caused large movements of population in and around the area. Some observers at the time and after argued that the "spark" that reignited yellow fever came in a slave ship from West Africa that arrived in Grenada in 1793, from whence the disease quickly spread to other islands and American ports.[55] All this may be true, but in Charleston, the "return" of epidemic yellow fever did not occur in 1793 but a year earlier. One can pinpoint a likely external source for this outbreak. French refugees fleeing the slave uprising in San Domingue (Haiti) began arriving in Charleston in the summer of 1792. Their arrival probably sparked the epidemic, much as a similar influx of refugees did in Philadelphia the following year. Many more refugees came to Charleston from San Domingue during the next two years, and they helped generate other epidemics in the city, combined with the simultaneous upsurge in the West Indian trade.[56]

This scenario is not incompatible with the suggestion that yellow fever may have visited Charleston on several occasions between the 1750s and 1780s. Because of the large number of immunes in the settled population during those years, cases would have been proportionally fewer and possibly less virulent than earlier in the century. The fever flared into recognition with an influx of susceptible sailors, immigrants, and visitors in the 1790s, perhaps combined with the arrival of a more virulent type of the virus from Africa via the West Indies.[57] In any case, yellow fever must have visited Charleston in the late eighteenth century to have produced the epidemiological results that followed in the 1790s and early 1800s. Nearly all of the victims in these epidemics were new arrivals to the city; the disease largely spared natives and long-term

---

[54] Benjamin B. Strobel, *An Essay on the Subject of Yellow Fever Intended to Prove its Transmissibility* (Charleston, 1840), 221; Hume, "Yellow Fever of Charleston," 22–23.

[55] McNeill, *Mosquito Empires*, 240–260. See also the works by David Geggus cited in the next note. Blake, "Yellow fever," 675; K. D. Patterson, "Yellow Fever" 856; Ramsay, *History of South Carolina*, 2: 47.

[56] Michael L. Kennedy, "A French Jacobin Club in Charleston, South Carolina, 1792–1795," *SCHM* 91 (1990), 6; David P. Geggus, ed., *The Impact of the Haitian Revolution in the Atlantic World* (Columbia: University of South Carolina Press, 2002), chaps. 8, 15.

[57] David Geggus raises this possibility for the West Indies and particularly San Domingue (Haiti) to explain, in part, the huge upsurge in yellow fever mortality there in the early 1790s that followed the large influx of susceptible soldiers from Britain and France. See Geggus, "Yellow fever in the 1790s: the British Army in occupied Saint Domingue," *Medical History* 23 (1979), 41–44. See also, David P. Geggus, "Slavery, War, and Revolution in the Greater Caribbean," in David B. Gaspar and David P. Geggus eds., *A Turbulent Time: The French Revolution and the Greater Caribbean* (Bloomington: Indiana University Press, 1998), 24–26.

residents. This could only have been because most of these people had already survived yellow fever, many of them as infants or young children.[58] In other words, the so-called putrid bilious fevers that killed newcomers between the 1750s and 1780s included many cases of yellow fever. The impact of these late colonial outbreaks was probably minimized by the fact that the majority of white immigrants into South Carolina after the 1750s went to the healthier backcountry from colonies to the north or moved there soon after they disembarked in or near Charleston. But after the Revolution, memories of the virulent epidemics of the early eighteenth century faded, and the city once again filled with susceptible people from Europe and other parts of the United States.

Other American ports were also affected by the resurgence of yellow fever in the 1790s, most notably Philadelphia. In 1793, yellow fever killed far more people there than it ever did in any Charleston epidemic, because Philadelphia was bigger and a much larger proportion of its population was susceptible to the disease. William Currie of Philadelphia was right when he said of the great epidemic of 1793, "we were strangers or newcomers to it to all intents and purposes, with this difference, that it was brought to us [by refugees from San Domingue] not us to it."[59] But whereas yellow fever gradually retreated from the North in the early nineteenth century, it continued to be a frequent visitor to Charleston. The city experienced more yellow fever epidemics in the antebellum period than any other major port on the Atlantic coast of the United States.[60]

Another complication must be addressed. Until 1799, Charleston's doctors did not call the epidemics of that decade yellow fever. The minutes of the Medical Society of South Carolina record epidemics of putrid bilious or malignant fevers every year between 1792 and 1799, except 1793 and 1798. In 1799, the society conceded that the disease might be yellow fever after all, and the following year they confirmed it. Some citizens, however, called it yellow fever almost from the start. In July 1794, the Medical Society issued a report denying rumors of a contagious malignant fever. The society's assurance did little good. In mid-August, Joseph Manigault wrote that many people feared that the city was being assaulted by yellow fever: "[I]t is very certain that one of a very putrid nature has carried off many people in a short space of time." Soon after Manigault wrote, the Medical Society conceded that a malignant fever was at large, but insisted that it was not yellow fever. In August 1796, the society again assured citizens that no dangerous contagious disease was present in the city. Within a few weeks, with hundreds dying, doctors were complaining that the daily beating of

---

[58] Thomas P. Monath, "Facing up to the re-emergence of urban yellow fever," *The Lancet* 353 (May 8, 1999), 1541; *Cambridge History of Disease*, 1103–1104.

[59] William Currie, *A Treatise on the Synochus Icteroides, or Yellow Fever, as it Lately Appeared in the City of Philadelphia* (Philadelphia, 1794), 12–13.

[60] Waring, *Medicine in South Carolina, 1670–1825*, 30–35, 157.

drums and the nightly noise made by blacks was causing "extreme inconvenience and distress to the sick."[61]

Why did the doctors deny the disease was yellow fever in the 1790s, while other local people insisted that it was? And why did the doctors reverse themselves in 1799? David Ramsay's writings may provide a clue. In an essay published in 1796, Ramsay denied that yellow fever was the disease that had struck Charleston in 1792 and 1794. It differed from yellow fever in two important ways, he claimed. It was not contagious and it did not affect anyone who had lived in Charleston "for any considerable time." He concluded that it was either a new disease or a type of typhus. Ramsay's conclusions were not entirely surprising. During the epidemics of the early eighteenth century, it was easy to conclude that yellow fever was contagious. Because few people among the white population had acquired immunity, it attacked large numbers in a short time. During the 1790s, the population contained a large number of immunes. Yellow fever was largely confined to newcomers and the districts they inhabited. It became easier to conclude it was not contagious. In 1797, the Medical Society discussed a member's paper arguing that yellow fever was a contagious disease. Most of those present thought it was not, a position the society's doctors were soon to agree on almost uniformly.[62]

Once again, Ramsay was not being entirely truthful in public. In 1799, the Medical Society's doctors declared that the disease that had been attacking Charleston since 1792 was yellow fever after all. Ramsay may have been privately leaning that way since 1794, when he read Benjamin Rush's account of Philadelphia's devastating epidemic the previous year. He wrote Rush that it was the same fever that had struck Charleston in 1792 and added, "but no public notice was taken of it, nor would there be this year but for the alarm created by your fever of 1793."[63] Why was "no public notice taken of" the Charleston epidemic of 1792? Did the local authorities purposely ignore it or did they think it too insignificant to concern them? Did they fear panic and a closed port if the words "yellow fever" appeared in official pronouncements? Despite his confession to Rush, Ramsay continued to deny publicly that yellow fever and the Charleston fever were the same disease. In an essay published in 1796, Ramsay was unequivocal: "Some persons [in Charleston]

---

[61] No one seems to have recorded the mortality for most of the epidemics of the 1790s, but in 1800, Ramsay stated that yellow fever had "raged with its greatest violence" in 1796 and 1797. If so, the fatalities must have numbered several hundred in each year, because he listed the number of deaths in 1799 as between two and three hundred, and claimed that the mortality was lower than in previous years. MSM, Sept. 28, 1793, July 26–27, Oct. 25, 1794, Aug. 10, Sept. 1, 1796; Joseph Manigault to Gabriel Manigault, Aug. 15, 1794, Manigault FP, SCL; David Ramsay, *A Review of the Improvements, Progress, and State of Medicine in the XVIIIth Century* (Charleston, 1800), 39; George Carter, *An Essay on Fevers* (Charleston, 1796), 22; Thomas Simons, "Observations on the Yellow Fever, as it occurs in Charleston," *Carolina Journal of Medicine, Science, and Agriculture* 1 (1825), 2.

[62] MSM, May 23, 1799; Ramsay, *Soil, Climate, Weather, and Diseases of South Carolina*, 23–24.

[63] Ramsay told Rush that Charleston's fever resembled the "endemial causus" of the West Indies recently described by British doctor Benjamin Moseley. But that was simply yellow fever by

die almost every year, with the bilious fever, whose skin is yellow before or after death, and some of whom discharge black matter by vomiting; but this is very different from what is commonly meant by the West-India yellow fever." Ramsay here echoed the views of many contemporary doctors that the disease "vulgarly called the yellow fever" was merely a highly virulent form of the intermittent and bilious fevers.[64] Perhaps he and the other Charleston doctors did not see yellow fever in the 1790s because they did not want to see it, given its frightful reputation and adverse effects on commerce. Perhaps officials and merchants, concerned with the economic vitality of the city, urged the doctors to consider another diagnosis or at least use another name. Perhaps the doctors were not that familiar with yellow fever. The physicians who had observed the acknowledged epidemics of the 1730s and 1740s were dead by the 1790s.

Whatever they called the disease, Charleston's doctors agreed that it was produced by the miasmas that also caused intermittent fevers.[65] That raised a problem. Intermittents were widespread every year but yellow fever was not. Why should this be the case when the environmental conditions appeared to be exactly the same? "In 1798," a puzzled Ramsay wrote, "we had none of it. In '99 we lost 259 strangers in the four sickly months and no obvious reason why we should escape the first year and suffer so much in the last." Something else puzzled the doctors: Yellow fever had a particular predilection for newcomers. Indeed, around 1800, many locals began to call it "strangers' disease."[66] That raised other questions. Why were strangers so vulnerable to it and natives largely exempt from it? To what extent were natives exempt? What should or could be done to combat this terrifying disease? The answers the doctors produced fit remarkably well with the concerns of the perceived needs of the local economy, and they made a bad problem worse.

another name. David Ramsay to Benjamin Rush, Oct. 14, 1794, in Brunhouse, *Ramsay*, 138–139; Benjamin Moseley, *A Treatise on Tropical Diseases* (London, 1792), 391, 395–397, 406; Benjamin Rush, *An Account of the Bilious Remitting Yellow Fever, as it Appeared in the City of Philadelphia in the Year 1793* (Philadelphia, 1794); MSM, May 17, 1808. Until 1793, Rush had considered yellow fever contagious and imported. See David Ramsay, *Eulogium upon Benjamin Rush, M. D.* (Philadelphia, 1813), 28–31.

[64] Ramsay, *Soil, Climate, Weather, and Diseases of South Carolina*, 23–24; Ramsay, "Extracts from an Address Delivered before the Medical Society of South Carolina," *Medical Repository* 4 (1801): 98–103; John B. Davidge, *A Treatise on the Autumnal Endemial Epidemic, Vulgarly Called the Yellow Fever* (Baltimore, 1798).

[65] Ramsay, *History of South Carolina*, 2: 54–55; Matthew Irvine, *Irvine's Treatise on the Yellow Fever* (Charleston, 1820), 18–22.

[66] *The Courier*, Aug. 3–Sept. 24, 1806; Ramsay, *History of South Carolina*, 2: 45–46; Ramsay to Benjamin Rush, Feb. 11, 1800, in Brunhouse, *Ramsay*, 150–151, 151n4; Ramsay, *Eulogium on Benjamin Rush*, 28–31.

5

Revolutionary Fever

> What will the world say now? ... They will ... revive a prophecy, broached a long time before the unfortunate issue of the campaign in 1781, that the triumph of Charles Town, portended the disaster at York[town]; and that from the laurels of Camden, would be extracted the bane of the British Empire on the Continent.
>
> "Themistocles," *A Reply to Sir Henry Clinton's Narrative*, 1783

> ... the miseries of ill health, to which all those are doomed who are to serve in those intensely hot and sickly climates, whose baneful influence is known only to those who have experienced it.
>
> George Hanger, 1801

FEVERISH CAMPAIGNS

At the beginning of the eighteenth century, John Archdale had declared that God had used disease to remove the Indians and make room for the English. During the southern campaigns of the American War for Independence, fevers proved to be an important ally of the revolutionaries. Fevers mauled both sides, but they hurt the British more. Military leaders on both sides recognized the perils of warm-weather campaigning in the southern coastal lands. That did not stop them from doing so. Revolutionary leaders mounted costly and fruitless summer campaigns against British in Florida and Georgia. Similarly, the British pursued a vigorous southern strategy in the later stages of the war. It produced their greatest victories to date but severely undermined the health of their forces and helped lead to their defeat. To secure control over the Carolinas and Georgia required stationing thousands of susceptible soldiers in the most fever-ridden area of the North American continent. Each summer and fall from 1779 to 1782, British forces in the region sustained heavy losses from disease, several times heavier than they suffered in the northern colonies. In April 1781, Lord Cornwallis cited saving his army from another Carolina fever season as one of the reasons for his decision to move north into Virginia.

Cornwallis's defeat at Yorktown that October may have secured American independence, but war in the Lower South continued to the end of 1782, and both armies continued to suffer severely from fevers. They are the forgotten casualties of the War for Independence.

With some exceptions, historians of the Revolution have either ignored or understated the influence of disease on the southern campaigns. A few historians mention disease as a major factor in the campaigns, and others point to instances when the sickness of a particular officer or unit may have affected the outcome of an engagement.[1] None has attempted to investigate the impact of disease on the conduct of the campaigns in a systematic way. Those involved in the war were keenly aware of the large role sickness played in the Southern campaigns. Disease alone did not determine the outcome of the campaigns, but it unquestionably affected their conduct and commanders' decisions in significant ways. Fevers killed and incapacitated large numbers of soldiers and felled key commanders at critical moments. Reading the evidence in contemporary accounts, it is hard to escape the conclusion that the biggest winners in the Southern campaigns were the microbes and the mosquitoes that transported so many of them from person to person. In terms of the outcome of the war, mosquito bites may have done more than partisan bullets to ensure an American victory.

The reason lies in what is called differential immunity. Most of the British, Loyalist, and German soldiers who served in North America had not served in the Caribbean or the southern colonies, and thus lacked immunity or resistance to the local fevers.[2] Most of their opponents had been born in or lived in the region for years and had acquired some immunity or resistance to the fevers. The difference may have been slight but it gave the revolutionaries

---

[1] The most systematic investigations of the relationship between disease and the Revolutionary War in the South are Peter McCandless, "Revolutionary Fever: Disease and War in the Lower South, 1776–1783," *Transactions of the American Clinical and Climatological Association*, 118 (2007), 225–249; and J. R. McNeill, *Mosquito Empires: Ecology and War in the Greater Caribbean, 1640–1914* (Cambridge: Cambridge University Press, 2010), chapter 6. Other works that emphasize to some degree the impact of disease on the southern campaigns include Sylvia Frey, *The British Soldier in the American Revolution* (Austin: University of Texas Press, 1981); Franklin and Mary Wickwire, *Cornwallis: The American Adventure* (Boston: Houghton Mifflin, 1970); John Pancake, *This Destructive War: the British Campaign in the Carolinas, 1780–1782* (Tuscaloosa and London: University of Alabama Press, 1985); Henry Lumpkin, *From Savannah to Yorktown: The American Revolution in the South* (Columbia: University of South Carolina Press, 1981); David K. Wilson, *The Southern Strategy: Britain's Conquest of South Carolina and Georgia, 1775–1780* (Columbia: University of South Carolina Press, 2005). On the role of smallpox in the Revolution, see Elizabeth Fenn, *Pox Americana: The Great Smallpox Epidemic of 1775–1782* (New York: Hill and Wang, 2001); Ann Marie Becker, "Smallpox in Washington's Army: Strategic Implications of the Disease during the American Revolutionary War," *The Journal of Military History*, 68 (2004), 381–430.

[2] James Lind, *An Essay on Diseases Incidental to Europeans in Hot Climates* (London, 1768), 36–37, 132–133, 148; McNeill, *Mosquito Empires*, 211–212; Hugh Bicheno, *Rebels and Redcoats: The American Revolutionary War* (London: Harper Collins Publishers, 2003), appendix B.

an edge. Some lowcountry revolutionaries understood their advantage and viewed disease as a potential ally. In the spring of 1776, the British sent a fleet and army to seize Charleston. In late May, patriot Richard Hutson predicted that if the British did not move against the city soon, it could breathe freely at least until November, "for it would be the height of madness and folly for them to come here during the sickly season."[3] Hutson's confidence was not misplaced. The British army commander, Sir Henry Clinton, fretted as June approached and the fleet sat off the South Carolina coast: "I had the mortification to see the sultry, unhealthy season approaching us with hasty strides, when all thoughts of military operations in the Carolinas must be given up."[4]

On June 28, Clinton's anxiety prevailed and the British fleet under Sir Peter Parker tried to force its way into Charleston harbor, only to be repulsed by cannon mounted in a hastily built and unfinished fort on Sullivan's Island. After the battle, Clinton insisted on moving his troops back north as quickly as possible. Their health was still excellent, probably because they had been camped on the beach of a local barrier island, well away from the malarial rice plantations. One of Clinton's officers, Francis Rawdon, reported that despite the heat, they had fewer sick "than might have been expected in a country town in England."[5] But Clinton's fears for the future were justified. In late September, Hutson wrote that the summer in Charleston had been "very sickly, and the mortality unusually great so early in the season."[6] Had the British captured Charleston in 1776, they would surely have suffered heavy casualties from fevers.

Some of the revolutionary leaders, notably William Moultrie, also cautioned against the perils of warm weather campaigning in the lowcountry. But commanders sometimes pursued offensive operations during the sickly months, with tragic results. The first took place in the late summer of 1776, after the Battle of Sullivan's Island. General Charles Lee, commanding the patriot forces in Charleston, ordered a land-based attack on the British at St. Augustine. His army of about 1,500 men never made it to Florida. Soon after they arrived in Savannah, Lee was ordered back to Philadelphia. The campaign floundered, and the patriots sustained large losses from fevers without being fired upon. At Sunbury, Georgia, the most advanced position they reached, the army buried about fifteen men a day, and nearly every officer of the South Carolina contingent became seriously ill.[7] In 1778, Lee's replacement, Robert

---

[3] Richard Hutson to Isaac Hayne, May 27, 1776, Richard Hutson Letterbook, Langdon Cheves III Papers, SCHS, 12/99/2.

[4] Henry Clinton, *The American Rebellion*, ed. by William B. Willcox (New Haven, CT: Yale University Press, 1954), 26, 28–29.

[5] Francis, Lord Rawdon to Francis, 10th Earl of Huntingdon, July 3, 1776, *Report of the Manuscripts of Reginald Rawdon Hastings, Esq.* 4 vols. (London:1934), 3: 177.

[6] Clinton, *The American Rebellion*, 375; Richard Hutson to John Godfrey, Sept. 26, 1776, Richard Hutson Papers, SCHS; see also, "Extracts from the Journal of Ann Manigault, 1754–1781," *SCHM* 21 (1920), 113; "Letters of Thomas Pinckney, 1775–1780," *SCHM* 58 (1957), 72–75.

[7] Edward McCrady, *History of South Carolina in the Revolution, 1775–1780* (New York: The Macmillan Co., 1902), 201–202; Charles E. Bennett and Donald R. Lennon, *A Quest for*

Howe, led another expedition against Florida. He did not leave Charleston until May, which was unusually hot. By early June, hundreds of men were sick. Because some militia contingents were late in arriving and Howe could not establish a unified command, the army sat stationary for weeks on the Altamaha River near Brunswick, Georgia. When they arrived at Fort Tonyn in northern Florida in early July, they found that the British had abandoned it without a fight. By then, about half the patriot army was dead or on the sick list, and less than a third of the 1,200 Continentals were fit for service. The commanders retreated before the army was totally destroyed, but by then they had lost 500 men. During the retreat, Charles Cotesworth Pinckney wrote Moultrie that "one campaign to the southward" was "more fatiguing than five to the northward."[8]

Pinckney blamed inadequate supplies for the disaster, namely a lack of canteens, medicines and especially tents, which forced men to sleep exposed to the damp night air. These wants hurt, but Moultrie pinpointed the fundamental mistake when he wrote Howe in late May that he was starting several months too late. Many people feared that the expedition would be "fatal to many of our men." Moultrie worried that the losses would not easily be made up because "our enlistments run out very fast, and we cannot induce the men to enter again." In June, he had advised Howe to retreat to save as many men as possible. Following the retreat, Moultrie told Henry Laurens that any future attempt to capture St. Augustine must take place in the winter.[9]

In the wake of Howe's expedition, the British took the offensive. Reinforced by forces from New York, they captured Savannah in December 1778. In the spring of 1779, British commander General Augustine Prevost, moved part of his army north and briefly threatened Charleston before retreating to Georgia. He withdrew in the face of two enemies: a larger patriot force under General Benjamin Lincoln and the advancing sickly season. He had good reason to be concerned about the danger of disease. Robert Jackson, a British army doctor who accompanied the expedition into South Carolina in 1779, wrote that many of the soldiers had come down with intermittent fevers the previous fall and suffered relapses during the fatiguing marches through the swamps. Prevost himself became ill. At the Battle of Stono Ferry just south of Charleston on June 20, the British commander, Lieutenant-Colonel John Maitland, had a force of 800 men, but only about 500 were fit for duty. As the British army sickened, Prevost decided he had no alternative but to

Glory: Major General Robert Howe and the American Revolution (Chapel Hill: University of North Carolina Press, 1991), 47–50.

[8] John Fauchereau Grimke, "Journal of the Campaign to the Southward, May to July 1778," *SCHM* 12 (1911), 61, 190–203; Moultrie, *Memoirs*, 1: 221–238; "Letters of Thomas Pinckney, 1775–1780," *SCHM* 58 (1957), 155–156; Bennett and Lennon, *Quest for Glory*, 72–82; McCrady, *South Carolina in the Revolution*, 321–324; Joseph Johnson, *Traditions and Reminiscences of the American Revolution in the South* (Charleston, 1851), 89; Harriott H. Ravenel, *Eliza Pinckney* (New York, 1925), 272.

[9] Moultrie, *Memoirs*, 1: 212–220, 227, 240.

withdraw. Lincoln's army pursued the British as far as the Savannah River, but both armies suspended major operations during July and August.[10] During the retreat, Prevost detached a large contingent under Maitland to Beaufort, because he was told it was the healthiest location in South Carolina. He hoped in that way to keep at least part of his army from sickness. Prevost informed Clinton that his own ill health was largely to blame for his failure to capture Charleston and predicted that the city would fall easily to "four thousand effective British troops."[11]

Prevost had about 4,000 men under his command, but many of them were far from effective in the summer of 1779. When he returned to Savannah in mid-July, he found the men he had left there suffering from widespread sickness. He informed Clinton that it was probable that the whole army would be ill within a few weeks. The army was badly lacking in officers, noncommissioned officers, and artillery men because so many of them were "always sick." Prevost listed about 28 percent of his force (1,189 of 4,271) as sick in the late summer. When he recalled a regiment of New York Loyalists to Savannah from Sunbury in September, almost half the men were too ill to march, and they were later captured by a handful of partisans. He anticipated great difficulties in mounting an adequate defense if the enemy moved against him but took some comfort in the fact that "in all probability the enemy will at least be as sick as we, if they attempt to keep the field."[12]

The revolutionaries also suffered badly from disease that summer. David Ramsay informed Benjamin Rush that for six weeks after Prevost's abortive attack, "we had the greatest mortality I ever knew."[13] Lincoln shared Prevost's fears of disease. He had assumed command of the Continental Army in the Southern Department in October 1778. The previous commander had resigned the job, arguing that he could not tolerate the southern climate.[14] Lincoln's own surgeon questioned his judgment in accepting the command, given the obvious health dangers. This warning, or his own frustrations and sufferings, led Lincoln to seek his recall in April 1779 on the grounds of ill health. He wrote to a friend: "I have been too long accustomed to a Northern climate to think of risking a seasoning at this time of life to a Southern one. I hope my friends will not suffer me to be kept here long." Replacing him would not have been easy, to judge by Edmund Pendleton's comment on learning of Lincoln's

---

[10] Robert Jackson, *A Treatise on the Fevers of Jamaica with some Observations on the Intermitting Fever of America* (London, 1791), 90–91; Charles Stedman, *The History of the Origin, Progress, and Termination of the American War* 2 vols. (London, 1794) 2: 119; Wilson, *Southern Strategy*, 270.

[11] Augustine Prevost to Sir Henry Clinton, July 14 and July, 30, 1779, PRO/30/55/17.

[12] Augustine Prevost to Sir Henry Clinton July 14 and July 30, 1779, PRO 30/55/17; Frey, *British Soldier*, 42–43; Wilson, *Southern Strategy*, 143, 273.

[13] David Ramsay to Benjamin Rush, Jan. 23, 1780, Robert L. Brunhouse, ed. *David Ramsay, 1749–1815: Selections from his Writings*, Transactions of the American Philosophical Society, N.S. 55: Part 4, 1965, 64.

[14] Bennett and Lennon, *Quest for Glory*, 50.

request: "We hear that General Lincoln has desired to be recalled ... if he is indulged, I imagine the appointment to succeed him in that unhealthy climate will not be anxiously sought after."[15] Congress eventually approved Lincoln's request, but by then he had decided to stay in the South, perhaps because he smelled a chance of victory.[16]

In the spring of 1779, Lincoln had proposed an offensive to Governor John Rutledge, arguing that conditions favored it: "Now seems the time for our greatest exertions – the weather is good, the season healthy, and the enemy not reinforced." Within less than two weeks, he decided that the fever season was too close for a protracted campaign. But Prevost's incursion into South Carolina that spring left him little choice but to keep his army in the field.[17] When the British retreated to Savannah in mid-July, Lincoln followed. In September, a French fleet and army under Admiral Count d'Estaing arrived, and the combined American and French forces besieged Savannah. The British defenders repulsed them, but Prevost lost one of his most talented officers, John Maitland, to a bilious fever.[18] His death was a serious blow for the British. As one historian asked: "Who knows what course of the southern campaign might have taken had this exceedingly capable officer lived?"[19] Prevost himself had been ill during much of the summer, and he appealed to Clinton to replace him.[20]

Prevost's invasion of South Carolina in 1779 had accomplished little beyond infuriating the patriots and feeding mosquitoes. But it helped convince the British government that a southern strategy could win the war. They agreed with Prevost that Charleston could be captured without great difficulty and believed that the city was the key to control of the Lower South. From there, they were convinced the British could draw on strong Loyalist support in the Carolinas. Clinton was determined that the operation should take place during the cooler months. He planned to leave New York in September and arrive in South Carolina in October. Had this happened, the British would have had about seven or eight relatively healthy months in which to subdue the Carolinas. But several unforeseen developments delayed his departure, including an outbreak of disease. On August 25, a British fleet arrived in New

[15] Edmund Pendleton to William Woodford, April 26, 1779, cited in David B. Mattern, *Benjamin Lincoln and the American Revolution* (Columbia: University of South Carolina Press, 1995), 237, n44.
[16] Browne to Benjamin Lincoln, Oct. 14, 1778, Lincoln to James Lovell, April 12, 1779, Everard Meade to Lincoln, May 6, 177, Benjamin Lincoln Papers, Boston Public Library, Microfilm, reels 2 and 3, I-II; Mattern, *Benjamin Lincoln*, 57–58, 68, 72–73.
[17] Lincoln to John Rutledge, April 1, 1779, Lincoln to James Lovell, April 12, 1779, Benjamin Lincoln Papers, Boston Public Library, reel 3-II; Mattern, *Benjamin Lincoln*, 69.
[18] Stedman, *American War*, 2: 133; Roger Lamb, *An Original and Authentic Journal of Occurrences during the Late American War* (Dublin, 1809, reprint, New York: New York Times and Arno Press, 1968), 290.
[19] Wilson, *Southern Strategy*, 143–144, 176.
[20] Clinton to Prevost, Sept. 9, 1779 (two letters), PRO 30/55/18; Henry Clinton to General Garth, Oct. 31, 1779, PRO 30/55/19.

York bringing reinforcements. "Jail fever" – probably typhus – was raging on the ships. It spread to Clinton's garrison on shore, and soon more than 5,000 men were sick. Uncertainty about the destination of the French fleet under d'Estaing also held up Clinton. He did not learn until October 8 that the French objective was Savannah, and it was December 10 before he learned that the siege of that town had failed and the French fleet had retreated. As a result, his army did not sail until December 24. The voyage was unusually long and stormy, and the expedition did not land in South Carolina until February 11, four months later than Clinton had planned. Those four months may have cost the British the war.[21]

Prevost joined Clinton with part of his army from Savannah, and soon the British had Charleston surrounded by 11,000 men. Lincoln, with about 5,000, had been preparing for a siege for several months, but his efforts had been frustrated by disease. An outbreak of smallpox in the winter of 1779–1780 made it harder to requisition slaves to work on the defenses, as their masters cited the epidemic as a reason not to send them to the city. Smallpox also discouraged militia units from coming to Charleston's defense. They feared the disease, General Moultrie wrote, more than the enemy. In late February, Lincoln protested that the fear was unreasonable, that smallpox was no longer in the city. Perhaps he was right, but it would soon return. Later in the spring, the lowcountry's unhealthy reputation contributed to a high rate of desertions among Virginia militia marching to the aid of the city. On the other hand, had they come to Charleston, they would have merely walked into a trap.[22]

Charleston's defenders held out until May 11, when Lincoln accepted Clinton's terms. It was the greatest British victory of the war to that point. One observer predicted that it would lead to "the submission of the Carolinas and maybe some other Provinces and terminate the rebellion ere the year is finished." He added that he had "feared the heats and the many other events that frequently defeat the best connected measures."[23] Despite his late start, Clinton had beaten the "heats" to capture Charleston. Ever careful of his own health, he returned to New York in June with about a third of the army, leaving Lord Cornwallis to finish the job. Given Clinton's concerns about the climate, it is hard to see how he could have been complacent about leaving thousands of troops in the lowcountry with the sickly season rapidly approaching. Many

[21] Clinton to Lord George Germain, Aug. 21, 1779, Germain to Clinton, Aug. 12, 1780, PRO 30/55/18, Clinton to Germain, Sept. 26, 1779, Germain to Clinton, Sept. 27, 1779, Clinton to Germain, Oct. 26, 1779, PRO 30/55/19; Clinton to Lord Auckland, Oct. 10, 1779, Auckland Papers, vol. 5, British Library, Add. Mss. 34416; Henry Clinton, *The American Rebellion*, ed. by William B. Willcox (New Haven, CT: Yale University Press, 1954), 140–152, 426–434; Wilson, *Southern Strategy*, 71.

[22] Moultrie, *Memoirs*, 2: 43–44, 48–49; 55–56; David Ramsay, *The History of the Revolution of South Carolina* (Trenton: Collins, 1785), 2:46; Benjamin Franklin Hough, *The Siege of Charleston, 1780* (Spartanburg, SC: The Reprint Co., 1975; originally published, Albany, NY, 1867), 37; Mattern, *Benjamin Lincoln*, 90; Wilson, *Southern Strategy*, 203–205, 218.

[23] G. Cressener[?] to Charles Jenkinson, June 29, 1780, Liverpool Papers, British Library, Add. Mss. 38214.

of the soldiers cannot have been happy about their prospects either, given the region's grisly reputation.[24]

The city and its hinterland were in prime condition for the spread of epidemics that summer. The region had suffered badly from the siege and years of privation and stagnant trade. The formerly wealthy inhabitants were often reduced to penury, the poor and slaves to utter destitution. In early July, James Simpson, a former resident whom the British had brought in to head the civil government, wrote Clinton, "Nothing but the evidence of my senses would have convinced me that one half of the distress I am witness to could have been produced in so short a time in so rich and flourishing a country as Carolina was when I left it. Numbers of families, who four years before had abounded in every convenience and luxury of life, are without food to live on, clothes to cover them, or the means to purchase either." Eliza Pinckney agreed with Simpson's assessment: "[S]uch is the deplorable state of our country from two armies being in it for near two years the plantations have been some quite, some nearly ruined."[25] Charleston was extremely filthy in the wake of the siege, and remained so for months, partly due to hygienic carelessness on the part of the soldiers.[26]

When the siege ended, smallpox was again circulating in the town and the region. Health conditions deteriorated through the summer and into the fall. General William Moultrie protested that many of his men who had been inoculated lacked adequate medicines or provisions.[27] Hundreds more prisoners of war arrived in Charleston after the British victory at Camden in August. Lieutenant Colonel Nisbet Balfour, the British commander, imprisoned many of them on ships in the harbor, where hundreds died of smallpox and malignant fevers. Revolutionary officers and doctors blamed the conditions the British had put them in. Moultrie demanded that they be moved to shore or another ship.[28] Balfour denounced Moultrie's letter as "violent" and "improper," and denied any general mortality or symptoms of malignant disease. He also claimed he had removed the prisoners to shore. In a letter to Cornwallis, however, Balfour reported that he was moving the rebel prisoners because their mortality was "truly shocking."[29]

[24] Lamb, *Late American War*, 294.
[25] James Simpson to Sir Henry Clinton, July 1, 1780, Great Britain, Historical Manuscripts Commission, *Report on American Manuscripts in the Royal Institution of Great Britain* 4 vols. (Boston: Gregg Press, 1972, reprint of original edition, London, 1904–1909), 2: 149–150; Eliza Pinckney to [?], Sept. 25, 1780, Charles Cotesworth Pinckney FP, Library of Congress, Washington, D.C., 1st ser., box 5. I owe the last reference to Elizabeth Fenn.
[26] Board of Police Proceedings, July 7, 1780, Jan. 5, 1781, CO5/519.
[27] Moultrie, *Memoirs*, 2: 112–113; Ramsay, *Medicine in the XVIIIth Century*, 41; James Wemyss to Cornwallis, July 11, 1780, PRO 30/11/2/269–270; Banastre Tarleton to George Turnbull, Nov. 5, 1780, PRO 30/11/4/63–64; Keating Simons to Cornwallis, Aug. 11, 1780, PRO 30/11/63/36–37; Josiah Smith, "Diary, 1780–1781," *SCHM*, 33 (1932), 21, 113; *Letters of Eliza Wilkinson*, arr. by Caroline Gilman (New York: 1839) 93; James Thacher, *A Military Journal of the American Revolution* (Boston, 1823), 294, 355.
[28] Moultrie, *Memoirs*, 2: 142–144.
[29] Balfour told Cornwallis he had put the prisoners on ships because he lacked proper facilities and sufficient men to guard the prisoners. Balfour to Cornwallis Oct. 22, 29, 1780,

At the same time, thousands of slaves were fleeing to the British lines in hopes of freedom and probably food. Many ran straight into the arms of death from smallpox and an unknown fever. In mid-July, Simpson reported that a malignant fever was "sweeping away" large numbers of blacks who had fled their plantations in hopes of gaining their freedom from the British. Whites seemed immune to the fever, although some of them, especially infants, were being attacked by smallpox, which had become more virulent since the spring.[30] By mid-July, the "Negro burying ground" was filled and blacks were being buried in various places around town. Whites were soon complaining that the burials were becoming "a public nuisance and extremely noxious to the inhabitants."[31]

PARTISANS AND PESTILENCE

In his July 16 report to Clinton, James Simpson found one thing to be pleased about: The British army was healthier than "could be reasonably expected" for the time of year and the inclemency of the weather, which had been unusually wet. Exactly what Simpson meant by "reasonably" is unclear. Certainly, some of the British soldiers had already had smallpox, either naturally or by inoculation. Some were already suffering from malarial fevers.[32] In any event, shortly after Simpson wrote these words, the army became extremely unhealthy and remained so throughout the fall. By December 1780, Simpson was reporting that smallpox and fevers had spread with unprecedented severity across the region.[33]

PRO 30/11/259–260 and 309–310; Cornwallis to Clinton, Dec. 3, 1780, PRO 30/55/27; Peter Fayssoux to David Ramsay, Mar. 26, 1785, *Documentary History of the American Revolution*, ed. Robert Wilson Gibbes (1853–1857; reprint, 3 vols. in 1, New York, 1971), 117–121.

[30] James Simpson to Sir Henry Clinton, July 16, 1780, PRO 30/55/24.

[31] Boston King, "Memoirs of the Life of Boston King, a Black Preacher," *The Methodist Magazine* 21 (March–June 1798): 107; Board of Police Proceedings, July 18, 1780, CO5/519; Alexander Innes to [John André], May 21, 1780, Henry Clinton Papers, 1730–1795, William L. Clements Library, University of Michigan, Ann Arbor; Eliza Pinckney [?] to [?], Charleston, Sept. 25, 1780, Charles Cotesworth Pinckney FP, Library of Congress; Josiah Smith to George Appleby, Dec. 2, 1780, Josiah Smith to George Smith, Dec. 5, 1780, "Josiah Smith Letter Book, 1771–1784," SHC; David Ramsay, *The History of the Revolution of South Carolina* 2 vols. (Trenton, 1785), 67; Ravenel, *Eliza Pinckney*, 272; "Letters of Eliza Pinckney," *SCHM* 76 (1975), 165–166. I owe the Innes and Smith references to Elizabeth Fenn.

[32] Simpson to Clinton, July 16, 1780, PRO 30/55/24; Robert D. Bass, *Swamp Fox: The Life and Campaigns of General Francis Marion* (New York: Henry Holt and Co., 1959), 61–62; Alex. Innes to [John André], May 21, 1780, Clinton Papers.

[33] James Simpson to William Knox, Dec. 31, 1780, *Documents of the American Revolution, 1770–1783*, Colonial Office Series, ed. K. G. Davies, 18: Transcripts, 1780, 268; William Burrows to ?, Feb. 27, 1781, PRO 30/11/105/4–5; William H. Hallahan, *The Day the Revolution Ended: 19 October 1781* (New York: Wiley, 2004), 260; S. Max Edelson, *Plantation Enterprise in Colonial South Carolina* (Cambridge, MA: Harvard University Press, 2006), 202, 251.

The spread of these diseases was facilitated by the constant movement of soldiers and residents. Following the surrender of Charleston, Clinton paroled the patriot militia and allowed them to go home. He also sent British forces inland to establish control and recruit Loyalists over the interior of the Carolinas. Neither of these goals was accomplished. British policies and actions were partly to blame for the outcome. Many people were not committed to either side; they simply desired to be left alone. Many of these neutrals and even some Loyalists were alienated by British attempts to force men to take loyalty oaths and then fight for the Crown. Atrocities committed by British and Loyalist soldiers also tarnished their cause, although both sides behaved with shameless brutality at times. Like many occupying armies trying to move quickly through hostile terrain, the British forces seized horses, cattle, and other provisions, sometimes by requisition, often by plundering.[34]

Despite these blunders, the British might have succeeded in their southern strategy had it not been for the diseases that struck their army during the summer and fall of 1780. On July 16, the same day that James Simpson wrote optimistically about the army's health, Cornwallis informed Clinton of a "most alarming" lack of medicine and medical staff in the Charleston hospital. He urged his commander to send help "as the sickly season is advancing." He had already sent one of his generals to New York because of ill health. Two days before he had informed Clinton that bringing the soldiers he had sent inland back to the coast before November "would be leading them to certain destruction."[35] Cornwallis had good reason for concern. The garrison at Charleston became increasingly sickly, with the Hessians suffering especially heavily.[36]

Surgeon Robert Jackson claimed that the most common illnesses the army suffered in 1780 were intermittents and malignant fevers. Others reported the presence of break-bone or dengue fever in the region. Dysentery was a problem as always. But the most commonly used terms in the British correspondence relating to the soldiers' sickness are "intermittents," "agues and fevers," "malignant fevers," "putrid fevers," and "bilious fevers," all of which point to malaria and possibly yellow fever and dengue. As the weather turned cooler in the fall, new cases of fever were few but often more severe, and relapses were common among the exhausted men, many of whom showed signs of dysentery and dropsy (edema, or swelling due to fluid retention). Jackson attributed

[34] Stedman, *American War*, 193n, 217n; H. H. Ravenel, *Eliza Pinckney* (New York, 1925), 290. On the atrocity issue, see Walter Edgar, *Partisans and Redcoats: the Southern Conflict that Turned the Tide of the American Revolution* (New York: Perennial, 2001).

[35] Cornwallis to Clinton, July 16, 1780, PRO 30/55/24; Cornwallis to Clinton, July 16, 1780, PRO 30/72/34–35.

[36] Balfour to Rawdon, Oct. 29, 1780, PRO 30/11/3/359–360; Balfour to Rawdon, Nov. 1, 1780, PRO 30/11/4/9–10; Balfour to Cornwallis, Nov. 17, 1780, PRO 30/11/4/152; *Revolution in America: Confidential Letters and Journals 1776–1784 of Adjutant General Major Baurmeister of the Hessian Forces*, tr. and ed. Bernhard A. Uhlendorf (New Brunswick, NJ: Rutgers University Press, 1957), 369.

these symptoms to the fevers, and he may have been correct: Malaria can produce severe diarrhea and edema. In treating these diseases, the British surgeons were hampered by inadequate medical facilities, supplies, and personnel. Many of them were themselves constantly ill. In November 1780, most of the surgeons' mates in Charleston were sent back to Britain because they were too ill to continue working.[37]

The situation in Savannah was similar. The commander there, Lieutenant-Colonel Alured Clarke, reported in early July that the heat and sickness was "beyond anything you can conceive." He had withdrawn troops from outlying posts at Ebenezer and Abercorn and moved all the regiments encamped outside into town because so many men had become ill. By late August, Clarke's force was so depleted that he was begging for reinforcements from South Carolina. In early October, he reported that the suffering of his men "in this vile climate is terrible." A Hessian regiment had lost "many men and some officers, and at present has not really above sixty men fit for duty." He had been severely ill himself.[38] Georgia's royal governor, Sir James Wright, urged Cornwallis to restore the posts at Ebenezer and other spots along the Savannah River. But the British commander refused, stating that "half of the men would die in three months" and the rest would be easily captured by the enemy.[39] Cornwallis's refusal meant in effect abandoning the hinterland of Georgia to the enemy. From Georgetown, about sixty miles north of Charleston, Major James Wemyss wrote on July 29 that his men were "falling down very fast" with intermitting fevers. A few days later, he reported that six men had died of putrid fevers within the past three days and thirty other men were ill. Cornwallis ordered Wemyss to move his men inland to the reputedly healthier Santee Hills.[40]

In August, Cornwallis wrote Clinton that his efforts to subdue the Carolinas were hindered not only by the rebelliousness of the people but by the "terrible climate." It was "so bad within an hundred miles of the coast, from the end of June to the middle of October, that troops could not be stationed [there] during that period without a certainty of their being rendered useless for some time for military service, if not entirely lost." An indication of the seriousness of the problem was that even South Carolina Loyalists were eager to abandon their plantations for Charleston during the summer: "[O]ur principal friends ... were extremely unwilling to remain in the country during that period, to assist forming the militia and establishing some kind of government." Cornwallis

---

[37] Jackson, *Fevers of Jamaica*, 301, 303; John McNamara Hayes to Cornwallis, Nov. 15, 1780, PRO 30/11/4/134; Alured Clarke to Cornwallis, Nov. 29, 1780, PRO 30/11/4/236; Wickwire, *Cornwallis*, 245–246.

[38] Alured Clarke to Cornwallis, July 10, 1780, PRO 30/11/2/258–261, Clarke to Cornwallis, Aug. 30, 1780, PRO 30/11/63/83–84; Clarke to Cornwallis, Oct. 5, 1780, PRO 30/11/3/86–87.

[39] Cornwallis to Balfour, Sept. 27, 1780, PRO 30/11/80/48–49.

[40] Wemyss to Cornwallis, July 29, 1780, PRO 30/11/2/389–390; Wemyss to Cornwallis, Aug. 4, 1780, PRO 30/11/63/17–18; Wickwire, *Cornwallis*, 245; Cornwallis to Wemyss, July 30, 1780, PRO 30/11/78/61–63.

must have wondered how people who left the area for fear of fevers expected the more vulnerable British soldiers to garrison it.[41]

The British leaders were not entirely surprised by the unhealthiness of the lowcountry. Its sickly reputation was well known. As they moved into the backcountry, however, they expected to find a healthier climate and large numbers of Loyalists. Both expectations were rudely shattered. They found far more rebels and a far unhealthier region than they had been led to believe. It is difficult to determine which was the more shocking, but disease, particularly malaria, reduced British fighting capacity more effectively than patriot bullets. From nearly every outpost and detachment in the backcountry of South Carolina and Georgia, Cornwallis received similar tales throughout the summer and fall: widespread and deadly sickness. The main British force, camped in and near Camden under Colonel Lord Rawdon, was also suffering. On August 1, Rawdon reported that he had sent many of his men to posts outside the town to what he believed were healthier locations. He had himself suffered a severe fever. Ironically, Cornwallis had picked Camden as a site for the main army partly because he was told it was "a tolerably healthy place" that could also be conveniently supplied from Charleston.[42]

Perhaps no British unit was more devastated by fevers than the 71st Highland regiment, and in no case were the consequences more serious for the British. During June, Cornwallis posted the 71st to Cheraw Hill, east of Camden, because it had a healthy reputation. By late July, fevers had incapacitated two-thirds of the force. Part of the reason for the high casualty rate among the 71st may have been a failure to listen to the advice of locals. The regiment camped near the banks of the Peedee River in a place where it was extremely sluggish, with stagnant pools. Experienced residents urged them to move into the nearby pinewoods, away from the river. British officers rejected the advice because they thought the woods too vulnerable to attack. According to Surgeon Jackson, the first battalion, which was camped furthest from the river, suffered far less than the second. The officers camped on the riverbank, and almost all came down with fevers. The ill officers included their commander, Major Archibald McArthur.[43]

McArthur remained at Cheraw longer than Cornwallis had intended him to because he believed it to be both secure and strategically important. But on July 24, he decided that it was imperative to change location. He marched his men to the east branch of Lynches Creek, from where many of the sick were removed to Camden. McArthur's move had serious political repercussions. Partisan leaders interpreted it as a retreat and a sign of weakness. In its

[41] Cornwallis to Clinton, Aug. 20, 1780, PRO 30/11/76/3–4.
[42] Balfour to Cornwallis, July 17, 1780, PRO 30/11/2/317–318; Rawdon to Cornwallis, July 17, 1780, PRO 30/11/2/329–330; Rawdon to Cornwallis, Aug. 1, 1780, PRO 30/11/63/3–4; Memorial from Officers of the Provincial Regiments, Aug. 25, 1780, PRO 30/11/2/362.
[43] Cornwallis to Clinton, Aug. 20, 1780, PRO 30/11/76; Cornwallis to Clinton, Aug. 10, 1780, PRO 30/55/25; Rawdon to Cornwallis, Aug. 1, 1780, PRO 30/11/63/3–4; Jackson, *Fevers of Jamaica*, 83–84; McArthur to Cornwallis, July 29, 1780, PRO 30/11/2/383–384.

wake, many people in the Peedee and Black River region took up arms against the British. Some locals who had joined the Loyalist militia switched sides and helped capture about 100 sick Highlanders McArthur had sent down the Peedee to get medical care in Georgetown. The move and the capture of McArthur's men was "a disaster," according to Cornwallis. Patriots captured more sick British soldiers a few days later. By early August, the British general was reporting that the backcountry was "in an absolute state of rebellion."[44]

At this point, Cornwallis learned that a patriot army under Horatio Gates was advancing south from Virginia. Cornwallis rushed to Camden to find that a large part of the British army was too ill to fight. The returns of August 13 show about 2,000 men fit for duty, perhaps 1,400 of them regulars, and more than 800 sick. Major George Hanger claimed that the whole army "was extremely sickly" when it went into battle. The 71st regiment was in the worst condition, with only 230 of their 700 men able to fight. Cornwallis thought that Gates had about 7,000 men, although it was probably only a little more than 3,000. Cornwallis might have retreated, but he later wrote that the sickness actually encouraged him to fight. To retreat, he argued, would have required leaving many of the sick to be captured by the enemy, along with magazines and supplies, with the probable loss of most of the state to the rebels.[45]

Cornwallis won a crushing victory at Camden. Gates and many of his men fled in disarray, and hundreds were killed or captured. But the battle did nothing to solve Cornwallis's two key problems: the partisan rising and the sickness in his army. Both were gaining strength. A few days after the battle, he reported that his army's "sickness was very great, and truly alarming." His officers were especially hard-hit, and the head surgeon and almost all of his assistants were ill. Every man on his staff was "incapable of doing his duty."[46] If his men did not get healthier, it would be impossible to accomplish anything. They did not get healthier for months. The 63rd regiment arrived in Camden a few days after the battle in a "very sickly state." In one unit, nearly half the men had died. The 71st regiment remained largely incapacitated by fevers.[47]

---

44 Cornwallis to Wemyss, July 30, 1780, PRO 30/11/78/ 61; Cornwallis to Rawdon, Aug. 1, 1780, PRO 30/11/79/2; Cornwallis to Clinton Aug. 6, 1780, PRO 30/55/25, Cornwallis to Clinton, Aug. 20, 1780, PRO 30/11/76; Cornwallis to Wemyss, July 30, 1780, PRO 30/11/78/61–64; Cornwallis to Rawdon, Aug. 1, 1780, PRO 30/11/79/2–3; Rawdon to Cornwallis, Aug. 1, 1780, PRO 30/11/63/3–4; Tarleton to Turnbull, Nov. 5, 1780, PRO 30/11/4/63; Banastre Tarleton, *A History of the Campaigns of 1780 and 1781 in the Southern Provinces of North America* (London, 1787), 152.

45 Return of the Army in Camden, Aug. 13, 1780, PRO 30/11/103/3; Cornwallis to Lord George Germain, Aug. 20, 1780, Aug. 21, 1780, PRO 30/11/76; James Martin to Lord George Germain, Aug. 18, 1780, CO5/176; Stedman, *American War*, 2: 205; Hanger, *Address to the Army*, 9n; Tarleton, *Campaigns of 1780 and 1781*, 137–138, 191; John Buchanan, *The Road to Guilford Courthouse: The American Revolution in the Carolinas* (New York: John Wiley and Sons, 1997), 157. Many of Gates' men were also ill, mainly with diarrhea, from the effects of fatigue and poor food. See Christopher Ward, *The War of the Revolution* 2 vols. (New York: The Macmillan Co., 1952), 724.

46 Cornwallis to Clinton, Aug. 23, 1780, PRO 30/55/25.

47 Cornwallis to Balfour, Sept. 12, 13, 18, 1780, PRO 30/11/80/16, 17, 20–21, 25–26; Cornwallis to Turnbull, Sept. 11, 1780, PRO 30/11/80/16; Cornwallis to Cruger, Sept. 12, 1780, PRO

The situation was complicated by the large number of prisoners from Gates's army captured in battle. Cornwallis decided to move them to Charleston as quickly as possible. Camden was "so crowded and so sickly" that he feared an outbreak of pestilential fever if the prisoners remained confined there. Cornwallis was not exaggerating the direness of the situation. Eliza Pinckney wrote to her son Thomas, a wounded prisoner, that she wished him "out of so sickly a place as Camden."[48]

Cornwallis wanted to get his own men out of Camden as well. Although he worried that many of his soldiers were too ill to march, he decided to move them northwest to the Waxhaws region on the border of North and South Carolina, which he was told was a much healthier place. From there, after a few days, he hoped to march into North Carolina to capitalize on his recent victory and rouse the Loyalists there. In early September, he marched the bulk of the army to the Waxhaws, leaving hundreds of sick behind in Camden. Some of the healthy troops he left there soon became ill from fevers or small-pox. At first, Cornwallis was pleased by his new location: "We have a pleasant camp, hilly and pretty open, dry ground, excellent water and plenty of provisions, and if that will not keep us from falling sick I shall despair."[49]

He soon began to sound desperate: So many of his men were sick that he decided they could not be moved. But while the army remained there, more men fell ill with fevers. In late September, he informed Clinton that the army's sickness had been increasing all month. A large part of the 71st regiment was still in Camden, too weak to march to the new camp. The 63rd was "totally demolished by sickness" and would need months to recover.[50] As fall approached, many men suffered relapses of their fevers, and the new cases of fever were more severe than before. Cornwallis grew increasingly frustrated. People had told him repeatedly that if he moved them a bit farther they would be healthy, but everywhere his army went fevers accompanied them. The continuing sickness in his army greatly delayed his intended advance into North Carolina in an effort to smash the patriot militias before they had time to regroup. One of his biggest problems was a chronic lack of wagons to move the soldiers who were too ill to march.[51]

30/11/80/19; Wemyss to Cornwallis, Aug. 28, 1780, PRO 30/11/63/79–80; Wemyss to Cornwallis, Sept. 3, 1780, *The Cornwallis Papers: Abstracts of Americana* comp. by George Reese (Charlottesville: The University Press of Virginia, 1970), 103; Wickwire, *Cornwallis*, 245.

[48] Cornwallis to Lord George Germain, Sept. 19, 1780, PRO 30/11/76/17; "Letters of Eliza Pinckney," *SCHM* 76 (1975), 163; Thomas Pinckney to Major J. Money, Sept. 22, 1780, PRO 30/11/3/84–85.

[49] Cornwallis to Clinton, Aug. 29, 1780, Charles Ross, ed. *The Correspondence of Charles, First Marquis Cornwallis* 3 vols. (London, 1859); Major England to Cornwallis, Oct.1, 1780, PRO 30/11/3/162–163; George Turnbull to Cornwallis, Oct. 2, 1780, PRO 30/11/3/172–173; Cornwallis to Balfour, Sept. 15, 1780, PRO 30/11/80/23.

[50] Cornwallis to Patrick Ferguson, Sept. 20, 1780, PRO 30/11/80/33; Tarleton, *Campaigns of 1780 and 1781*, 196; Cornwallis to Clinton, Sept. 22, 1780, PRO 30/11/72/ 53.

[51] Cornwallis to Wemyss, Oct. 7, 1780, PRO 30/11/81/26–27; Cornwallis to Turnbull, Oct. 7, 1780, PRO 30/11/81/30; Cornwallis to Major England, Sept. 20, 1780, PRO 30/11/80/31; Archibald McArthur to Cornwallis, Oct. 7, 1780, PRO 30/11/3/199–200.

Before he moved his army into North Carolina, Cornwallis decided to establish a post at the border town of Charlotte. Disease once again thwarted him. He ordered Lieutenant Colonel Banastre Tarleton, commanding the cavalry of the British Legion, to reconnoiter and clear the army's route of hostile forces. But after thinking that Tarleton had gone, Cornwallis learned that he was prostrated by a fever at Fishing Creek across the Wateree River. Cornwallis was frantic at the news and asked for constant updates on Tarleton's condition. His greatest fear was that Tarleton might be captured. His cavalry was in a dangerously exposed position, without infantry support, more than twenty miles from the main army. Tarleton was the army's eyes and ears and its most vigorous and feared commander. But he could not be moved, and Cornwallis hesitated to send the Legion without him, for fear he would be captured by the enemy. To make matters worse, all but one officer of the British cavalry were sick. Cornwallis wanted to move to their support. To do so, however, would require leaving many of his sick behind to be captured because he lacked wagons to move them.[52] Tarleton's illness, he wrote, was "of the greatest inconvenience" because he not only lost his services but that of his men. They had to remain with him to protect him. Cornwallis was convinced that he could not safely advance on Charlotte "unless the Legion can advance to clear the country of all the parties who would certainly infest our rear."[53]

Finally, on September 22, Tarleton was moved to a safer location, and Cornwallis ordered an advance guard of the Legion under Major George Hanger to secure Charlotte. As they entered the town on September 24, the British met fierce resistance from rebel militia. Cornwallis had to order the infantry to disperse a force the cavalry should have handled easily. Shortly afterward, Hanger and five other Legion officers were prostrated by a malignant fever. Hanger later claimed it was yellow fever and that it was the same disease that had struck Tarleton. Hanger barely survived, his health so shattered he was sent to Bermuda to recover, and finally back to Britain. The other officers who became ill with Hanger died within a week.[54]

By the time the British entered Charlotte, Tarleton was recovering, but he remained ill for several weeks. His sickness helped the partisans gain one of their most important victories. On October 7, Isaac Shelby's "Over Mountain

---

[52] Cornwallis to Clinton, Sept. 22, 1780, PRO 30/11/72/54; Cornwallis to Major England, Sept. 20, 1780, PRO 30/11/80/31; Cornwallis to Archibald Campbell, Sept. 20, 1780, PRO/30/11/80/29; Cornwallis to Patrick Ferguson, Sept. 20, 1780, PRO 30/11/80/33; Robert Bass, *The Green Dragoon: The Life of Banastre Tarleton and Mary Robinson* (London: Alan Redman, 1957), 106; Bass, *Swamp Fox*, 72–73.

[53] Cornwallis to Balfour, Sept. 21, 1780, PRO 30/11/80/35; Cornwallis to Clinton, Sept. 22, 1780, PRO 30/11/72/54–55; Bass, *Green Dragoon*, 106; Robert Bass, *The Gamecock: The Life and Campaigns of General Thomas Sumter* (New York: Holt, Rinehart, and Winston, 1961), 86.

[54] Cornwallis to Clinton, Sept. 22, 1780, PRO 30/11/72/56; Hanger, *Life, Adventures, and Opinions*, 172, 179–181; Hanger, *An Address to the Army*, 68–70; Stedman, *American War*, 2: 216; Buchanan, *Road to Guilford Courthouse*, 186–190.

Men" destroyed a Loyalist force under Colonel Patrick Ferguson at King's Mountain. Cornwallis had been fretting about Ferguson's exposed position for days and requested Tarleton to go to his aid. Tarleton replied that he was too ill to ride, and Cornwallis was reluctant to send the Legion without Tarleton in command. Their performance at Charlotte had convinced him that the Legion "are different when Tarleton is present or absent."[55] After the war, Tarleton blamed Cornwallis for the disaster by not sending Ferguson reinforcements. After reading Tarleton's account, Cornwallis protested, "My not sending relief to Colonel Ferguson ... was owing to Tarleton himself: he pleaded illness from a fever, and refused to make the attempt, although I used the most earnest entreaties."[56]

There may have been another reason for the failure to reinforce Ferguson, and the chaos that followed. When Cornwallis learned of the disaster on October 9, he was severely ill from a fever himself and may not have been thinking clearly at this critical time. He remained extremely ill for weeks, leaving a leadership vacuum. Balfour, now commanding at Charleston, had long feared this eventuality. After the victory at Camden, he wrote Cornwallis, "For God's sake do not get sick." During the earl's illness, Lord Rawdon assumed command and repeatedly emphasized in letters to subordinates that Cornwallis was not seriously ill. In fact, he was virtually incapacitated. For more than two weeks, he was unable to write and sometimes unable to move. Rawdon had decided to play down the severity of the situation to prevent panic. After Cornwallis recovered, Balfour wrote, "we never knew how ill you were, until you [were] greatly better."[57]

A few days after King's Mountain, Cornwallis called in his exposed detachments and ordered his men to move back to Winnsboro, South Carolina, to regroup. Reeling from attacks by partisans and fevers, the army that seemed invincible a few weeks before was stopped in its tracks and rolled back. The retreat from Charlotte was chaotic, and the troops suffered terribly. It rained constantly for several days, and they had no tents and very little rum, which many doctors considered requisite in feverish climates. The soldiers drank foul water, which Charles Stedman claimed was "frequently as thick as a puddle."

[55] Cornwallis to Balfour, Oct.1, 1780, PRO 30/11/81/2; Cornwallis to Ferguson, Oct. 6, 1780, PRO 30/11/81/23; Cornwallis to Balfour, Oct. 7, 1780, PRO30/11/81/25; Cornwallis to Ferguson, Oct. 8, 1780, PRO 30/11/81/31; Bass, *Green Dragoon*, 107–108; Wickwire, *Cornwallis*, 195; W. J. Wood, *Battles of the Revolutionary War, 1775–1781* (Chapel Hill, NC: Algonquin Books, 1990), 197.

[56] Ross, *Correspondence of Charles, First Marquis Cornwallis*, 59n.

[57] J. Money to Balfour, Oct. 10, 1780, PRO 30/11/81/34; Balfour to Cornwallis, Aug. 31, 1780, PRO 30/11/63/87–88; Balfour to Cornwallis, Oct. 10, 1780, PRO 30/11/3/205–206; Rawdon to Turnbull, Oct. 19, 20, 21, 22, 1780, PRO 30/11/3/241–242, 245–246, 251–252, 257–258; Rawdon to Balfour, Oct. 21, 1780, PRO 30/11/3/253–254; Rawdon to Alexander Leslie, Oct. 24, 1780, PRO 30/11/3/267–270; Rawdon to Cruger, Oct. 26, 1780, PRO 30/11/3/285–286; Balfour to Rawdon, Oct. 26, 1780, PRO 30/11/3/289–290; Rawdon to Clinton, Oct. 28, 1780, PRO 30/11/3/297–298; Alexander Innes to Cornwallis, Oct. 31, 1780, PRO 30/11/3/344–345; Balfour to Cornwallis, Nov. 5, 1780, PRO 30/11/4/27–34.

Many Loyalists deserted. The 7th regiment was "reduced to nothing by sickness." Smallpox struck the blacks working on the defenses of Camden; many died or fled. The commander there, George Turnbull, asked to be relieved due to illness. "Only a northern climate," he claimed, could reestablish his "constitution."[58]

The army's health finally began to improve in November. Cornwallis found Winnsboro to be "a healthy spot" and told Clinton he would remain there until he was joined by reinforcements coming from Virginia under General Alexander Leslie. Things were improving in Charleston, too. The chief surgeon informed Cornwallis that "health once more begins to shine upon us."[59] But the effects of the fevers lingered into the colder months, as soldiers suffered relapses or long periods of convalescence. At the end of November, Lieutenant Colonel John Cruger at Ninety-Six informed Cornwallis that his garrison was "still plagued with the fever and ague." In mid-December, Rawdon reported that he was unable to send a trusted officer to attack General Francis Marion because he had "not yet conquered his ague."[60] Patrick Tonyn, governor of British East Florida, effectively summed up the campaign of 1780 when he wrote, "sickness and disease have made more havoc in the neighboring colonies than the sword."[61]

In January 1781, reinforced by 2,000 men under Leslie, Cornwallis resumed his march into North Carolina, pursuing a reinforced patriot army under General Nathanael Greene. In March, Cornwallis won a Pyrrhic victory at Guilford Court House. Greene's army remained intact and the country hostile. The British had sustained heavy losses and were short of supplies. Cornwallis retreated southeast toward Wilmington to get reinforcements, supplies, and some hoped-for Loyalist support. He arrived in early April. Meanwhile, Greene had moved behind him into South Carolina to attack Lord Rawdon's force at Camden. Cornwallis faced a major decision. Should he return to South Carolina to help Rawdon or go elsewhere? On April 10, he wrote Clinton that he had decided to march north into Virginia and link up with a British army corps there. He argued that he was too far away to reach Rawdon in time, and that the Carolinas could be subdued only when Virginia was securely under British control. But he gave another reason for his choice: Only by moving north could he "hope to preserve the troops, from the fatal sickness, which so

[58] Stedman, *American War*, 2: 224–225, 225n, Rawdon to Clinton, Oct. 28, 1780, *Documents of the American Revolution*, 18: Transcripts, 1780, 215; Turnbull to Cornwallis, Nov. 3, 4, 1780, PRO 30/11/4/14–15, 25–26; Rawdon to Balfour, Oct. 21, 1780, PRO 30/11/3/253–254; Turnbull to Cornwallis, Nov. 10, 1780, PRO 30/11/4/93–94. Rawdon to Cornwallis, Nov. 15, 1780, PRO 30/11/4/132–133; Buchanan, *Road to Guilford Courthouse*, 242.

[59] John McNamara Hayes to Cornwallis, Nov. 15, 1780, PRO 30/11/4/134.

[60] Cruger to Cornwallis, Nov. 1780, PRO/30/11/4/225–226; Clarke to Cornwallis, Nov. 29, 1780, PRO 30/11/4/236; Rawdon to Cornwallis, Dec. 17, 1780, PRO 30/11/4/343–344.

[61] Tonyn to Lord George Germain, Dec. 9, 1780, *Documents of the American Revolution*, Transcripts, 1780, 18: 253; Josiah Smith to James Poyas St. Augustine, Dec. 5, 1780, Josiah Smith Letter Book, 1771–1784, SHC. I owe the last reference to Elizabeth Fenn.

nearly ruined the army last autumn."[62] No doubt Cornwallis was concerned about preserving his own health, too, after his close call in the fall. Perhaps he recalled Balfour's words on his recovery in the fall: "[I]f fortune puts you another summer in this climate more care will be absolutely necessary for your health."[63]

THE LAST FEVERISH CAMPAIGNS

On April 25, 1781, Cornwallis began the march north that led to his fateful encounter at Yorktown. Ironically, malaria would contribute to his defeat there that fall. Although most histories of the Revolutionary War follow Cornwallis on the road to Virginia, we will leave him there, and follow General Greene into South Carolina. Rawdon defeated Greene's army at Hobkirk's Hill in April 1781, but sustained heavy losses and soon withdrew his garrisons from Camden, Ninety-Six, and other backcountry posts. Both sides limited their campaigning that summer. Rawdon, who claimed to be suffering from fever, retreated to Orangeburg in June. The bulk of Greene's army consisted of southerners and was thus probably less vulnerable to malaria than Rawdon's. But Greene's men were not wholly immune, only resistant, and Greene himself was from Rhode Island. A former comrade of Greene's wrote to him about the same time, praying that God would protect the general while he remained in the "sickly South." He moved his men to the High Hills of Santee for several weeks that summer. General Thomas Sumter wrote Greene several times excusing his own inaction on the grounds of ill health. Even the legendary Swamp Fox, Francis Marion, complained of suffering from fever that September. Whether all these men were as ill as they claimed to be, the ubiquitous fevers gave them a ready reason for avoiding battle.[64]

The last major battle in the Carolinas, at Eutaw Springs in September 1781, was essentially a draw. Soon after it, the British lost another highly capable officer and hero of the battle, Major John Marjoribanks, to fever. By the end of 1781, British forces controlled only Charleston, Savannah, and their immediate perimeters. In July 1782, they evacuated Savannah. Minor battles and skirmishes continued in South Carolina until the end of the year. The last took

---

[62] Leslie to Cornwallis, Jan. 8, 1781, PRO 30/55/27; Cornwallis to Clinton, April 10, 1781, PRO 30/11/5/207–208; Clinton, *American Rebellion*, 231, 508–510; *The Clinton-Cornwallis Controversy*, ed. by Benjamin Franklin Stevens, 2 vols. (London, 1888), 1: 395–399; Cornwallis to Major Gen. Phillips, April 10, 1781, in Ross, *Correspondence of Charles, First Marquis Cornwallis*, 87–88; Themistocles, *A Reply to Sir Henry Clinton's Narrative* (London, 1783), 14n; Stedman, *American War*, 2: 353–355; 247.

[63] Balfour to Cornwallis, Nov. 7, 1780, PRO 30/11/4/57–58.

[64] McNeill, *Mosquito Empires*, 220–234; Bass, *Swamp Fox*, 202; "Letters of Brig-Gen. Thomas Sumter and Major-Gen. Nathanael Greene, 1780–83," *Charleston Yearbook*, (Charleston, 1899), 27, 53, 124; *The Papers of General Nathanael Greene*, 11 vols., ed. by Dennis M. Conrad (Chapel Hill and London: The University of North Carolina Press, 2000), 9: 305, 383, hereafter, *NGP*.

place on John's Island just south of Charleston in November 1782, two weeks before the British evacuated the city.[65] None of these engagements was decisive, which may account for their disappearance from most works of history. But the southern campaigns of 1781 and 1782 produced immense suffering for both armies and the civilian population. Disease was responsible for most of it. Commanders on both sides tried to avoid active campaigning in the sickly season, and to move their men to what they believed were healthy locations when they could. But fevers badly mauled their armies anyway. Governor Edward Rutledge had urged an all-out assault on Charleston in the fall of 1781. His reasoning showed an appreciation of the epidemiological reality. If Greene's army did not take the city before the next summer, Greene would have to abandon the lowcountry. To keep the army there for another fever season was to risk its destruction. Rutledge may have been more concerned about protecting the property of the planter elite than the lives of the soldiers, but he had a point.[66] Greene did not follow Rutledge's advice, and his army remained encamped in the lowcountry for another year and a half, losing hundreds of men to fevers. By early October 1781, most of the surgeons were too ill to perform their duty, including their head, Charleston's Dr. Peter Fayssoux. Greene complained that the southern climate required more physicians and medical supplies than that of the North, and that his army suffered terribly from lack of them, especially bark.[67]

The British were in worse shape. Their officers continued to be felled by disease or left to restore their health. In August 1781 Rawdon sailed for England, pleading a broken constitution. General Paston Gould, who replaced Rawdon, was incapacitated by fevers from the time he arrived in Charleston in June.[68] At the end of 1781, Gould's replacement, Alexander Leslie, reported that his army had been severely weakened by battle and "great sickness." Leslie's reports to his superiors during the next year constantly emphasized sickness, his own as well as that of his army. He repeatedly asked to be relieved of command because the climate and demands of his job had ruined his constitution. One of his generals was totally useless due to constant ill health. Another sailed to Britain in June 1782 on the advice of his physician.[69]

---

[65] Walter Edgar, *South Carolina: A History* (Columbia: University of South Carolina Press, 1998), 236–237.

[66] "Letters to General Greene and Others," *SCHM* 17 (1916), 4–5.

[67] *NGP*, 9: 440–441, 482, 485, 602.

[68] Rawdon to Cornwallis, March 7, 1781, PRO 30/11/69/7–11; Cornwallis to Rawdon, May 20, 1781, PRO 30/11/69/41; Cornwallis to Clinton, June 30, 1781, PRO 30/55/30/3582; Cornwallis to Balfour, July 16, 1781, PRO 30/11/88/20–21; Cornwallis to Rawdon, July 23, 1781, PRO 30/11/88/46–47; Cornwallis to Balfour, Aug. 27, 1781, PRO 30/11/89/25; Lamb, *Late American War*, 307; Roderick Mackenzie, *Strictures on Lt. Col. Tarleton's History of the Campaigns of 1780 and 1781 in the Southern Provinces of North America* (London, 1787), 126; Edward McCrady, *History of South Carolina in the Revolution, 1780–1783* (New York: The Macmillan Co., 1902), 384n; *NGP*, 9: 493, n2.

[69] Leslie to Clinton, Nov. 30, 1781, PRO 30/55/33; Leslie to Sir Guy Carleton, June 10, 20, Aug. 2, 1782, PRO 30/55/42, 45; Great Britain, Historical Manuscripts Commission, *Report on*

In July, disease was raging so widely among his men that he was forced to reduce the size of the garrison at a key post a few miles from the city. In August, more than 600 Hessian soldiers and 22 officers were down with what a German officer called malignant fevers. The number of ill was so great that Leslie barely had enough men to relieve his posts. Greene had moved closer to the city, and Leslie concluded that he was about to attack. If Greene did not attack, Leslie thought, fevers and the fear of them might cause the revolutionary army to disintegrate.[70]

Leslie's reasoning made sense, but he underestimated Greene's ability to hold his army together, at least at this point. The revolutionary army, reinforced by Pennsylvania and Maryland regiments after the British surrender at Yorktown, harassed British outposts and conducted skirmishes but never assaulted Charleston. Greene's strategy was to wear down the British and force them to evacuate. Perhaps he expected disease to work in his favor. Eventually the strategy worked, but American losses from disease were also heavy. In June 1782, many men in Greene's army came down with fevers. When the British evacuated Savannah in July, Greene urged General Anthony Wayne in Georgia to send most of his men to Carolina as fast as possible because "our army is getting exceedingly sickly." Greene feared that Leslie would take advantage of his weakness and attack with reinforcements from Savannah. But Leslie was not eager to move either.[71] On July 11, Greene moved his army from Bacon's Bridge near present-day Summerville down the Ashley River to Ashley Hill, only fifteen miles from Charleston. He was not preparing to attack the city as Leslie thought, only hoping to improve the health of his troops. Locals had told him it was a healthy site.[72] When they arrived at the new camp, Colonel Lewis Morris, an aide to Greene, exuded confidence: "This is a fine commanding position we are now in. They say it is healthy.... The British may be disappointed in their human expectations, and notwithstanding the violence of the season we may oppose to them the countenance of energy and health instead of the emaciated picture of disease."[73]

It was not to be. A few days after they arrived at Ashley Hill, large numbers of men came down with fevers. According to Walter Finney of the Pennsylvania Continentals, "intermitting fevers struck two-thirds of the men within three days." These men must in fact have been infected before the move, because the incubation period for malaria is nine-to-seventeen days, depending on

American Manuscripts in the Royal Institution of Great Britain 4 vols. (Boston: Gregg Press, 1972, reprint of London edition of 1904–1909), 2: 434, 450, 457, 543, 3: 24; Mackenzie, *Strictures*, 120–122.

[70] Great Britain, *Historical Manuscripts Commission, Report on American Manuscripts*, 3:28, July 19, 1782, 3:51, August 2, 1782; *Confidential Letters and Journals 1776–1784 of Adjutant General Major Baurmeister of the Hessian Forces*, 529, October 6, 1782; NGP, 11: 397.
[71] NGP, 11: 359–361, 382, 444, 447, 455, 482.
[72] NGP, 11: 435–436; McCrady, *South Carolina in the Revolution, 1780–1783*, 669.
[73] "Letters of Colonel Lewis Morris to Miss Ann Elliott," *SCHM* 40 (1939), 122.

the type of plasmodium. Most likely, they were infected with the less deadly *vivax* malaria, because both Finney and Greene state that the attacks at this point were rarely fatal. By August, however, the fevers were operating "differently," according to Finney. A "great mortality" ensued that "struck a damp into all the survivors." The most likely cause was an outbreak of *falciparum* malaria, the malignant autumnal fever. The Pennsylvanians suffered the worst losses, surely because they had little or no experience with southern fevers. Another Pennsylvania soldier declared that they had 376 men in hospital with fevers and more than half in camp were sick: "We are scarcely able to relieve our guards." Greene was slow to admit the seriousness of the situation. On September 1, he reported that many men were ill but few were dying: "[T]he fevers of this country are more troublesome than dangerous." He soon changed his views. By the middle of September, fever deaths were frequent and in November he reported, "we have buried upwards of 200 of our fine fellows.... This has been one of the sickliest seasons known this thirty years." In August and September, more than half his army was sick. Greene himself came down with fever. As commanders in this region often did, he found some consolation in the fact that the British and their Hessian mercenaries had suffered a similar calamity. Informers had told him that many soldiers and people in Charleston were sick and dying rapidly.[74]

One can get some sense of the revolutionary soldiers' predicament from the journal of Major Ebenezer Denny. A Pennsylvanian, he was sent to South Carolina in November 1781. He and most of his fellows remained healthy until the following summer. Soon after the army moved to Ashley Hill in July, he came down with fever. He was sent to the hospital, a "very disagreeable place – all sick, and some continually dying." He noted that the Ashley River was very low and full of alligators. The alligators were not a serious problem, but the lack of flow undoubtedly was. The river's sluggish pools were ideal for breeding the mosquito carriers of malaria. In August, Denny noted that both armies seemed "disposed to be quiet; ours is in no condition for doing much." By September, the hospitals were crammed, and a great many in the camp were sick. Death became so common that funeral ceremonies were no longer observed. By October, deaths were less frequent, but the ranks had been "thinned very much." By the time the British evacuated Charleston in December, the three Pennsylvania regiments had been reduced by death and desertion to one regiment of 600 men.[75]

Greene declared that his failure to defeat the British that fall was due largely to the widespread sickness in his army. He may have been right. Many of his men had died, many were still sick, and most of those listed as fit for duty in

---

[74] *NGP*, 11: 398n6, 614, 639, 671; Henry Lee, *The Campaign of 1781 in the Carolinas* (1824; Spartanburg, SC: The Reprint Co., 1975), appendix, xxvi.

[75] *Military Journal of Major Ebenezer Denny* (1859; reprint, The New York Times & Arno Press, 1971), 45–49; McCrady, *South Carolina in the Revolution, 1780–1783*, 668–670; Gregory D. Massey, *John Laurens and the American Revolution* (Columbia: University of South Carolina Press, 2000), 224.

the monthly returns were in fact convalescents unable to perform active service. In October, he reported that the army was so sickly, they "cannot move for some days."[76] Many of Greene's officers were incapacitated for lengthy periods of time.[77] Among them was Greene's aid Lewis Morris, who had been so confident of the healthiness of Ashley Hill a few weeks before. Morris recovered very slowly. A few days before the British evacuated Charleston in December, he wrote that he was still extremely weak. In April, Morris wrote that he believed he could not survive in the lowcountry and that he must leave the region before the coming sickly season.[78] Many of his fellow soldiers came to the same conclusion. Illness continued to haunt the patriot army after it occupied Charleston. Greene begged Congress for extra funding on the grounds that illness was a far greater problem in the South – he estimated five times greater – than in the North. On December 10, he wrote that the whole army had "been in the hospital, more or less, and the mortality great."[79] They were soon on the verge of mutiny. In early April 1783, Greene requested Washington to allow him to march his men north, for two reasons: They could be used to attack the British in New York and they were "extremely dissatisfied" with their location. Their fear of the climate, Greene claimed, was far greater than their fear of the enemy. He declared that if he did not lead his army north soon, it might disintegrate. A regiment of cavalry had already set off for Virginia, but they were convinced to come back. One of his officers had written him that nothing was "more dreadful to the soldiers than the thoughts of continuing in this country another autumn." He predicted that many of them would rather face the risks of a military court than those of "this destructive climate." They did not have to face either, as the British agreed to peace terms that spring. [80]

Let us conclude by returning to Henry Clinton, whose fears of campaigning in South Carolina proved well founded. In December 1781, he wrote to Lord Germain that he expected an attack on New York or Charleston in the spring. If it was Charleston, he declared, he would go there unless it began "later than the beginning of April."[81] His choice of date was clearly due to fear of disease. In 1776, he had insisted on moving his soldiers north to preserve their health. In 1780, he had gone north after Charleston surrendered to preserve his own. Unfortunately for the British cause, he left thousands of his men to battle pestilence as well as partisans, a combination that virtually ensured their defeat. Of the two enemies, pestilence may well have been the most important.

[76] *NGP*, 12: 20, 55–56.
[77] *NGP*, 12: 67–68, 317.
[78] *NGP*, 11: 564–565, 577, 593, 614, 624–625, 627–628, 652, 663, 682–683, 695, 12: 573; "Letters of Colonel Lewis Morris to Miss Ann Elliott," *SCHM* 41 (1939), 10.
[79] *NGP*, 12: 274, 313.
[80] *NGP*, 12: 545, 553, 567.
[81] Clinton to Germain, Dec. 26, 1781, *Documents of the American Revolution*, calendar, 1781–1783, 19: 234.

6

Strangers' Disease

Our knowledge of this fever is very limited. It appears that there is a certain something in the air of Charleston that is comparatively harmless to the inhabitant, but the source of disease and death to the stranger. What is that something?

David Ramsay, September 1799

At Madame D'Orvals they have sent to the hospital. The poor Irish woman they say with the yellow fever – she waited on them; perhaps she will die there by strangers buried and by strangers mourned.

Vanderhorst diary entry, September 1838

"CHARLESTON'S YELLOW FEVER"

"The mortality is beyond anything known for many years. There are very few strangers ... escaping. Those who did not make a seasonable flight have found an untimely grave in a land which they had visited for wealth or pleasure." The author of these words, Joshua Whitridge, was describing an epidemic of yellow fever in Charleston in 1817.[1] Whitridge was himself a stranger, a doctor who had recently migrated from New England, perhaps lured like others by the fact that the city had been virtually free of the fever since 1807. He had just recovered from the disease and was treating its victims with great success, or so he claimed. Whitridge's observations and experiences reflected the new view of yellow fever as mainly a disease of people who had recently come to the city. Although some came for "wealth or pleasure" most were poor folk looking for work.

As we have seen, around 1800, yellow fever underwent a paradigmatic transformation in Charleston. Once viewed as a disorder that threatened almost everyone, it was now seen as endemic to the city and of little danger to acclimated inhabitants. By the time local doctors decided around 1800 that they were dealing with yellow fever, they had also concluded that

[1] Joshua B. Whitridge to William Whitridge, Sept., 1817, Whitridge Papers, SCHS.

earlier views of its nature had been mistaken. The scenario went something like this. The 1790s: This is not yellow fever, because it does not behave like yellow fever. It isn't contagious or imported and it is not dangerous to locals. After 1800: This is yellow fever, but accepted views of yellow fever are wrong. It is a disease of domestic origins, not imported and not contagious. By the early 1800s, yellow fever was becoming accepted as a regular part of the Charleston scene. Doctors began to refer to it as the "endemial" or "endemical" fever, a disease generated locally when atmospheric conditions were right. Dr. John Shecut called yellow fever "the proper endemic of the city of Charleston." People sometimes referred to it possessively as "Charleston's yellow fever."[2]

Indeed, for many Charlestonians, the new view of yellow fever had a comforting side. The settled population seemed to be virtually immune to it. In the epidemic of 1794, Martha Laurens Ramsay recorded that "the reigning disorder is said to be confined to strangers and those who live irregularly."[3] In 1796, an upcountry resident wrote that Charleston had recently suffered terribly from an epidemic fever, in which most of the victims were strangers. He had heard that nearly all of nineteen newcomers who had arrived by ship from London in August had died.[4] The doctors of the Medical Society declared in 1799 that hardly any cases during the last seven years had been among the permanent residents of Charleston. The disease's predilection for newcomers soon became common knowledge, and the realization affected how Charlestonians thought of themselves – and others. It contributed to a feeling that they were different from people "from off."[5]

David Ramsay, as so often, publicized the good epidemiological news. After the epidemics of 1799 and 1800, he noted that the mortality was less than expected, given the fearsome reputation of the disease: "[I]ts ravages were by no means so extensive as represented by common fame." Moreover, it had not killed any adults "who had been long used to the air of the city." It was largely confined to the neighborhoods where country people and sailors lived.[6] The

---

[2] Tucker Harris, "Yellow Fever of Charleston," *Philadelphia Medical and Physical Journal* 2 (1805), 21; *The Courier*, Sept. 3, 1806; Samuel Henry Dickson, *Philadelphia Medical and Physical Journal* 3 (1821–1822), 250, cited in Waring, *Medicine in South Carolina, 1670–1825*, 157n; Waring, *Medicine in South Carolina, 1825–1900*, 35; "The Letters of Charles Caleb Cotton, 1798–1802," *SCHM* 51 (1950), 224; MSM, May 17, 1808; Shecut, *Medical and Philosophical Essays*, title page of "Essay on the Prevailing Yellow Fever of 1817".

[3] David Ramsay, *Memoirs of the Life of Martha Laurens Ramsay* (Boston, 1812), 132–133.

[4] "S.A." to Henry Rugeley, Oct. 20, 1796, Rugeley Family Papers, X 311/155, Bedfordshire Record Office, Bedford, England.

[5] MSM, Aug. 24, 1799; Harris, "Yellow Fever of Charleston," 28.

[6] David Ramsay to Benjamin J. Morse, Sept. 6, 1799, in Robert L. Brunhouse, ed., *David Ramsay, Selections from His Writings*, Transactions of the American Philosophical Society, N.S. 55, Part 4 (Philadelphia: American Philosophical Society, 1965), 150; David Ramsay, "Extracts from an Address delivered before the Medical Society of South Carolina, on the 24th of September 1799," *Medical Repository* 4 (1801), 99–100; David Ramsay, "Facts concerning the yellow fever, as it appears at Charleston (South Carolina)" *Medical Repository* 4 (1801), 217–218.

pattern continued. In 1802, of ninety-six deaths ascribed to yellow fever, not one was a native of Charleston. Most of the victims were sailors.[7] In 1804, the fever claimed about 150 victims, again all strangers. Ramsay blamed their deaths partly on the fact that the disease had largely spared the city in 1803, encouraging many of them to remain in Charleston.[8] In 1807, he reported 176 deaths from yellow fever, nearly all strangers. The number of deaths was probably higher. Joseph Johnson, who became president of the Medical Society that year, claimed that September 1807 had been "the blackest month" in the history of Charleston. He recorded 328 deaths that month, although he ascribed many of them to influenza.[9] After 1807, Charleston was largely free of yellow fever for a decade. *The Courier* declared in 1817 that the city had been free of the fever since 1807 except for a minor outbreak in 1812.[10] The hiatus in epidemics between 1807 and 1817 may have occurred for several reasons: a drop in the number of susceptible strangers in the city; the end of the legal slave trade in 1808; and a decline in the Caribbean trade resulting from the embargo and non-intercourse acts against Britain and France, and the War of 1812. All these developments probably combined to reduce the chances of epidemics. According to a later writer, Charleston's West Indies trade during the war was handled by Cuban ships, whose crews were "habituated" to yellow fever.[11]

Whatever caused the apparent retreat of yellow fever, it returned with the end of the war and the economic boom that followed. In 1817, an epidemic killed 274 people in Charleston and an unknown number in other communities across South Carolina and Georgia. It killed one-sixth of the population of Beaufort, more than 900 people in Savannah, and attacked some inland communities. Again, most of the Charleston victims were strangers. Dr. Samuel Henry Dickson recalled that large numbers of northern and foreign sailors had been recruited in 1817 to go up the rivers as boatmen. Many of them, he claimed, had contracted country fevers that changed to yellow fever when they were taken to hospitals in Charleston. One explanation of Dickson's observation may be that the sailors contracted malaria in the

---

[7] David Ramsay, *Charleston Medical Register for 1802* (Charleston, 1803), 3–5, 21.

[8] David Ramsay, "Facts concerning the yellow fever which prevailed in Charleston (South Carolina), during the hot season of 1804," *Medical Repository* 2d ser. 2 (1805): 365–367; Ramsay to Benjamin Rush, Sept. 27, 1804, in Brunhouse, *Ramsay*, 157.

[9] David Ramsay, "Remarks on the yellow fever and epidemic catarrh, as they appeared in South Carolina during the summer and autumn of 1807," *Medical Repository* 2d ser. 5 (1808), 234; Joseph Johnson, *An Oration Delivered before the Medical Society of South Carolina at their Anniversary Meeting December 24, 1807* (Charleston, 1808).

[10] According to Ramsay, Edisto Island, about thirty miles south of Charleston, experienced yellow fever in 1811. Ramsay to John Coakley Lettsom, Oct. 29, 1808, in Brunhouse, *Ramsay*, 163; *The Courier*, Sept. 17, 1817; MSM, Nov. 1, 1811, Oct. 1, 1812.

[11] William Hume, "The Yellow Fever of Charleston, considered in its relation to West India commerce," *Charleston Medical Journal and Review* 15 (1860), 25; Benjamin B. Strobel, *An Essay on the Subject of Yellow Fever Intended to Prove Its Transmissibility* (Charleston, 1840), 221.

country, then yellow fever once in Charleston. They could also have contracted yellow fever on the boats.[12]

Major epidemics occurred in Charleston again in 1819 and 1824. In the
latter year, port physician Thomas Simons claimed that yellow fever "raged in
violence equal to any period in the annals of this country."[13] It continued to
visit the city until 1876, with particularly severe epidemics in the 1830s and
1850s. Some years were relatively or entirely free of yellow fever, particularly
in the 1840s, but in most years, doctors reported some cases. The city's death
records reveal that between 1821 and 1858, yellow fever killed more people in
Charleston than all other fevers combined – almost 3,000. The great majority
of deaths from yellow fever – and all fevers – were among strangers. Of the
more than 4,700 recorded fever deaths in the city during that period, almost
3,400 came from other countries, other parts of the United States, or other
parts of South Carolina. The number of deaths officially attributed to yellow
fever very likely understated the reality, given the city government's reluctance to admit the presence of the disease in the early stages of an epidemic.
How many people died of yellow fever in communities outside of Charleston
is impossible to know. To confuse matters further, during epidemics, other
diseases might be misdiagnosed as yellow fever. As one doctor put it, "let
the existence of the disease be once fairly established and every thing, even
a common cold, is yellow fever."[14] Yellow fever could easily be overlooked in
the early stages of an epidemic, or in mild outbreaks, but the number of cases
during a major epidemic could also have been exaggerated.

COMPARATIVE IMMUNITIES

The idea that yellow fever was more dangerous to strangers than natives or
long-term residents did not suddenly emerge around 1800. In the 1750s, John
Lining had argued that the disease was especially deadly to newcomers from
cold climates.[15] Lining claimed that whites' immunity came from having survived yellow fever. His colleague James Kilpatrick noted that people who
had survived the epidemic of 1732 were immune in that of 1739. Another
Charleston doctor, John Moultrie, Jr., agreed that the fever's chief victims

[12] Samuel Henry Dickson, *Essays on Pathology and Therapeutics* 2 vols. (Charleston, 1845),
1: 335; Hetty Heyward to Mother, Oct. 9, 1817, Heyward and Ferguson Family Papers,
COCSC; Jeffery R. Young, *Domesticating Slavery: The Master Class in Georgia and South
Carolina* (Chapel Hill and London: University of North Carolina Press, 1999), 183.
[13] Strobel, *Yellow Fever*, 221; Thomas Y. Simons "Observations on the Yellow Fever, as It Occurs
in Charleston, South Carolina," *Carolina Journal of Medicine, Science, and Agriculture* 1
(1825); MSM, Sept. 1, 1818, Aug.–Sept. 1819.
[14] Ramsay, *History of South Carolina*, 2: 239; Hume, "Yellow Fever of Charleston in Relation
to West Indian Commerce," 22; *Report of the Committee of the City Council of Charleston
upon the Epidemic of Yellow Fever, of 1858* (Charleston, 1859), 47–65; Strobel, *Yellow Fever*,
204; MSM, 1810–1858; Waring, *Medicine in South Carolina, 1825–1900*, 30–35.
[15] John Lining, "A Description of the American Yellow Fever," *Essays and Observations,
Physical and Literary* 2 (1756), 370–395.

were newcomers, but that it sometimes attacked Europeans who had resided in the city for years. Their observations were not mutually exclusive. There was a key difference between surviving a case of the disease and simply residing in the fever-prone area for a certain period of time.[16] Lining perceived correctly that vulnerability to yellow fever came not from being a stranger to Charleston, but from being a stranger to the disease. That distinction was not always appreciated. After 1800, many Charlestonians concluded that merely having lived in the city for many years conferred immunity. Others thought that age by itself was a protective factor. In 1801, Alice Izard declared "that the disorder attacks the young and vigorous" but "seldom commits any ravages on any subject past 40." Mary Izard claimed that she did not avoid Charleston during the warm season because she was "too old for the yellow fever." They were partly right. Yellow fever is most fatal among adolescents and young adults, and people who had resided in the city for a long time had a good chance of having attained immunity through infection.[17] But certainty was impossible.

In 1802, John Drayton noted that yellow fever was particularly dangerous to three classes of people: country people, locals who had avoided the city during the fever season, and foreigners at first arrival.[18] Dr. John Shecut explained the fever's discrimination by declaring that natives were assimilated to the "specific gaseous poison" that caused the fever. The unassimilated – foreigners and native children – were susceptible to the full force of the causative agent. Thus, climatic conditions that produced malignant yellow fever in strangers caused only a common bilious remittent or break-bone fever in Charlestonians. Anyone, he added, could assimilate to yellow fever by residing in the city for a certain amount of time, about nine to twelve years for both strangers and native children.[19] Such views became common and persisted in the face of contrary evidence. As late as 1851, Dr. Thomas Y. Simons maintained that "all natives [of Charleston] arriving at adult age are exempt from this disease, as well as those strangers who have had the disease." He added that people who had resided in the city for many years and had never had yellow fever were also immune.[20]

Natives and long-term residents did not always accept the idea that they were safe from yellow fever. David Ramsay thought that the immunity of the local population might prove to be limited in some way. In 1799, he cautioned against complacency. He noted that in a recent epidemic, the fever had

[16] James Kirkpatrick, *The Analysis of Inoculation* (2d ed. London: 1761), 64; Waring, "John Moultrie, Jr.," 773–774.

[17] Mary Izard to "Mrs. Gen. Pinckney," June 29, [?], R. F.W. Allston Collection, series 12/21/17, SCHS; Alice Izard to Mrs. Gabriel Manigault, Aug. 31, 1801, Manigault Family Papers, SCL, both quoted in Joyce Chaplin, *An Anxious Pursuit: Agricultural Innovation & Modernity in the Lower South, 1730–1815* (Chapel Hill: The University of North Carolina Press, 1993), 100.

[18] John Drayton, *A View of South Carolina* (Charleston, 1802), 27–28.

[19] J. L. E. W. Shecut, *Medical and Philosophical Essays*, (Charleston, 1819), 92, 108–110, 115.

[20] Thomas Y. Simons, *An Essay on the Yellow Fever in Charleston* (Charleston, 1851), 10.

attacked some local children as well as strangers. Should the exciting cause achieve "one grade more of malignity," he predicted, "the distinction in favor of inhabitants which has heretofore prevailed will probably be done away with."[21] In fact, yellow fever may already have afflicted Ramsay's acquaintances and family. During the epidemic of 1794, his wife Martha recorded that a young friend had died in September after a six days' illness. Martha's sister, Mary Pinckney, died that same month after a few days' illness. In early November, Martha nearly succumbed to an illness that lasted seven days and produced "a state of deplorable weakness." Martha never used the term "yellow fever" but at that time her husband and the Medical Society were assuring everyone that disease was not present in the city.[22] During the epidemic of 1799, planter John Ball reported the death of a friend who was "no stranger to the air of Charleston." Ball was unsure of his own immunity. He avoided the city during the epidemic, although the rest of his family was there, and remained at his plantation on the advice of his wife and doctors. He felt trapped and helpless, forced to remain in the malarial countryside, with his family in the city, "where death stalks ghastly with gigantic strides."[23]

In 1817, fears about the vulnerability of some local inhabitants materialized. Dr. Joshua Whitridge noted with surprise that the disease had attacked some old residents and "even natives."[24] Roger Pinckney reported that the epidemic had been "fatal to natives, who were never before attacked." Natives had in fact never been wholly exempt. Some native children had died in epidemics since the 1790s. But in 1817, natives suffered more severely than they had in living memory: "[T]here is scarcely a family but what has a death in it, in some instances every child has been snatched from their parents." Pinckney's daughter and his youngest son both became ill but survived. Pinckney noted that the disease primarily attacked people aged one to twenty-five but "seldom after that." It is not surprising that many victims of the epidemic were children because no epidemic had occurred in Charleston in ten years. Added to an influx of strangers, the young children gave the virus sufficient fuel. Samuel Henry Dickson recalled that "the mothers of Charleston long remembered with tears the unhappy summer of 1817." Charles Kershaw reported that many families had suffered losses. Most of his own children came down with yellow fever but survived. One of his acquaintances had lost two children.[25]

[21] David Ramsay, "Extracts from an Address Delivered before the Medical Society of South Carolina, on the 24th of September 1799," *Medical Repository* 4 (1801), 103.

[22] Ramsay, *Martha Laurens Ramsay*, 136–137.

[23] John Ball Sr., to John Ball, Jr., Sept. 7, Oct. 29, 1799, Ball Family Papers, SCHS, 11B.

[24] Joshua B. Whitridge to William Whitridge, Sept.19–21, 1817, Whitridge Papers, SCHS; *The Courier* Aug. 14, 1817.

[25] Roger Pinckney to his aunt, Oct. 2, 1817, Roger Pinckney Correspondence, SCHS; Samuel Henry Dickson, *Essays on Pathology and Therapeutics* 2 vols. (Charleston, 1845), 1: 353; J. H. Easterby, ed., *The South Carolina Rice Plantation* (Columbia: University of South Carolina Press, 2004; 1945), 364–365, 372.

Nevertheless, the view that Charlestonians were immune to yellow fever persisted. Pronouncements on that score were often contradictory. In September 1838, the merchant house of Lewis and Robertson assured planter Robert Allston that natives of Charleston were "perfectly exempt" from the current epidemic. At the same time, the Medical Society was reporting that yellow fever was attacking "an unusually large number of children of the natives ... and at an age, which in preceding epidemics, afforded them immunity." Some Charleston natives getting the fever were in their twenties, including one man of twenty-five who had never left the city in his life. The doctors added that the disease had invaded parts of the city where it had never been known before, which may explain why it attacked some older natives.[26]

Because many people believed that immunity to yellow fever was related to residence in the city, some Charlestonians believed that they could lose their immunity if they resided elsewhere for any length of time. Roger Pinckney knew of a family that did not dare to go into Charleston during the epidemic of 1817, even though their house was only half a mile away. They had not lived in the city for many years and so considered themselves "strangers." To make such a trip "would surely be fatal to them," he agreed.[27] Frederick Rutledge cautioned his absent brother not to return to Charleston in September because the yellow fever was raging there and might "treat you as a stranger if you go there too early." Some doctors concurred. Samuel Henry Dickson argued that people could lose immunity to yellow fever if they left Charleston for too long. He was wrong about that, but people could lose resistance to malaria by moving out of the region for more than a few months, and that may have confused the issue.[28]

Young people who had left the city for long periods of time were believed to be especially vulnerable. One student feared that spending years at Yale University might leave him prey to yellow fever when he returned. Another local recounted a tale of two young children who got yellow fever after being forced from Sullivan's Island into the city by a hurricane. One of them died, and this happened because "neither of them has ever resided in the city during the summer months." During the epidemic of 1817, Charles Kershaw advised Charlotte Allston that her son Robert should not land in Charleston, but go to New York until the epidemic ended.[29] In 1856, Charles Manigault made light of the danger to some of his family, but not to others. On October 11, he reported that the fever was "still confined to strangers" and people with "bad habits, etc." His family "did not think any thing of it." But in the

[26] Easterby, *South Carolina Rice Plantation*, 407; MSM, Sept. 1, 1838.

[27] Roger Pinckney to his aunt, Oct. 2, 1817, Roger Pinckney Correspondence, SCHS.

[28] Frederick Rutledge to John Rutledge, Sept. 22, 1804, John Rutledge Papers, SHC, quoted in Chaplin, *Anxious Pursuit*, 100; Dickson, *Pathology and Therapeutics*, 1: 343–344.

[29] Thomas Legare to Jedediah Morse, Aug. 24, 1811, Thomas Legare Papers, section A, Duke University Library, Seth Lothrop to Sylvanus Keith, Sept. 23, 1804, Sylvanus and Cary Keith papers, folder 1 Cabinet 78, Duke University Library, both quoted in Chaplin, *Anxious Pursuit*, 101; Easterby, *South Carolina Rice Plantation*, 364.

case of his son Louis, then coming to Charleston from the North, Charles showed much greater concern. Because Louis had spent much time in Europe, Charles reasoned that his son had "got a stock of foreign health" and might be susceptible to yellow fever. He insisted that Louis not return to Charleston before mid-November, or until the city had experienced a "black frost." A week later, Charles reversed himself. Although the epidemic had not abated, the family had concluded that Louis could return immediately because he had "so decided a Southern Constitution, and [has] passed so many summers here (several of them during yellow fever)." Perhaps Louis was safe but there was no way to be sure. People who believed that they or their loved ones were immune simply by having lived in the city for a certain number of years were sometimes proven wrong. The occasional deaths of Charleston natives – especially young ones – exposed what Benjamin Strobel (see Figure 6.1) called the "delusion of trusting to what is commonly called acclimatization." He concluded, "if 20 years do not acclimatize, a whole life will not." Strobel perceived that the absence of epidemic yellow fever for several years rendered some young natives vulnerable to it: "[C]ould such a thing occur as that yellow fever should not exist in Charleston for thirty years, and then an irruption should take place, nearly every person in the community under that age would be liable to an attack."[30]

"SWEEPING OFF THE STRANGERS"

Yellow fever did visit Charleston frequently enough that its victims were mostly strangers. Englishman John Davis marveled at the "incredibly great" mortality yellow fever caused among Europeans in Charleston.[31] Francois Andre Michaux, a French botanist who visited the city about the same time, calculated that 80 percent of the foreigners who got yellow fever died. Michaux added that rural South Carolinians were as vulnerable as foreigners, and that even those who lived close to the city were not always immune. People from the countryside were reluctant to go to Charleston during the yellow fever season, which meant that for several months a year, communications were "nearly cut off between the country and the town." When Michaux returned to Charleston in October 1802, he did not meet anyone on the "most populous road" going to or returning from there "for a space of three hundred miles." No one he met thought it prudent to go to the town during the fever season.[32] Michaux may have exaggerated, but not much.

[30] James M. Clifton, ed., *Life and Labor on Argyle Island: Letters and Documents of a Savannah River Plantation, 1833–1867* (Savannah, GA: The Beehive Press, 1978), 228–230; Strobel, *Yellow Fever*, 201–202.

[31] John Davis, *Travels of Four Years and a Half in the United States of America, 1798–1802* (London, 1803), 112, 114–115.

[32] Francois Andre Michaux, *Travels to the West of the Alleghany Mountains* (London, 1805), in Reuben Gold Thwaites, ed. *Travels West of the Alleghanies* (Cleveland, 1904), 118–121.

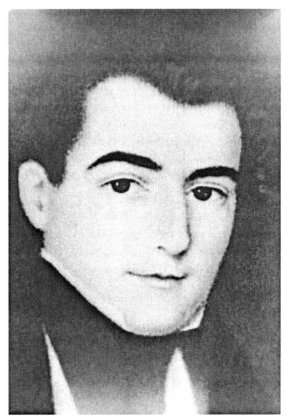

FIGURE 6.1. Benjamin Strobel, M.D., Charleston's yellow fever maverick (Courtesy of the Waring Historical Library, MUSC).

Newcomers sometimes convinced themselves that they would not be in great danger from the disease, but reality could shake their confidence quickly. Charles Caleb Cotton arrived in Charleston in the summer of 1799 and got a job teaching at the College of Charleston. He had been told that it was much healthier than cities to the north. After a few weeks, he was reporting that yellow fever was killing ten to twenty people a day. The rapid and nauseating effects of the disease horrified him: "[P]utrefaction frequently commencing before the unhappy patient has breathed his last." It raged especially among seamen who had recently come from Europe, killing most of the crew on some ships.[33] Cotton survived and soon left for Canada, but other members of the college faculty were not so lucky. In the summer of 1800, the new headmaster, Robert Woodbridge, ignored suggestions that he retreat to Sullivan's Island to avoid yellow fever. He died of the "prevailing disorder" that September. His

[33] "Cotton Letters," *SCHM*, 51 (1950), 224.

brother-in-law, recently hired as an assistant master, took heed and resigned his appointment.[34] Michaux thought he could avoid the disease through a regimen that would prevent "effervescence of the blood" but quickly learned his mistake. He, too, ignored advice to retreat to Sullivan's Island and contracted yellow fever, but survived. After his experience, he cautioned travelers not to come to the city between July and October. Even inland areas were not free from the disease. One had to move "two hundred miles, and even two hundred and fifty, from the ocean" to be completely safe from the fever.[35]

Strangers often obeyed warnings to avoid Charleston during the fever season, though it is impossible to know how many did so. In 1808, David Ramsay ascribed a drop in yellow fever mortality in part to the fact that fewer strangers than usual came to the city that year. As we have seen, there may have been other reasons. But whenever the fever subsided for a few years, many strangers no doubt concluded or hoped that the city was safe. Others knew nothing of the danger, learned about it too late, heard it was exaggerated, or simply took their chances. After a few years, the number of strangers in the city would build up and the fever would reap a rich harvest of victims. Sometimes one or two fever-free years would be enough to encourage an influx of strangers. The severe epidemic of 1817 was followed by another, almost as severe, in 1819. Shortly before the latter epidemic, John Shecut noted that there were "an immense number of strangers in Charleston." A few weeks later, a local planter reported that yellow fever was "sweeping off the strangers."[36]

Yellow fever was particularly lethal during the antebellum period among the city's small but expanding Roman Catholic community. The reason is that such a high percentage of Catholics were recent immigrants. During the epidemic of 1838, Catholics accounted for almost one-third of the deaths ascribed to yellow fever, but made up only 5 percent of the population. Astonishingly, more than 40 percent of the deaths among Charleston's Catholics between 1800 and 1860 were ascribed to yellow fever. Ethnically, the majority of the antebellum victims were Irish and Germans who had recently arrived by ship and often lived in crowded urban locations near the docks. In August 1838, one observer noted that most yellow fever victims were sailors, Germans, and Irish. Many of the latter two groups had recently come to work on rebuilding parts of the city destroyed by a major fire that spring. In the 1850s, another brief surge of Irish and German immigration was followed by renewed epidemics. The new arrivals were densely packed into squalid housing, making them easy prey for the virus-carrying mosquitoes.[37] During the epidemic of 1854, the

[34] J. H. Easterby, *A History of the College of Charleston* (Charleston, SC, 1935), 46–47.

[35] Michaux, *Travels West of the Alleghanies*, 300.

[36] Shecut, *Medical and Philosophical Essays*, 106; Gabriel Manigault to Charles I. Manigault, Sept. 15, 1819, Manigault FP, SCL.

[37] Thomas Y. Simons, "A Report on the Epidemic Fever as it occurred in Charleston in 1852," *Charleston Medical Journal and Review*, 8 (1854), 365; J.W. Cheesborough, ALS, Aug. 28, 1838, SCL; Walter J. Fraser, *Charleston! Charleston! The History of a Southern*

nearly completed Roper Hospital was opened as an emergency yellow fever hospital. Most admissions were recent immigrants, and of those received by October 1, more than one-third died, 62 of 180.[38] Because it was particularly deadly among young adults, yellow fever left many orphans in its wake, especially among the immigrant poor. Charleston's Orphan House, established in 1790, was enlarged in the 1850s. The timing was probably not coincidental.[39]

Many victims of yellow fever came to Charleston unaware of the danger they were courting. Inability to read warnings may have doomed some people. Others may have been misled or confused by the terminology used to describe yellow fever. In one sense it may not matter what people call a disease. What matters is whether one gets sick or dies. Words mattered, however, when some deterred people from entering the infected area and others did not, when some triggered quarantine and others did not. The term "strangers' disease" should have been troubling to newcomers – if they heard it – but it may not have conveyed the same terror as "yellow fever." Other common names in the early nineteenth century such as "endemial fever" and "prevailing fever" probably conveyed little meaning to many immigrants and visitors. Charleston newspapers often used these as euphemisms for a disease that dared not speak its name.[40] During the epidemics of 1807 and 1817, hundreds died from yellow fever, but not one death listed in the *Charleston Times* was attributed to it. During the epidemic of 1824, the *Charleston Mercury* reported that yellow fever had killed many people in New Orleans, but when reporting fever deaths in Charleston, it used "prevailing fever," "bilious fever," or "short but painful illness." In 1827, the *Mercury* reported one death due to "yellow fever." The city death records list sixty-two deaths due to the disease that year.[41]

Perhaps the newspapers can be excused to some extent. Local doctors were often divided about whether the disease was present and what they should

City (Columbia: University of South Carolina Press, 1989), 236. I owe the Simons and Cheesborough references to David Brown.

[38] Susan S. King, *Roman Catholic Deaths in Charleston, South Carolina, 1800–1860* (Columbia, SC: SCMAR, 2000); Charles S. Bryan, "Yellow Fever and the Church," *Journal of the South Carolina Medical Association* 99 (2003), 60–61; Charleston Death Records, 1850–1859; *Report of the Committee of the City Council of Charleston upon the Epidemic Yellow Fever of 1858* (Charleston, 1859), 47–65; *Report of the President of the Howard Association of Charleston* (Charleston, 1858), 11; Frederick Law Olmsted, *A Journey in the Seaboard Slave States* (New York, 1856), 404; MSM, Oct. 2, 1854.

[39] Basil Hall, *Travels in North America in the Years 1827 and 1828* 3 vols. (Edinburgh, 1829), 3: 166; Fraser, *Charleston!*, 179.

[40] *Yellow Fever of 1858*, 27; *The Courier*, Nov. 11, 1807; Charleston *City Gazette*, Sept. 15, 1819; "Marriage and Death Notices from the *City Gazette and Daily Advertiser*," SCHM 31 (1930), 260–262, 33 (1932), 210–215.

[41] MSM, Aug. 1, Sept. 1, 4, 1817; *Marriage and Death Notices from the (Charleston) Times*, comp. by Brent Holcomb (Baltimore: Genealogical Publishing Co., 1979), 172–181, 318–323; *Marriage and Death Notices from the Southern Patriot, 1815–1830* comp. by Teresa E. Wilson and Janice L. Grimes (Easley, SC, 1982), 53–55, 121–124; *Marriage and Death Notices from the (Charleston, South Carolina) Mercury, 1822–1832*, comp. by Brent Holcomb (Columbia, SC: SCMAR, 2001), 70–79, 148.

call it. In 1806, the Medical Society of South Carolina debated the question: "[I]s yellow fever only a higher grade of the common intermittent?"[42] In 1812, the society's minutes declared that "bilious remittents" were by far the most numerous diseases, and that in the case of strangers, the remittents had "terminated in yellow fever." Two things are indicated here: The doctors were assuming that yellow fever was a higher grade or more virulent form of malaria, and that strangers were the most susceptible to this complication. In September 1817, the minutes refer to the presence in the city of an epidemic of "yellow fever *or* aggravated bilious fever."[43]

John Shecut tried to explain the problem of terminology, but only indicated how confused the doctors' diagnoses were. In certain years, a small number of cases of a virulent fever occurred, which some doctors called "sporadic yellow fever." Others argued that it was merely a "high grade of our autumnal remittent." The sporadic fever occurred in years in which atmospheric conditions were not conducive to "true yellow fever." To muddy things further, many doctors held that changing atmospheric conditions could alter the type of fever during an epidemic. In 1817, Shecut noted, the disease began to abate after a heavy rain with some distant thunder. The predominant form of fever changed to catarrhal (perhaps influenza), and in some cases the symptoms were so mixed "as to produce a doubt, which of the types predominated." In mid-October, after strong thunderstorms, the fever transformed into another type of fever "or rather formed or blended itself along with most other types of fever." According to Shecut, the other types included intermitting, remitting, nervous, worm, and country fevers. The other fevers probably included malaria or dengue, or perhaps both. Doctors sometimes confused these fevers with "legitimate" yellow fever. Shecut claimed that the difficulty of discriminating between true yellow fever and other fevers deterred even experienced doctors from declaring the presence of the former until they were absolutely sure, to prevent unnecessary panic.[44]

Another Charleston doctor was less indulgent than Shecut. In 1840, Benjamin Strobel rebuked his colleagues for sowing confusion about yellow fever's origins and spread. This arose, he charged, from "the want of accuracy in describing, and the blunders and mistakes which have been made, in calling it by such a variety of names, as for instanced, *Petechial Typhus, High Bilious, Putrid Malignant*, etc. etc." Through "ignorance or design," some doctors had contributed to yellow fever mortality. He told the story of one doctor, "endowed with more *whiskers* than brains" who was asked in the midst of an epidemic "if he had seen any cases of yellow fever? And who replied – No, I have seen some of violent fevers, which some doctors no doubt would *call* yellow fever – but I consider them only *high bilious*." Such doctors, Strobel fumed, "are the bane of the community, and the curse of our profession."[45]

[42] MSM, May 1, 1806.
[43] MSM, Nov. 1, 1812, Sept. 1, 1817; Waring, *Medicine in South Carolina, 1670–1825*, 30–35.
[44] Shecut, *Medical and Philosophical Essays*, 101, 106, 121–122.
[45] Strobel, *Yellow Fever*, 204.

The reluctance of many doctors to declare the presence of yellow fever in the early stages of an epidemic – or in years of "sporadic fever" – meant that Charleston's death records, which began in 1819, surely underestimated the ravages of the disease. In 1825 and 1826, yellow fever was blamed in only two deaths, but bilious and country fevers allegedly claimed eighty-three lives. In 1827, sixty-four deaths were ascribed to yellow fever, but another fifty-six were attributed to bilious and country fevers. In 1828, yellow fever was listed as the cause of twenty-six deaths; bilious and country fever accounted for forty-one. Dengue fever, which appeared in the death records for the first time that year, was said to have killed twelve people, most of them in the weeks just before yellow fever deaths appeared. Dengue did not make another appearance in the death records until 1850, when it was listed as "brake bone" fever and blamed for nineteen deaths. Because classic dengue resembles yellow fever but is rarely fatal, some deaths ascribed to dengue were probably due to yellow fever. Charles Manigault claimed that "broken bone" fever was present along with yellow fever in the fall of 1856. He noted that among strangers, breakbone and other fevers could "incline towards the type of yellow, or strangers' fever (which are the same thing)." As we have seen, many doctors believed that one disease could mutate into another under certain circumstances. During the yellow fever epidemic of 1839, Dr. Thomas Simons claimed that "a peculiar fever resembling dengue appeared, [and] the yellow fever began to disappear."[46]

The city death records contain other oddities. After 1848, bilious fever disappeared as a cause of death, except for a few cases in 1858. Country fever, commonly listed as a cause of death in the 1820s and 1830s, also disappeared after 1848. Perhaps the upsurge in reported yellow fever deaths in the following decade was due in part to the mysterious disappearance of bilious and country fevers. The upsurge of the 1850s may be misleading in another way. In 1849, Charleston Neck, where about 15,000 people lived, was officially made part of the city. Deaths in that area were henceforth included in the city's mortality reports. The population of the older part of the city had also grown in the 1840s, though slowly. During the 1830s and 1850s, the population actually declined slightly. Yellow fever was one of the reasons, by both killing and deterring strangers.[47]

MISLEADING ASSURANCES

During the early nineteenth century, many people accused Charleston's leaders of deliberate attempts to mislead outsiders about the danger of yellow fever

[46] Charleston Death Records, 1821–1829; *Yellow Fever of 1858*, 47–65; *The Courier*, Sept. 11, 20, 1827; Clifton, *Life and Labor on Argyle Island*, 229; Simons, *Yellow Fever*, 11.

[47] Charleston Death Records, 1821–1829; *Yellow Fever of 1858*, 47–65; Daniel Horlbeck to Judge Glover, Oct. 29, 1858, MSS 945, WHL; MSM, Sept. 1, 1829; Peter Coclanis, *Shadow of a Dream* (New York and Oxford: Oxford University Press, 1989), 115, Table 4–4.

in the city. In September 1803, Andrew Jamison, chairman of Charleston's committee of health, declared that anxious rumors of a malignant fever being present in town were baseless. False reports had terrified inhabitants, led many people to flee the city, and injured its commerce. He predicted that in a few days the city's safety would be clear, country people would come to the markets, and citizens would resume their normal routines. Perhaps people were unduly alarmed. Yellow fever killed "no more than 59" people that year, according to David Ramsay. The real number was probably higher and would have been higher still if more "fugitive citizens" and country folk had been in the city.[48]

Charleston newspapers often complained that the press in other cities published misleading articles about the danger of yellow fever in the city. During the epidemic of 1817, The Charleston *Courier* complained that "northern papers" were full of "exaggerated statements of the fever now prevalent in this city." But northern papers were not alone in accusing Charleston's officials of hiding the true state of affairs. North Carolina's *Fayetteville Observer* claimed that printers in Charleston were "forbidden to publish the full extent of the dreadful mortality." The Charleston Board of Health had reported the mortality returns of the previous week as sixty-two, but "a gentleman of that city" had informed the *Observer* that the number of deaths had been almost three times that great. The newspaper accused the health board of the "cruel act" of luring strangers to Charleston by greatly understating the mortality. The unfortunate strangers, the newspaper predicted, would become "certain victims of the yellow fever very soon after their arrival." The Charleston *Courier* denounced the article as "injudicious and unwarrantable" and denied that the Board of Health's report was inaccurate or that printers were forbidden to publish anything on the subject of the epidemic. The editor then added, as if it were relevant, that yellow fever was raging in New Orleans. Ironically, *The Courier* itself had contributed to the sense of crisis. A few weeks before, the editor had asked Charleston natives to subscribe to a fund to help newcomers – "industrious mechanics" – who were forced to flee for their lives. They needed the aid of Charleston natives who were "happily exempt from the influence of this malignant disease."[49]

Just before yellow fever exploded again in 1819, *The Courier* protested that almost every paper in the country had been erroneously reporting its existence in Charleston. The editor mocked such articles as sensational filler, designed "to excite the enquiries of those who find it pleasant to be alarmed." Reports of yellow fever were "extremely injurious" to commercial towns and should never be published "without the most substantial proof." The offenders included a rival Charleston newspaper. On August 11, *The Courier*'s editor chided the *Southern Patriot* for reporting the existence of the fever. He assured his readers that the few cases were anomalous and nothing to be alarmed

[48] *The Courier*, Sept. 26, 1803; Ramsay, *History of South Carolina*, 2: 47.
[49] *The Courier*, Sept. 20, Aug. 9, 1817.

about. They certainly did not justify flight from the city. The next day, *The Courier* announced that the city was "free of contagion ... and as healthy as any large maritime city in the Union." During the next week, the newspaper continued to deny that any serious problem existed. On August 21, the Board of Health reported four cases of yellow fever and in the following week reported that thirty-six people died of it. The final official death toll was 177, nearly all of them strangers. It would have surely been higher had not many of them fled once the epidemic was acknowledged. A letter to the *Southern Patriot* charged *The Courier* with recklessly encouraging strangers to stay in the city by denying the presence of yellow fever.[50]

In the fall of 1821, the *New York Commercial Advertiser* charged that Charleston doctors were hiding the existence of yellow fever. The doctors were calling it "country fever" to avoid repelling visitors. The editor of the *Carolina Gazette* promptly denied the charge: "We may pardon a man for not distinguishing between yellow fever and country fever, or for confounding sporadic cases with an *epidemic*. But we assure the editor, that the gentlemen composing the Board of Health in Charleston would never disguise so important a fact as the existence of epidemic disease, nor are they in the habit of making a weekly report of *falsehoods*." Charleston was "the healthiest city in the world."[51] Indeed, the number of fatalities officially diagnosed as country fever in 1821 was not large, only twenty-one. Another thirty-three deaths were attributed to bilious fever, and twenty-four to other fevers. No deaths were ascribed to yellow fever, which naturally aroused skepticism given the severe epidemics in recent years. Of the seventy-eight fever deaths that summer and fall, the great majority (fifty-nine) were among natives, an indication that strangers were avoiding the city. A similar pattern occurred during the next two years. But the number of strangers began to increase again, and in 1824, epidemic yellow fever definitely returned. Deaths officially ascribed to the disease outnumbered deaths from other fevers, 235 to 46. Fever deaths of strangers of all kinds also greatly exceeded those of Charleston natives, 214 to 67. The death toll would probably have been higher had the *Charleston Mercury* not informed its readers in early August that yellow fever might be present and urged strangers to leave town "at least until the nature of the apprehended disease may be fully developed."[52]

Such warnings often came too late, because city officials and newspapers were reluctant to declare the presence of yellow fever until it could not be denied. In August 1838, *The Courier* announced the disease's arrival for the benefit of "the great number of persons now residents here who are subject to its attacks" and called on the city authorities to "caution strangers not to visit the city until they can do so without peril." The editor had good reason

[50] *The Courier*, July 20, Aug. 11 to Sept. 3, 1819; Easterby, *South Carolina Rice Plantation*, 372.
[51] *Carolina Gazette*, Oct. 27, 1821; Waring, *Medicine in South Carolina, 1670–1825*, 67, 163.
[52] *Charleston Mercury*, Aug. 11, 1824; Charleston Death Records, 1821–1829; MSM, Aug. 12, 1824.

to know: He explained that he would have issued the warning earlier, but that he had been "at Death's door" himself for the past ten days. Perhaps his experience had awakened his sympathy to other potential victims. The Mayor's Office issued the desired announcement the next day and declared that the disease had been present in the city for at least three weeks. City officials excused the late announcement by claiming that the number of cases had been fewer than usual at that date in previous epidemic years. Now "avalanches of rain" were producing conditions more favorable to its propagation. With the reality of the situation clear, *The Courier*'s editor issued an interesting piece of advice. He urged "temporary residents" to leave the city immediately. But he offered the opposite advice to those who "intend making Charleston their home, and the home of their families." They should never leave, but "manfully meet the crisis, trust to Providence, the skill of their physicians, and the kindness of their friends, and they will, probably, in a few short weeks, be equally prepared with the natives, to aid the sick, and the stranger, in their turn."[53] This was a convoluted, obscure way of saying, "stay, and if you get yellow fever and manage to survive, you will never need to worry about it again." Members of the local elites uncertain of their own susceptibility often ignored such helpful advice. The Trustees of the College of Charleston certainly could not advise students and faculty to remain. The college, which had closed in 1836 for lack of students and money, had recently reopened as a municipal institution. The trustees were trying to attract faculty and students from outside the city, and could not afford to lose them to yellow fever. In late August, they announced that classes would be suspended until October 15, because the faculty and some students were "strangers to our climate." During the following years, the college changed its calendar to reduce the danger of yellow fever, beginning the summer vacation in August and ending it in October. The change may have reduced the danger but could not eliminate it. That would have required a six months' vacation.[54]

As *The Courier* continued to chide newspapers in other cities for circulating "exaggerated" and "ridiculous" reports about the epidemic of 1838, the death toll continued to mount. In the second week of September, more people died of yellow fever than in any week for which records existed. To the editor, the main reason for the mortality was obvious: "[A]t no previous period, were there ever congregated here such a number of strangers." A major fire that had destroyed about one-third of the city in April had attracted a large number of "mechanics and laborers" to rebuild and improve the city. The editor blamed the epidemic and the high mortality largely on the workers' "loose habits," which we may translate as frequenting taverns and brothels, along with living in overcrowded and run-down tenements, as poor immigrants were generally forced to do. As so often in history, the alleged immorality of the poor and foreign provided both a ready explanation for an epidemic and how it chose its

[53] *The Courier*, Aug. 22, 24, 25, 30, Sept. 7, 13, 19, 26.
[54] Easterby, *College of Charleston*, 88–95, 136.

victims. The editor predicted that the mortality would soon drop because so many of the susceptible, disreputable characters had already been infected or fled the city. In fact, the number of deaths shot up the following week. It seemed that many susceptible, disreputable people had failed to leave or could not afford to do so. Moreover, and to the surprise of many, some natives and old residents were dying, and in respectable parts of the city and other areas that had previously been considered safe from the fever. "The only hope left for relief," the puzzled editor concluded, was "an early frost."

The number of deaths declined in late October, and *The Courier* began to encourage those who had fled to return. The editor admitted that some cases of the disease were still occurring and would occur until a hard frost took place, but assured the timid that the number of cases would "be so few that none need fear, and can hardly arise among such as take ordinary care of their health." He added, in his usual breezy manner, that a few deaths a week should not be alarming to anyone, any more than a few deaths from "apoplexy or any other ordinary disease." When ice was observed in parts of the city on October 31, he exulted *"Charleston herself again!"* as if the Charleston of the epidemic was an anomaly. On November 2, the Board of Health announced that the yellow fever epidemic was officially over. Its effects, however, lasted much longer. A decade later, Joseph Johnson remarked that the city had not yet recovered. He claimed that many people had left the city permanently after the fire and epidemic, and indeed, its population declined slightly during the 1830s.[55]

During the 1840s, yellow fever gave the city a reprieve. Between 1841 and 1848, only one death in the city was officially blamed on it, in 1843. In that year, however, the fever was declared to be epidemic in the area to the north of the city limits known as Charleston Neck. It is odd that this was the first recorded occasion in which the Neck experienced an epidemic when the disease was not epidemic in the city. The deaths in the Neck were not tabulated, because it was not then within the city limits. Nevertheless, the 1840s seem to have been relatively free of yellow fever, perhaps because it was also a decade in which the city's maritime commerce stagnated or declined.[56]

The confusing and suspicious pattern of reporting deaths, coupled with official and press denials of the danger, continued. Charleston's leaders and press continued to complain that other port cities were spreading exaggerated tales about yellow fever in the city. In 1849, Dr. Eli Geddings of the Medical College of South Carolina applauded the city's efforts to prevent publication of yellow fever deaths as a way of reducing panic. Preventing panic was a commendable goal, but obscuring the presence of yellow fever sacrificed the

---

[55] *Charleston Mercury*, Aug. 11, 1824; *The Courier*, Aug. 22–Nov. 3, 1838; Joseph Johnson, "Some Account of the Origin and Prevention of Yellow Fever in Charleston, South Carolina," *Charleston Medical Journal and Review*, 4 (1849), 157–158; Fraser, *Charleston!*, 217.

[56] William Hume, "Report to the City Council of Charleston, on a Resolution of Inquiry, relative to the Source and Origin of Yellow Fever," *Charleston Medical Journal and Review* 9 (1854), 156–157; MSM, Oct. 2, 1843, 151; Coclanis, *Shadow of a Dream*, Tables, 120–124.

lives of susceptible persons. Moreover, once the disease became widespread, denial of its presence was futile and only increased distrust of the city's assurances and the local doctors' skills and ethics. It is not surprising that some observers accused Charleston's doctors of gambling with human lives for the sake of commercial interests. Thomas Y. Simons, the port physician, bristled at such charges. The claim that doctors would falsify medical reports for the "sake of commercial prosperity" was an insult to the medical profession, the merchants, and city officials. He added that the yellow fever in Charleston was "in such a form as to be easily controlled," a claim that must have raised some eyebrows among his medical colleagues.[57]

Being proved wrong repeatedly did not deter the city's officials, doctors, and newspapers from denying the presence or danger of yellow fever. The 1850s brought Charleston's worst epidemics in terms of absolute numbers killed. In August 1854, with an epidemic already underway, *The Courier* declared that "at present, Charleston is the healthiest city in the Union" and that rumors to the contrary existed "only in the minds of evil disposed people." The *Charleston Mercury* reported on epidemics in other southern cities while ignoring the one on its doorstep. On September 18, the editor of the *Mercury*, no longer able to ignore the situation, announced that the epidemic appeared to have peaked and was about over. In the next three days, the moribund epidemic killed sixty-three people. The official death toll for yellow fever was more than 600 that year.[58]

In 1858, the official number of deaths exceeded 700, the largest recorded mortality from one yellow fever epidemic in the city's history. Charleston newspapers again denied reality and accused other newspapers of spreading false rumors. Soon, scores of people were dying every day, more than fifty on some days. The dead included one of *The Courier*'s editors and many natives. Novelist William Gilmore Simms lost two sons in one day. The unfortunately named George Coffin, president of Charleston's philanthropic Howard Association, unhelpfully declared that the city's epidemic was "light" compared to one in New Orleans that year. That may have been true in terms of the absolute numbers of victims, but Charleston's image as a graveyard for strangers may have been worse than that of New Orleans. In 1860, Frederick Law Olmsted declared Charleston the unhealthiest city in the United States for white newcomers.[59] Olmsted may have been wrong, but the city's mendacious reputation in respect to yellow fever was firmly established. During

[57] Thomas Y. Simons, "A Report on the Epidemic Fever as it occurred in Charleston in 1852," *Charleston Medical Journal and Review* 8 (1854), 375–376. I owe this reference to David Brown; MSM, Sept. 1849; Simons, *Report on Yellow Fever*, 22–23.

[58] *The Courier*, Aug. 23, 1854; *Charleston Mercury*, Sept. 18–21, 1854; Easterby, *South Carolina Rice Plantation*, 120; Charleston Death Records, 1854.

[59] *Report of the President of the Howard Association of Charleston* (Charleston, 1858), 9–10; Frederick Law Olmsted, *The Cotton Kingdom* (New York, 1861), 259; M. Foster Farley, *An Account of the Stranger's Fever in Charleston South Carolina, 1699–1876* (Washington, DC: University Press of America, 1978), 114–120.

Charleston's last major epidemic in 1871, *The Courier* denied the disease was present and accused newspapers in other cities of spreading "false rumors." The nonexistent epidemic claimed more than 200 lives.[60]

The city's pattern of denying the danger of yellow fever was a part of a broader pattern, one that included planters' denials that their slaves suffered severely from the local diseases. There was a tension between the two sorts of denials, however. Charleston's leaders wanted to attract trade and immigrants and so they tended to downplay the threat to whites from disease. Planters wanted to justify slavery, increasingly under attack after 1820, so they stressed that only blacks could work effectively in the unhealthy low-country. Doctors helped both causes, by denying the presence or danger of yellow fever in Charleston and by denying that blacks suffered much from the region's diseases. Death, however, would not be denied.

---

[60] *The Courier*, Sept. 1, 2, 1871; *Yearbook, City of Charleston*, 1880, 30–33, 39, 75–77; Waring, *Medicine in South Carolina, 1825–1900*, 67; E. Chernin, "The Disappearance of Bancroftian filariasis from Charleston, South Carolina," *American Journal of Tropical Medicine and Hygiene* 37 (1987), 111–114.

7

"A Merciful Provision of the Creator"

> The flux which prevailed amongst [the slaves], could not be stopped by the most able of our physicians. From this disorder 13 are now dead and some still not out of danger and the best that remain in a poor and meager condition.
>
> Henry Laurens, 1756

> Here the negro enjoys better health in the vicinity of the rice fields, and arrives at greater longevity than he does in the mountains. He requires not to be acclimated, but is constitutionally at home along the shores of our sluggish rivers, and in situations adapted to the culture of indigo, cotton, and rice, where a similar exposure would prove fatal to the white man. Short-sighted men may ascribe all this to accidental causes and the results of blind chance; we confess, however, we view it in a different light – we see in it evidences of design – we regard it as a merciful provision of the Creator in imparting to the human constitution the tendency to produce varieties adapted to every climate and every country.
>
> John Bachman, The Doctrine of the Unity of the Human Race, 1850

> Stoke Martha is sick. Rock Sena has some fever. Harcules is sick. Driver Simon is sick. Stoke Hetty is sick. Stoke Mudlong is sick. Marcia is sick. Saby is sick. Duckey's Tom is sick.
>
> Thomas Sinkler, overseer, Stoke Plantation, August 1833

RICE, SLAVERY, AND DEATH

The combination of rice and slavery did more than anything else to make the lowcountry the richest and deadliest region in British North America. Today, many people wax lyrically about the halcyon days of "Carolina gold," as the best lowcountry rice was known. Few people have understood or perhaps wished to confront how ghastly the business of rice cultivation was. Most of this book describes the effects of disease on the white population for the simple reason that they left abundant written records. But the fact that black voices are seldom heard in these sources should not obscure their enormous suffering from disease. Contrary to the views of apologists for slavery, blacks endured as much or more sickness than whites. This was especially true of the great majority who cultivated rice. Many whites could avoid the rice fields and their disease vectors in the warm months. Blacks (and some whites) had no such option. Moreover, many blacks did not enjoy the disease immunities some whites comfortably ascribed to them.

In 1826, architect Robert Mills attributed the lowcountry's unhealthiness to the faulty development and then abandonment of rice cultivation in the interior swamps. The region would have been healthier, Mills claimed, had the swamps been left in their natural state.[1] He was surely right, even if he did not know the reason, that the removal of trees and the creation of rice ponds and fields had increased potential breeding places for the local mosquito vector of malaria, which prefers stagnant, sunlit water. Nor did he know that the importation of Africans to create and work on the plantations had brought *falciparum* malaria as well. In hindsight, the adoption of rice cultivation seems a perverse choice. In the early eighteenth century, however, it made economic sense to many landowners. For decades, they had been trying to find a staple that could fetch good prices on world markets. Rice proved to be that staple, aided as it was by British mercantilist policies.[2] It seemed a quick road to opulence, and for many planters it was. Often it brought them and their family members an early death as well. To almost everyone else in the region, the choice of rice brought immense suffering (see Figure 7.1).

Cultivating and processing rice was an arduous and unhealthy business, especially in the eighteenth century. The backbreaking labor of clearing woodland swamps and then growing, harvesting, and threshing the crop weakened the workers' resistance, especially given an often inadequate diet. In a letter to the Royal Society of Arts in London in 1755, Dr. Alexander Garden detailed the debilitating nature of rice cultivation. Masters who overtasked their slaves often paid dearly for their "inexpressible avarice" and "barbarity" by the loss of many "valuable Negroes." To Garden, it was obvious why this happened: "[T]he poor wretches, forced to work incessantly to accomplish their task," often became overheated. Subsequent exposure to "bad air" or the drinking of cold water brought on "dangerous pleurisies and peripneumonies, which soon rid them of cruel masters, or more cruel overseers, and end their wretched being here."[3] Garden may have had his exact causation wrong, but he was definitely onto something. The large numbers of slaves who died of respiratory disorders in the fall and winter probably had their immune systems weakened by malaria and dysentery, as well

[1] Robert Mills, *Statistics of South Carolina* (Charleston, 1826), 140.
[2] Peter A. Coclanis, *The Shadow of a Dream: Economic Life and Death in the South Carolina Low Country, 1670–1920* (New York and Oxford: Oxford University Press, 1989); Peter A. Coclanis, "Tracking the Economic Divergence of the North and the South," *Southern Cultures* 6.4 (2000), 83–85.
[3] "Correspondence between Alexander Garden, M.D. and the Royal Society of Arts," ed. by Joseph I. Waring, *SCHM* 64 (1963), 16–17.

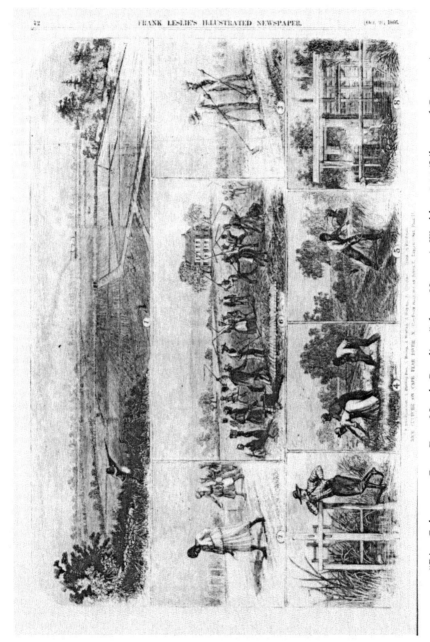

FIGURE 7.1. "Rice Culture on Cape Fear, North Carolina," from *Harper's Weekly*, 1866 (Library of Congress).

as by overwork and poor nutrition. In 1756, Henry Laurens reported that "parapneumonia" was killing many blacks.[4]

In the early 1770s, the author of *American Husbandry* called the cultivation of rice in South Carolina "dreadful." It was difficult to imagine any work more "fatal to health." The "poor wretches" were forced to work while standing in water and mud, "exposed all the while to a burning sun." He compared laboring in this "furnace of stinking putrid effluvia" to that of digging in the notorious silver mines of Potosi. Slaves employed in other work might increase in numbers, but those engaged in rice production decreased in numbers, "and it would be miraculous were it otherwise."[5] New Englander Elkanah Watson, who came to South Carolina on a mission for the new American government in 1777–1778, was astonished that any rice slaves survived given their "wretched" diet and intense labor in a torrid sun.[6] Another New Englander who came to Charleston in the 1770s declared that threshing, "the excessive hard labor of beating the rice in mortars to separate it from a hard stiff hull which adheres to it," was responsible for killing "great numbers every winter."[7]

Englishman Francis Hall, who passed through the lowcountry in 1816, conceded the common planter argument that whites could not "support the labour of [rice] cultivation." He argued, however, that blacks engaged in such work suffered heavily from disease.[8] His countryman Basil Hall, who arrived a decade later, claimed that the rice plantations were so lethal they sucked large numbers of slaves from the healthier states of Virginia and North Carolina: "[T]he cultivation of rice thins the black population so fast, as to render a constant fresh supply of negroes indispensable, in order to meet the increasing demand for that great staple production of the country." A Savannah doctor told Hall of a friend who lost 40 out of 300 slaves in the previous year, mainly from pulmonary diseases. Hall's observations of rice cultivation changed his views of slavery. Prior to his visit, his objections to slavery had been primarily moral. But now he added "a long catalogue of diseases and death, which thin the ranks of the unhappy sufferers." Just before the Civil War, Frederick Law Olmsted repeated these observations and noted in particular the extremely high infant mortality among the slaves on rice plantations. It proved that they were not immune to "the subtle poison" of the

---

[4] Elizabeth Donnan, ed., *Documents Illustrative of the Slave Trade to America* 4 vols. (Washington, DC: Carnegie Institution of Washington, 1930–1935), 4: 343.

[5] The silver mines of Potosi in Bolivia were notorious for producing high mortality among the slaves the Spanish forced to work there from the mid-sixteenth century to the late eighteenth century. Carman, *American Husbandry*, 276–278; see also, Mark Catesby *The Natural History of Carolina, Florida, and the Bahama Islands* 2 vols. (London, 1771), 1: xvii.

[6] Elkanah Watson, *Men and Times of the Revolution; or Memoirs of Elkanah Watson*, ed. by Winslow C. Watson (New York, 1856), 54–55.

[7] *Life in the South, 1778–1779: The Letters of Benjamin West*, ed. by James S. Schoff (Ann Arbor, MI: The William L. Clements Library, 1963), 30–31.

[8] Francis Hall, *Travels in the United States and Canada* (Boston, 1818), 245.

marsh miasmas. The widespread view that southern blacks suffered less from disease than whites was absurd: "They may be less subject to epidemic and infectious diseases, and yet be more liable to other fatal disorders, due to such influences, than whites."[9]

Records from nineteenth-century rice plantations show them to have been highly lethal for the slave inhabitants. On the Ball family plantations, slaves born between 1800 and 1849 had a life expectancy of 19.8 years for males and 20.5 years for females. About half of the children did not live to adulthood. Sickness among the slaves was a constant refrain in the letters of overseers to their employers.[10] At the Manigault plantation at Gowrie on the Savannah River between 1833 and 1861, nearly twice as many slaves died as were born. Ninety percent of children born at Gowrie did not survive to age sixteen. Most of the infant and child deaths seem to have been due to malaria, neonatal tetanus, and enteric or bowel disorders such as dysentery and typhoid. The English actress Fanny Kemble was appalled by the high child mortality on the plantation of her husband, Pierce Butler, in the late 1830s. Nine slave women she talked with had given birth to fifty-five children, of whom only fourteen survived. William Dusinberre notes that "recent demographic studies remind one of what everyone knew in the eighteenth century, that slaves died much faster in the rice region than elsewhere in the American South." A conservative estimate suggests that at least 55 percent of the children born on nineteenth-century rice plantations did not survive beyond age of fifteen. Dusinberre thinks the true percentage was closer to two-thirds dead by fifteen.[11]

It is not possible to quantify with exactness morbidity and mortality rates on eighteenth-century rice plantations. It was probably higher than in the nineteenth century, because, as Dusinberre notes, "slavery in the eighteenth century was an even grimmer institution" than in the antebellum period.[12] Mortality was probably highest among newly imported African slaves. In the Chesapeake and West Indies, for which more reliable statistics exist, they died at very high rates indeed: More than one-third of imported Africans

[9] Basil Hall, *Travels in North America in the Years 1827 and 1828* 3 vols. (Edinburgh, 1829), 3: 188, 196, 205; Frederick Law Olmsted, *The Cotton Kingdom* (New York, 1861), 1: 235, 2: 258–259.

[10] Cheryl Ann Cody, "Slave Demography and Family Formation: A Community Study of the Ball Plantations, 1720–1896," Ph.D. diss., University of Minnesota, 1982, 215–219, 239, 244, 255, 405–409.

[11] William Dusinberre, *Them Dark Days: Slavery in The American Rice Swamps* (Athens: University of Georgia Press, 2004), 50–55, 70–75, 80, 236–245; Jeffrey R. Young, "Ideology and Death on a Savannah River Rice Plantation, 1833–1867: Paternalism Amidst a 'Good Supply of Disease and Pain,'" *Journal of Southern History* 59 (1993), 673–706; Richard Steckel, "Slave Mortality: Analysis of Evidence from Plantation Records," *Social Science History* 3 (1979), 86–114; James M. Clifton, ed., *Life and Labor on Argyle Island: Letters and Documents of a Savannah River Plantation, 1833–1867* (Savannah, GA: The Beehive Press, 1978). For Kemble's account, see Frances Anne (Fanny) Kemble, *Journal of a Residence on a Georgia Plantation, 1838–1839* (Athens: University of Georgia Press, 1984).

[12] Dusinberre, *Them Dark Days*, 80.

died within three years of arrival. They could hardly have fared much better on lowcountry rice plantations and probably suffered worse than those put to growing tobacco in Maryland and Virginia. The cultivation of indigo, an important lowcountry product from the 1740s to the 1780s, was probably just as dangerous as rice growing. Indigo was cultivated on rice plantations and, like rice, required the impoundment of standing water. The strong smell of the fermented indigo plants also attracted myriads of flying insects.[13]

THE LUCKY SLAVES

In 1834, James Louis Petigru recorded the results of a cholera epidemic that broke out in rice plantation areas along the Savannah River and then spread south into Georgia: "[T]here are probably near 1000 negroes less on the Savannah and Ogeechee since the 1st of September." On Petigru's plantation, 2.5 percent of the slaves had died, but on some plantations, the disease had killed up to 20 percent of the slaves. Petigru felt fortunate to have gotten "off so well, still I am a great loser."[14] Unfortunately, we have no record of the slaves' views of their losses. The black majority was virtually silenced by bondage and illiteracy, and we are overwhelmingly dependent on the white elite for information about their world. These sources are often biased and seldom linger over slaves' sufferings. Sometimes, however, they cannot help but convey it, even if inadvertently. To read through the Diary and Account Book of Hanover, the plantation of Rene and Henry Ravenel, with its endless record of the deaths of slave children, provides a chilling sense of what the least fortunate inhabitants must have endured.[15] Planters sometimes professed distress at the diseases and deaths of slaves that went beyond concern for their economic loss. Eliza Lucas Pinckney wrote anxiously to her daughter Harriott in June 1778 about some ill slaves on one of her plantations. They were falling to a "distemper" that had recently struck a neighbor's slaves: "We lost George and Phebe in a few days, and before I heard they were sick. Abram and little Toby lay at the point of death on Saturday, some more down." A few days later, she wrote to a doctor she had hired to care for her slaves, "Pray God put a stop to this raging disease."[16]

One may debate whether Pinckney's anguish was over people or her investment in them. In any case, many planters possessed a comforting response to

---

[13] Coclanis, *Shadow of a Dream*, 44–45; Wood, *Black Majority*, 77–85; Judith A. Carney, *Black Rice: The Origins of Rice Cultivation in the Americas* (Cambridge, MA and London: Harvard University Press, 2001), 118; Philip D. Morgan, *Slave Counterpoint: Black Culture in the Eighteenth-Century Chesapeake and Lowcountry* (Chapel Hill: University of North Carolina Press, 1998), 92, 152–153, 163, 444.

[14] *Life, Letters and Speeches of James Louis Petigru: The Union Man of South Carolina* (Washington, DC: W. H. Lowdermilk and Co., 1920), 164.

[15] Diary and Account Book of Rene and Henry Ravenel of Hanover, 1731–1860, Thomas Porcher Ravenel Collection, SCHS, 12/313/1.

[16] "Letters of Eliza Pinckney," *SCHM* 76 (1975), 154.

death and disease among their slaves: that they suffered far less than would whites subjected to similar labor in the hot and humid climate. During the antebellum period, it became an axiom of white thinking in the South that blacks – as a "race" – were largely immune to the fevers that ravaged whites. This "fact" became part of the proslavery argument, but it persisted long after the abolition of slavery as a defense of the peculiar institution. Samuel Gaillard Stoney summarized it neatly in 1939: "Luckily, a few hundred millennia of life in African jungles had given the negroes immunity to [malaria]. They throve where their masters perished and they lived comfortably enough on the plantations while white men dared not be caught there within an hour of night-fall."[17] By Stoney's day, the idea that the African or black "race" possessed immunities to malaria and yellow fever had become deeply entrenched in white thinking. It had wide academic acceptance and has proved enduring. In the 1950s, historian John Duffy claimed that blacks' ability to resist malaria, yellow fever, and smallpox was what "made them so valuable to the planters in the Carolina lowlands." The only odd thing about his claim was his inclusion of smallpox.[18] Over the years, I have heard many people repeat the claim about black immunities, or ask me "is it true?" Putting aside the racist origins of racial categories, the reality is that people of African origins were not "racially" immune to these disorders, though many possessed some form of genetic resistance to malaria and perhaps yellow fever. Others acquired immunity or resistance through suffering from these diseases, but whites could acquire that as well. Moreover, imported Africans met European and some African diseases to which they had no previous experience and no immunity or resistance. Since the nineteenth century, however, pronouncements on immunities have tended toward a simple declaration of black-white racial differentiation. They are a heritage of nineteenth-century racialism and more social than biological in origin. Interestingly, an early dissenter from the racialist view was a South Carolina historian. In 1945, J. Harold Easterby of the College of Charleston concluded that the high mortality rate among slaves on rice plantations "does not support the general belief that Negroes enjoyed almost complete immunity from the diseases of the [South Carolina] Rice Coast."[19] When and how this "general belief" originated is complex.

During the slavery era, whites often had no idea what diseases were sickening and killing blacks. Large numbers of blacks died from an unidentified fever during the Revolutionary War. Some years later, David Ramsay declared that blacks on the local plantations sometimes suffered outbreaks of an unknown fever. These isolated epidemics had been "so destructive at different times of

---

[17] Samuel Gaillard Stoney, *Plantations of the Carolina Low Country* (Charleston, SC: The Carolina Art Association, 1939), 34.

[18] John Duffy, "Eighteenth-Century Carolina Health Conditions," *Journal of Southern History* 18 (1952), 300.

[19] Easterby, *South Carolina Rice Plantation*, 30; Joseph L. Graves, *The Emperor's New Clothes: Biological Theories of Race at the Millennium* (New Brunswick, NJ and London: Rutgers University Press, 2001).

negro property, as to add much to the uncertainty of planters' estates." In the summer of 1803, a fever killed seventeen blacks in the village of Pineville and on a nearby plantation, but "scarcely affected white people." From the description of the symptoms, the disease could have been yellow fever: violent headache, pain in the back, low pulse, great weakness, and delirium. But if it was yellow fever, why did it affect very few whites? One possibility is that the whites had acquired immunity from suffering from the disease. Neither Ramsay nor other doctors who mentioned these idiosyncratic fevers had any idea what they were, and we will probably never know. A cynic might conclude that the fact one dies is more important than what one dies of. Nevertheless, doctors did get more specific – if not more accurate – in their diagnoses of "black" diseases as the nineteenth century progressed.

Colonial planters did not cite specific immunities to justify slavery. They did not need to. By the time the Carolina colony was founded in 1670, African slavery was firmly established throughout much of the Americas. Planters of sugar and other staples in hot climates had decided that black labor was both cheaper and easier to obtain than white labor. Even in the temperate northern colonies, some people used African slaves to help with agricultural and other tasks, and certainly not because of any immunity to tropical fevers the Africans may have possessed. The Barbadian planters who helped establish the Carolina colony in the 1670s brought black slaves with them as a matter of course, not because they believed the place to be especially unhealthy. During the eighteenth century, planters sometimes justified slavery in general constitutional terms. In the early 1780s, planters told Charles Stedman, a British army commissary, that it would be impossible to cultivate rice and indigo without blacks, "the whites not being able to bear the heat of climate."[20] The case for African labor was succinctly put by Alexander Hewatt in the late 1770s: "The utter ineptitude of Europeans for the labour requisite in such a climate and soil, is obvious to every one possessed of the smallest degree of knowledge respecting the country; white servants would have exhausted their strength in clearing a spot of land for digging their own graves." The rich lands would have "remained a wilderness, had not Africans, whose natural constitutions were suited to the clime and work," been employed in cultivating it. The arduousness of the work of raising, beating, and cleaning rice was such that even if it were possible to obtain European labor to do it, "thousands and ten thousands must have perished."

Hewatt was not an apologist for slavery. He viewed it as a moral evil and advocated the use of free black labor. But he believed that constitutional differences between blacks and whites advantaged the latter when it came to work like rice cultivation in the hot southern swamps.[21] David Ramsay, who

---

[20] Charles Stedman, *The History of the Origin, Progress, and Termination of the American War* 2 vols. (London, 1794) 2: 217n.

[21] Alexander Hewatt, *Rise and Progress of South Carolina and Georgia* 2 vols. (London, 1779) 1: 120, 123, 2: 92, 94.

also opposed slavery when he came to South Carolina in 1774, soon concluded that black labor was essential to the cultivation of the local soils. In 1780, he wrote to Benjamin Rush that "Providence intended this for a negro settlement. Their constitution is undoubtedly better suited to the climate, and all planters tell us that their lands cannot be cultivated by white men and that no education will bring up a white boy [equally] capable of labor in our lands with the blacks."[22]

These arguments for slavery, it bears repeating, rested on the idea that blacks' constitutions enabled them to work more effectively in the hot, moist climate than whites. They did not depend on claims to specific African immunities. The first lowcountry person to make such a claim in print was John Lining in the 1750s, who argued that Africans were immune to yellow fever. Lining did not use that claim to justify slavery, nor apparently did anyone else during the colonial period. It would have been of limited use anyway, because yellow fever was then largely confined to Charleston. It was also unnecessary. The general claim that Africans were physically more able to labor in the local environment than Europeans was sufficient for most whites. Another reason why few people claimed that blacks were immune to yellow fever may be that medical theory had not yet accepted the concept of specific diseases with specific causes. This was particularly true of fevers. Most doctors believed that all fevers were fundamentally similar in their causes and cures. They arose from miasmas or corrupted air, not specific organisms or toxins. General causes produced general diseases. Nervous, intermittent, bilious, and yellow fevers were types of a generic fever. Atmospheric changes could transform one type into another, which might be more or less virulent. Doctors also tended to think of disease in general climatic and constitutional terms. African bodies, designed for a hot climate, were better fitted than European ones to withstand labor in the lowcountry.[23] Benjamin Franklin summarized these views in a letter to John Lining in 1758: "May there not be in negroes a quicker evaporation of the perspirable matter from their lungs and skin, which by cooling them

---

[22] Robert L. Brunhouse ed., *David Ramsay, 1749–1815: Selections from His Writings*, Transactions of the American Philosophical Society, N.S. 55, Part 4 (Philadelphia: The American Philosophical Society, 1965), 65. Despite his opposition to slavery, Rush's writings also provided ammunition for later apologists for slavery, as in his claim that black skin was due to leprosy and that as a result Africans were largely impervious to pain from hard labor and physical punishment. See Mark M. Smith, *How Race Is Made: Slavery, Segregation, and the Senses* (Chapel Hill: University of North Carolina Press, 2006), 18.

[23] Richard Dunn, *Sugar and Slaves: the Rise of the Planter Class in the English West Indies, 1624–1713* (Chapel Hill: University of North Carolina Press, 1972); Philip D. Curtin, *The Rise and Fall of the Plantation Complex* (New York: Cambridge University Press, 1998), 79–81; Philip D. Curtin, "Epidemiology and the Slave Trade," *Political Science Quarterly* 83 (1968), 190–216; Seymour Drescher, "White Atlantic: The Choice for African Slave Labor in the Plantation Americas," in *Slavery in the Development of the Americas*, ed. by David Eltis, et al. (New York: Cambridge University Press, 2004), 60–61; Winthrop Jordan, *White over Black: American Attitudes toward the Negro, 1550–1812* (Baltimore: Penguin Books, 1969), 260–264; Peter Wood, *Black Majority: Negroes in Colonial South Carolina from 1670 through the Stono Rebellion* (New York: W.W. Norton and Co, 1975), 83–84, 88, 90–91.

more, enables them to bear the sun's heat better than whites do? ... if that is a fact, as it is said to be; for the alleged necessity of having negroes rather than whites, to work in the West-India fields, is founded upon it."[24] Such an explanation did not require a concept of specific diseases.

It is perhaps no accident that the first detailed argument for the superiority of African labor in the lowcountry came from Georgia in the 1730s. The reason why such an argument was made in this case was that the Georgia Trustees initially banned slavery. Their goal was to establish a colony of free whites that would protect the southern borderlands of British North America against the Spanish in Florida. The idea appealed to members of the British government, who believed that the slave majority in South Carolina was its Achilles' heel, rendering it vulnerable to attack. In the end, the pursuit of wealth trumped the quest for security. Soon after Georgia was established, a group of planters sought to overturn the ban on slavery by arguing that white labor could never make the colony profitable. The Malcontents, as they were called, received some support from South Carolina. Samuel Eveleigh argued that the Georgia Trustees' decision to ban slave labor from the new colony was economically unsound: "Without negroes," he declared, "Georgia can never be a colony of any great consequence." Although it possessed excellent land for rice, white people would not be able to cultivate it successfully, because "the work is too laborious, the heat very intense, and the whites can't work in the wet at that season of the year as [negroes] do to weed the rice." The Malcontents argued that whites were unsuitable for field labor because they would suffer too much from disease: "[I]nflammatory fevers ... tormenting fluxes; most excruciating cholicks, and dry belly aches; tremors, vertigoes, palsies, and a long train of painful and lingering nervous distempers." The list of diseases is notable for being vague and including some that killed many blacks, especially fevers and dysentery.[25]

The Malcontents differed from antebellum defenders of slavery in an important respect. The former admitted that plantation labor was extremely hard and dangerous even for blacks. In effect, they argued that no one would wish to do such work, but someone had to if the fields were to be tilled, and blacks could do it more profitably than whites. Nowhere in the Malcontents' argument – or anywhere else in the eighteenth century – does one find the healthy, happy "negro" of antebellum proslavery propaganda. For eighteenth-century planters generally, the main argument for slavery was that blacks were more able than whites to labor in the hot climate because blacks were habituated to such a climate. Only after the antislavery movement gained strength, especially after 1820, did writers justify slavery by claiming that blacks were immune to specific diseases.[26]

[24] *The Papers of Benjamin Franklin,* ed. Leonard Labaree (New Haven, CT and London: Yale University Press, 1965) 8: 111.
[25] Wood, *Black Majority,* 84–85, 105, note 35; Hewatt, *South Carolina and Georgia,* 1: 110.
[26] Clarence ver Steeg, ed. *A True and Historical Narrative of the Colony of Georgia by Pat. Tailfer and Others* (Athens: Georgia University of Georgia Press, 1960), 50–51, 79, 139; Julia

Some eighteenth-century observers argued that the advantages of black labor were exaggerated, and that white bodies could tolerate working in hot and humid climates. The Georgia Trustees declared this, at least initially. One of them, Lord Egmont, denounced the Malcontents' arguments. He pointed to the Salzburger community at Ebenezer on the Savannah River as proof that whites could do hard labor in Georgia without suffering excessively from sickness. In fact, malarial fevers caused problems for the Salzburgers, but their settlement generally prospered until slavery became established in the region in the 1750s. Egmont conceded that agues were common in Georgia in the warm seasons, but that the Malcontents exaggerated their effects on white servants' ability to work. To Egmont, the claim that whites could not labor in the lowcountry was merely an excuse for "idle people who want to see their work done by others." The Trustees' opposition to slavery was supported by the Salzburgers and some Scots settlers at Darien, but to no avail.[27]

Other observers argued that whites could work effectively in tropical climates. British naval surgeon James Lind acknowledged the danger of fevers to Europeans who engaged in heavy outdoor labor in low, swampy locations. He added, however, that the danger was much greater to recent arrivals than long-term white residents. Over time, European constitutions could become seasoned to warm climates, if not too badly weakened by repeated bouts of disease after their arrival. Those who achieved this state were "generally subject to as few diseases abroad as those who reside at home; in so much as that many persons, dreading what they may again be exposed to suffer from a change of climate, choose rather to spend the remainder of their lives abroad, than to return to their native country." In other words, Europeans could gradually acclimate to work in the tropics. Lind was correct, although the seasoning process required much suffering and posed a high risk of death. His argument also threatened to undermine one key rationale for black slavery. The idea that they might eventually become like blacks was surely disturbing to many whites as well.[28]

In 1802, South Carolina governor John Drayton tried to plant slavery on a firm philosophical basis. He argued that it was based on "nature's unerring laws." Drayton cited Alexander Pope's *Essay on Man* (1734), with its faith in God's benevolent design. Everything that exists does so for a purpose, and the purpose must be a good one. As Pope put it, "Whatever is – is right." The claim derived most immediately from the optimistic philosophy of Wilhelm

---

F. Smith, *Slavery and Rice Culture in Georgia, 1750–1860* (Knoxville: University of Tennessee Press, 1985), 17–23; Betty Wood, *Slavery in Colonial Georgia, 1730–1775* (Athens: The University of Georgia Press, 1984), 24–25, 44–45; Jordan, *White Over Black*, 262.

[27] ver Steeg, *True and Historical Narrative*, 50–51, 79, 139, 159; Robin Blackburn, *The Overthrow of Colonial Slavery* (London and New York: Verso, 1988), 146; Joyce E. Chaplin, *An Anxious Pursuit: Agricultural Innovation and Modernity in the Lower South, 1730–1815* (Chapel Hill and London: University of North Carolina Press, 1993), 117–120.

[28] James Lind, *An Essay on Diseases Incident to Europeans in Hot Climates* (London, 1768), 146–147.

Leibnitz (1646–1716) and, much farther back, Aristotle. In the fourth century
B.C., Aristotle had defended slavery on the grounds that some people were natural slaves. Nature had designed them for that purpose, just as it had designed
others to be philosophers or kings. For those individuals tempted to exploit
their fellow humans – a large class of people to judge by history – the natural
slave argument has always provided a convenient justification, encompass-
ing both hierarchy and teleology. Nature, Drayton claimed, had been kind to
South Carolina. Had the state not been "furnished" with African slaves, like
manna from heaven, she would have cut a poor figure in the world: "[I]n the
scale of commerce and importance, she would have been numbered among
the least respectable states of the union." Without Africans to till the soil,
"the best lands of this state [the rice lands] would have been rendered useless"
because they were "particularly unhealthy and unsuitable to the constitutions
of white persons; whilst that of a negro is perfectly adapted to its cultivation."
The introduction of African slaves enabled the "planting interest" to cope
with "the dangers, and climate, of the country." God was on the side of the
planters, but also on the side of the Africans because He had designed them for
their work, whereas He had designed the planters for supervising the slaves.[29]
When Englishman Basil Hall traveled through the region in the late 1820s, he
heard the same refrain everywhere: Cultivating the land with white labor was
"visionary" and "impossible." Planters, doctors, and merchants, even some
who claimed to oppose slavery, agreed that the lowcountry must be cultivated
by blacks or abandoned. Hall agreed, but rejected the view that slavery was
therefore justified. He was appalled by the slave system. But he had nothing
at stake.[30]

   To establish the view that blacks were benevolently designed for working
on the rice plantations, it was necessary to dispose of some inconvenient evidence. During the eighteenth century, some observers had argued that blacks
were not immune to lowcountry fevers. In the 1760s, Dutch surveyor John De
Brahm declared that agues and fevers were prevalent among both Europeans
and Africans.[31] Lord Adam Gordon, an officer in a Highland regiment stationed in South Carolina during the same period, maintained that poverty,
not race, was the common denominator that produced high morbidity and
mortality there, assisted by the swampy terrain and rice cultivation. The "fall
fevers and agues, dry gripes and other disorders ... are often fatal to the lower
sort of people, as well white as black."[32] Johan David Schoepf, a German who
visited the region in 1784, agreed that warm countries were more natural and

[29] John Drayton, *A View of South Carolina*, (Charleston, 1802), 146–149, 160; Chaplin, *Anxious
     Pursuit*, 122. For Aristotle's theory of slavery, see the *Politics*, Book 1, chapters 3–7.
[30] Hall, *Travels in North America*, 3: 194.
[31] John G. W. De Brahm, *Report of the General Survey in the Southern District of North America*
     ed. by Louis De Vorsey, Jr. (Columbia: University of South Carolina Press, 1971), 79.
[32] *Journal of Lord Adam Gordon*, in Newton D. Mereness ed., *Travels in the American Colonies*
     (New York: The Macmillan Co., 1916), 399.

agreeable to blacks than whites. Despite this advantage, he claimed that black deaths were disproportionately high: "It is sufficient proof of the bad situation in which [the blacks] find themselves here that they do not multiply in the same proportion as the white inhabitants."[33] Schoepf may have erred in claiming that blacks grew more slowly in numbers than whites. He came right after the Revolutionary War, a period of exceptionally high mortality for blacks. But he raised a legitimate issue. Why were blacks dying at such high rates in a region supposedly agreeable to their constitutions?

Statistical evidence for black immunities in eighteenth-century South Carolina is either lacking or decidedly mixed. Let us consider yellow fever, because epidemics of that disease often killed so many people in a short time that observers sometimes recorded the numbers of deaths. After the epidemic of 1699, Hugh Adams reported that 162 Europeans, 16 Indians, and 1 black had died in Charleston.[34] Hundreds of blacks died in epidemics during 1711–1712. Some sources say that as many as three-fourths of the dead were black. But the causes of the mortality at that time included several diseases: smallpox, influenza, yellow fever, malaria, and dysentery may all have been involved.[35] Alexander Hewatt wrote that a yellow fever epidemic in 1728 killed many people, "both white and black," but he was writing fifty years later. In the epidemic of 1732, Governor Robert Johnson informed the Board of Trade that 130 whites had died, and "many" blacks.[36] Most accounts of eighteenth-century epidemics simply noted that yellow fever had killed a lot of people, a lot of strong and healthy men, or a lot of newcomers.[37]

Another kind of evidence indicates that many whites did not consider blacks to be immune to yellow fever. The quarantine laws of colonial South Carolina were largely designed to prevent the importation of malignant fevers from Africa, an indication that the framers thought that Africans could get the disease. The act that legalized slavery in Georgia in 1750

[33] Johann David Schoepf, *Travels in the Confederation, 1783–1784* (reprint, New York: Burt Franklin, 1968), 221.

[34] Extract of a letter from Hugh Adams to Samuel Sewell, Feb. 23, 1700, in Diary of Samuel Sewell, 2: 11–12, April 22, 1700, Massachusetts Historical Society, *Collections* 5th series, 6: 11–12.

[35] Klingberg, *Johnston*, 98; Klingberg, *Le Jau*, 104, 108; Benjamin Dennis, Feb. 26, 1711/12, SPG Letterbooks, A7: 402–403.

[36] Hewatt, *History*, 1: 316–318; *SCG*, July 15, Aug. 5, 12, 19, Sept. 2, 15, 23, Oct. 20, Dec. 16, 1732; *Collections of South Carolina Historical Society* 5 vols. (Charleston, 1897), 3: 317–318; Johnson to Board of Trade, Dec. 15, 1732, BPRO/SC 16:4.

[37] Thomas Hasell, Sept. 6, 1707, SPG letters, A3: 281–282, cited in John Duffy, "Eighteenth-Century Carolina Health Conditions," *Journal of Southern History* 18 (1952), 289–302; Andrew Leslie, Jan. 7, 1739, SPG Letter Books, B7: 243–244; John Fordyce, Nov. 4, 1745, SPG Journals, 10: 129; Charles Boschi, Oct. 30, 1745, SPG Letter Books, B12; *SCG*, Sept. 15, Oct. 7, Nov. 11, 1745, Sept. 6, 1748; *JCHA*, 6:12; E. Merton Coulter, ed., *The Journal of William Stephens, 1743–1745* (Athens: University of Georgia Press, 1959), 243, 250; Message of Gov. James Glen, Journal of the Upper House of Assembly, Dec. 5, 1745, SCDAH; Journal of His Majesty's Council, Oct. 5, Nov. 6, Dec. 5, 7, 1745, SCDAH.

explicitly made that claim. It established a quarantine system there, because to send the "blacks on shore when ill of contagious distempers (particularly the yellow fever) must be of the most dangerous consequence."[38] The belief probably derived from the experience of South Carolina or another British colony. Descriptions of Caribbean epidemics show that some whites believed Africans were susceptible to yellow fever. John Oldmixon reported that large numbers of blacks died in the Barbados epidemics of the 1690s.[39] James Clark, a British doctor who witnessed a yellow fever epidemic a century later on Dominica, claimed that it attacked almost all newcomers to the island, and killed most of them, irrespective of color: "[T]he new negroes, who had been lately imported from the coasts of Africa, were attacked with it." The only blacks who escaped the disease were those who had long resided in the town, or on the island.[40]

Contrary views were common. Benjamin Moseley, former surgeon-general of Jamaica, noted that on British expeditions against the Spanish in Nicaragua in 1780, few of the blacks brought along became seriously ill. More than 75 percent of the British perished. At the taking of Fort Omoa, "half of the Europeans who landed died within six weeks, but very few negroes; and not one, of 200, who were *African* born." Most of the blacks who became ill were born in the Americas. Colin Chisholm, a British doctor who described the introduction of yellow fever into Grenada in 1793, declared that the disease attacked some blacks on the plantations near town, but did not spread much or produce a high fatality rate. Only about 25 percent of the blacks were infected, and of those only one in eighty-three died, compared to almost universal infection among whites, with a death rate ranging from one in three to one in fifteen.[41] Robert Jackson, a British army surgeon who served in the American South and Jamaica, claimed that blacks who came from Africa never got yellow fever. He added, however, that the disease seldom attacked anyone, European or African, who had resided for "any length of time in a tropical country." In other words, anyone could acquire immunity, something we now know to be true.[42]

---

[38] Donnan, *Slave Trade*, 4: 610–611.

[39] Jack Greene, *Imperatives, Behaviors, and Identities: Essays in Early American Cultural History* (Charlottesville: University Press of Virginia, 1992), 38; Sheldon Watts, "Yellow Fever Immunities in West Africa and Beyond: A Reappraisal," *Journal of Social History* 34 (2001): 962.

[40] James Clark, *A Treatise on the Yellow Fever as it Appeared on the Island of Dominica in Years 1793–96* (London, 1797), 2; Richard B. Sheridan, *Doctors and Slaves: A Medical and Demographic History of Slavery in the British West Indies, 1680–1834* (Cambridge: Cambridge University Press, 1985), 186–187, 213.

[41] William Currie, *A Treatise on the Synochus Icteroides, or Yellow Fever, as it Lately Appeared in the City of Philadelphia* (Philadelphia, 1794), 13–14; Colin Chisholm, *An Essay on the Malignant Pestilential Fever* (Philadelphia, 1799), 97–101.

[42] Benjamin Moseley, *A Treatise on Tropical Diseases* (London, 1792), 147n; Robert Jackson, *A Treatise on the Fevers of Jamaica* (Philadelphia, 1795), 162–163.

TOWARD A THEORY OF RACIAL IMMUNITIES

By the end of the eighteenth century, no clear medical consensus existed concerning black immunities. Nevertheless, during the early nineteenth century, some local doctors began to argue that blacks as a group possessed immunities to malaria and yellow fever. David Ramsay, as usual, had good news for the planters: Blacks suffered less from summer and fall fevers than whites, the maladies that predominated during the months labor was most in demand on the plantations. "Unseasoned negroes" – newly arrived Africans – were sometimes infected by yellow fever, but when treated "properly" were readily cured. Blacks often contracted "common intermittents" but they were mild and "easily cured." To be sure, blacks were more vulnerable than whites to respiratory disorders. But like people who blamed the poor for getting yellow fever, Ramsay declared that blacks themselves were partly to blame for this difference: They were "incorrigibly careless" in matters of health. They wantonly exposed themselves to the elements. They did not try to avoid getting minor illnesses, but saw them as a chance to get out of work. Moreover, they knew their owners would pay for their medical care. Why they would look forward to some time off at the price of bleeding, purging, and vomiting Ramsay did not say.[43]

Ramsay was a transitional figure. His views of black immunities were not radically different from those of colonial physicians, but they were somewhat more specific. John Lining had claimed that Africans possessed an inherent immunity to yellow fever. But he argued that they were as susceptible as whites to "bilious fever."[44] What he meant by that is not clear. As we have seen, bilious fever was a highly malleable term that many physicians used to describe any fever that produced a jaundiced appearance. Lining's colleague, Lionel Chalmers, agreed with him that blacks were immune to yellow fever. He argued, however, that they were as vulnerable as whites to most other diseases, and more vulnerable to some, especially pneumonia and pleurisy. Moreover, Chalmers never claimed that differences in disease vulnerabilities of blacks and whites were racial, but rather socio-cultural and environmental. For example, he noted that blacks were less prone to gout than whites, but added that if they lived like whites, they would be just as liable to gout. To Chalmers, as to many Enlightenment thinkers, the human body was much the same everywhere, "differing only in being more braced in one climate, and laxer in another." Whites and blacks lived in a climate of seasonal extremes that differed from both Europe and Africa: Their bodily "fibers" were alternately and severely braced in winter and lax in summer. The strains this alteration put on their bodies meant that all the inhabitants suffered heavily from

[43] David Ramsay, *History of South Carolina* (Charleston, 1858) 2: 51–52, 294.
[44] John Lining, "A Description of the American Yellow Fever," *Essays and Observations, Physical and Literary* 2 (1756): 374.

disease. Chalmers's analysis implied that over time, black and white bodies would both adapt to the climate they lived in. Bodies were bodies. Chalmers's argument was potentially subversive because it implied that slavery would someday be unnecessary.[45]

The idea that blacks were immune to yellow fever was widely debated during and after the devastating Philadelphia yellow fever epidemic of 1793. Benjamin Rush and other doctors initially assumed that blacks were immune to yellow fever. Some black leaders agreed and mobilized their community to nurse the sick. But as the epidemic progressed, large numbers of blacks became ill, and 300 died. Rush and the black leaders reconsidered their belief that people of African descent enjoyed full immunity. The idea that blacks were resistant to the disease persisted, however. Philadelphia doctor William Currie claimed that blacks were liable to yellow fever, "though not in the same proportion as whites."[46]

As we have seen, Ramsay agreed that blacks got yellow fever less often than whites, and that their cases were usually mild. His explanation, like Chalmers', was essentially environmental. Most white victims of yellow fever, Ramsay claimed, were "strangers" from Europe or other parts of North America and had no experience with the disease. Conversely, most Charleston blacks had "the advantage of old [white] residents" of having lived in the city all of their lives or having come from places where yellow fever was common. Rural blacks appeared to be more susceptible to the disease than those who lived in the city. Few of them came from the country while the disease was known to be in Charleston. Ramsay also concluded that blacks who had recently come from Africa were much less likely to get yellow fever than white strangers, and seldom died of it. He ascribed this to their coming from a climate similar to that of South Carolina. Blacks and whites who had resided in the West Indies for many years were also largely exempt from yellow fever.[47]

During the early nineteenth century, the argument about black immunity to yellow fever became increasingly racialized. In 1802, visiting natural-ist Francois Andre Michaux declared that all blacks in South Carolina were immune to yellow fever, a view he surely picked up locally. In 1819, Dr. John Shecut conceded that black newcomers to Charleston could contract yellow fever, but in a milder form than white strangers and white children. He did not explain what he meant by "black newcomers," but as the legal slave trade

[45] Lionel Chalmers, *An Account of the Weather and Diseases of South Carolina* 2 vols. (London, 1776) 1: 31; Chalmers, *An Essay on Fevers* (Charleston, 1768), v–vi.

[46] Wood, *Black Majority*, 82, note 70; Currie, *Treatise on the Synochus Icteroides, or Yellow Fever*, 13–14; John Harvey Powell, *Bring Out Your Dead* (Philadelphia: University of Pennsylvania Press, 1949), 100–107, 271.

[47] David Ramsay, *The Charleston Medical Register for the Year 1802* (Charleston, 1803), 21; David Ramsay, "Remarks on the yellow fever and epidemic catarrh, as they appeared in South Carolina during the summer and autumn of 1807," *Medical Repository*, second ser. 5 (1808), 233–236; Ramsay, *History of South Carolina*, 2: 47; Duffy, "Eighteenth-Century Carolina Health Conditions," 300.

had ended, he must have meant blacks from other parts of the United States. The Medical Society of South Carolina proclaimed much the same view.[48] In 1827, Samuel Henry Dickson, professor at the new Medical College of South Carolina, declared that he had "never known an *African* negro to be attacked" with yellow fever. His stress on "African" indicates that he believed blacks born in America did sometimes get it, and thus it was not a racial immunity. In the 1840s, however, he presented a more detailed and explicitly racialist view. He acknowledged that yellow fever had infected large numbers of blacks in the Americas, but he claimed that the disease was less common and less fatal in them than among whites. Mulattoes occupied a middle position between whites and blacks in terms of susceptibility to yellow fever. Then he went much farther: Differences in susceptibility went beyond black and white to encompass "the various tribes and races of white men." He posited a complex ethnic hierarchy of susceptibility. The Irish, Germans, and "Scotchmen" were most susceptible to yellow fever, followed by the English, New Englanders, and Americans from states to the West. The Spanish, French, and Italians were the least susceptible of European types.[49]

If nothing else, the fact that Dickson was a teetotaler and that the Europeans he considered most susceptible to yellow fever had a reputation for heavy alcohol consumption should raise a red flag. At this point – if not before – one could be forgiven for becoming skeptical about the whole enterprise of trying to relate yellow fever immunities to something as culturally malleable as nineteenth-century racialism. Many antebellum doctors nevertheless racialized immunities, ascribing to *all* blacks what *some* of them – and it should be added, some whites as well – possessed. Southern doctors in particular gradually dropped environmental explanations of black disease immunities in favor of explicitly racial ones: There was something about blacks as a group that made them less likely than whites to die from the local fevers.[50] As we have seen, John Lining had made the same claim about yellow fever in the 1750s, while declaring that whites could only acquire immunity by surviving the disease. Right or wrong, Lining was making an observation, however, not providing a justification for slavery. Later southern physicians went much farther. They proclaimed that any immunity a black possessed was a gift from a benevolent God who had

[48] Michaux, *Travels West of the Alleghanies*, 119; Thomas Y. Simons, "Observations on the Yellow Fever, as it Occurs in Charleston," *Carolina Journal of Medicine, Science, and Agriculture* 1 (1825), 3; MSM, Nov. 1, 1824, 252.

[49] John L. E. W. Shecut, *Shecut's Medical and Philosophical Essays* (Charleston, 1819), 108–109; Samuel Henry Dickson, "Account of the Epidemic which prevailed in Charleston, S. C. during the summer of 1827," *The American Journal of the Medical Sciences* (1828), 2: 7; Samuel Henry Dickson, *Essays on Pathology and Therapeutics* 2 vols. (Charleston, 1845), 1: 345, 353.

[50] Trevor Burnard, "The Country Continues Sicklie': White Mortality in Jamaica, 1655–1780," *Social History of Medicine* 12 (1999) 71–72; Kenneth F. Kiple and Virginia H. Kiple, "Black Yellow Fever Immunities, Innate and Acquired, as Revealed in the American South," *Social Science History* 1 (1997), 425–428.

designed blacks for the purpose of toiling happily in places where whites could not work except at grave peril. Meanwhile – with one of those leaps of logic that takes one's breath away – whites tended to assume that *any* immunity *they* possessed to local fevers was acquired rather than inherited. Whereas blacks passively "received" inherited immunities, whites actively "earned" them by suffering through the "seasoning" process. This view was illogical and conveniently ignored the massive toll diseases of all kinds inflicted on the black population. Much if not most of the immunity blacks "enjoyed" from malaria and other fevers was "earned" at a high cost in sickness and death from constant enforced residence and hard labor in disease-prone areas. It is true that whites often noted that blacks were highly susceptible to certain diseases, notably respiratory disorders and dysentery. But among antebellum planters, those susceptibilities did not undermine arguments that blacks were inherently better suited for plantation labor than whites. One could argue that this was because most deaths from respiratory disorders occurred *after* the harvest season, but the evidence is circumstantial.[51]

Contrasting the inherited immunities of blacks with the acquired ones of whites was not only a form of racial boasting or a purely medical debate. It was also a matter of economics, politics, and ethics. In the antebellum era and beyond, arguments about differential racial immunities provided a rationale and justification for plantation slavery and the "southern way of life." The rapid growth of abolitionism after 1820 inspired spirited defenses of slavery. Advocates of what became known as the pro-slavery argument rejected the old view that slavery was a necessary evil and declared it a positive good. They supplied religious, political, economic, and ethical arguments for African bondage. It is hardly surprising that medical arguments also appeared, one of which centered on the differences between black and white susceptibilities to malarial and yellow fevers. The medical arguments survived slavery to buttress racial segregation in the idea that blacks "carried and transmitted" many diseases without suffering much from them, if at all. Paradoxically, after emancipation, some whites also began to argue that blacks were doomed to extinction.[52]

ENTER UNCLE REMUS

In the 1820s, some doctors began to add specific disease immunities among blacks to the justification for slavery. The timing was hardly coincidental. The concept of specific diseases with specific causes was gaining ground in medical thought. It is not surprising that some southern doctors – many of them also

---

[51] Chaplin, *Anxious Pursuit*, 102, 108, 117–122; Wood, *Black Majority*, 78.
[52] Jeffery Robert Young, *Domesticating Slavery: The Master Class in Georgia and South Carolina* (Chapel Hill and London: University of North Carolina Press, 1999); Jordan, *White over Black*, 260; Jill Dubisch, "Low Country Fevers: Cultural Adaptations to Malaria in Antebellum South Carolina," *Social Science Medicine* 21 (1985), 645–647.

planters – began to use the concept to refine the general constitutional and cli-matic arguments in favor of African labor. It is also hardly surprising that low-country doctors should be among the first to do so, given the region's reputation as a charnel house for whites and Charleston's position as a major cultural cen-ter in the South. In 1825, Thomas Y. Simons stated the medical argument for slavery succinctly: "[I]n this country, intersected with immense bodies of swamp lands, and reserves of water kept back for the culture of rice, all [whites] who are exposed to the miasma, arising from these sources, are victims of remit-tent and intermittent fevers, and their sequelae diseased liver and spleen ... It is somewhat singular that this state of things is confined to the white population." The happy, healthy slave enters the scene, suitably contrasted to a fever-wracked bundle of white misery: "While the white man is seen shivering with ague, his countenance cadaverous and his temper splenetic, the black, is fat, plump and glossy, in the full enjoyment of health and vigor."[53]

Another local physician, Philip Tidyman, presented a more detailed and nuanced picture. Tidyman claimed that blacks were protected by their con-stitutions "from the unhealthiness of hot climates, which are so inimical to the whites, especially among those who may be necessitated to labour in low swampy situations, and inhale a deleterious atmosphere. Under such circum-stances, negroes are seen working with cheerfulness and alacrity, when the white labourer would become languid and sink from the effects of a torrid sun." In part this was the old constitutional argument updated to present blacks as not only able but happy to do their tasks: Blacks' color and copious perspiration allowed them to withstand high temperatures and a scorching sun with fewer ill effects than whites, and helped them ward off many diseases that whites could not withstand. But Tidyman became more specific. Blacks, he claimed, suffered little from certain diseases. They were "generally" immune to intermittent and remittent bilious fevers (malaria). Intermittent fever was only a minor irritant, and they were largely immune to bilious fevers. They were virtually immune to yellow fever: "Nature has, with special regard to the safety of the blacks, rendered them almost proof against the insidious attacks of this terrible disease." Tidyman conceded that nature did not pro-tect blacks from all diseases. They were susceptible to a fatal type of dys-entery. Overall, however, the health of the slaves was "remarkable." Blacks who worked on rice plantations were as healthy as they would have been if living in the mountains.[54] In 1850, the Lutheran minister and accomplished

---

[53] Thomas Y. Simons, "Case of the Derangement of the Spleen and Liver," *Carolina Journal of Medicine and Science and Agriculture* 1 (1825), 141–142. For a thorough and sympa-thetic analysis of proslavery thought, see Elizabeth Fox-Genovese and Eugene D. Genovese, *The Mind of the Master Class: History and Faith in the Southern Slaveholders' Worldview* (New York: Cambridge University Press, 2005). See also, *The Ideology of Slavery: Proslavery Thought in the Antebellum South, 1830–1860*, ed., with an introduction, by Drew Gilpin Faust (Baton Rouge: Louisiana State University Press, 1981).

[54] Philip Tidyman, "A Sketch of the Most Remarkable Diseases of the Negroes of the Southern States," *Philadelphia Journal of the Medical and Physical Sciences* 12 (1826), 306–330.

naturalist John Bachman merged the medical views of Simons and Tidyman with Drayton's neo-Aristotelian claim that slavery was a product of benevolent design. Blacks lived healthy and long lives in the lowcountry – longer and healthier than slaves in the mountains – because they were adapted to the climate and work. The difference was providential. A loving deity had designed "varieties adapted to every climate and every country."[55]

The idea that blacks were designed for plantation labor became widely accepted in America, along with other elements of nineteenth-century racism. But there were dissenters. In 1845, Daniel Drake, an Ohio physician who also worked in Kentucky, claimed that intermittent and remittent fevers were the greatest killers of slaves. His observations agreed with those of colonial physicians such as Garden and Chalmers: Many blacks who survived autumnal fevers were weakened and died the following winter of respiratory infections. Drake denied that blacks were immune to yellow fever. He agreed that it was not a major killer of blacks, but maintained that was mainly because most of them did not live in urban areas where the disease was prevalent.[56]

The happy, healthy slave of Simons, Tidyman, and Bachman was a caricature. Those who argued for black immunities to malaria and yellow fever were not entirely wrong, however, even if their arguments and interests coincided. Modern biology has confirmed that many Africans and people of African ancestry possess some genetic immunity or resistances to malaria. Some of them may also possess a genetic resistance to yellow fever. Many are immune to *vivax* malaria due to the absence in their blood of the Duffy antigen. This genetic trait prevents the plasmodia from entering blood cells. Duffy-negative people can be infected but show no symptoms at all, and the trait seems to cause them no harm. The ability of many blacks to work in the rice fields during the hot summer months may have owed much to the widespread genetic immunity of West Africans to *vivax* malaria, which tends to peak in the summer. The slaves were more vulnerable to the "fall fever," *falciparum* malaria. Although many of them possessed some acquired or genetic resistance to that disease, infections could lower their resistance to respiratory and other diseases as the weather turned colder in the late fall and winter.

Some genetic traits provide partial immunity – or rather resistance – to *falciparum*. The most famous and most important of these results from the inheritance of the sickle cell (Hemoglobin S) gene, but several others provide some measure of resistance, such as G6PD deficiency, which seems to provide some protection to heterozygous females, but not to males. These are not racial traits, however; they are not confined to sub-Saharan Africans. Some people of Mediterranean, Middle Eastern, or South Asian ancestry

[55] Although Bachman defended slavery as a positive good, he refuted racial polygenesis and argued that whites and blacks belonged to one race. John Bachman, *The Doctrine of the Unity of the Human Race, Examined on the Principles of Science* (Charleston, 1850), 209.
[56] Daniel Drake, "Diseases of the Negro Population," *Southern Medical and Surgical Journal*, NS 1 (1845), 342.

possess them. Neither are they necessarily benign. They may also produce dangerous and even fatal conditions such as severe anemia and metabolic disorders. Sickle cell anemia predisposes its victims to pneumococcal infections. If these genetic traits helped some blacks survive malaria, they brought suffering and early deaths to others. It would be absurd to emphasize this kind of "protection" unduly. Moreover, some enslaved Africans lacked immunities of any kind, genetic or acquired, to certain strains of malaria. Today, most of the 1–2 million people who die of malaria every year are African, the great majority of them children. Many millions more are debilitated and immunologically compromised by the disease. In this context, claims of an "African" immunity to malaria seem perverse indeed.[57]

The most important malarial immunity – or rather resistance – for blacks was not genetic but acquired from frequent exposure to the disease. Anyone who survives malaria, however, may acquire that immunity. People who reside constantly in endemic areas without prophylaxis will be regularly infected by the parasite. They may not become dangerously ill, but may suffer periods of debility, fever, chills, and lowered immunity to other infections. In such a situation, the disease is fatal mainly to young children. In order to maintain this less than ideal state, however, people must remain in the endemic area. If they leave it for an extended period, they may lose their hard-earned acquired immunity, regardless of race.[58] This happened to whites who left the region for an extended time. Charles Pinckney died of malaria in 1758 soon after his return from a five-year absence in Britain. Peter Manigault, who was educated in Britain, suffered repeated attacks of malaria after his return to South Carolina in the 1750s. The disease undermined his health and destroyed a promising political career. In 1773, he returned to England where he died the same year.[59]

Paradoxically, one reason blacks tolerated local fevers somewhat better than many whites was that they could not leave for their health or education. When blacks left their plantations, it was because their owners sold them or

[57] Herbert M. Gilles and David A. Warell, *Bruce-Chwatt's Essential Malariology*, 3d edition (New York: Oxford University Press, 1993), 60–64; Leonard Jan Bruce-Chwatt, *Essential Malariology*, 2d edition (New York: John Wiley and Sons, 1985), 85–89; Kiple, *Cambridge History of Disease*, 857; Margaret Humphreys, *Malaria: Poverty, Race, and Public Health in the United States* (Baltimore: Johns Hopkins University Press, 2001), 18–20; Kenneth Kiple, *The Caribbean Slave: A Biological History* (1984), 16–17; Todd Savitt, *Medicine and Slavery: The Diseases and Health Care of Blacks in Antebellum Virginia* (Urbana: University of Illinois Press, 1978), 20–22; Keith Wailoo, *Dying in the City of the Blues: Sickle Cell Anemia and the Politics of Race and Health* (Chapel Hill and London: University of North Carolina Press, 2001), 55–56.

[58] Gilles and Warell, *Bruce-Chwatt's Essential Malariology*, 64–65; Bruce-Chwatt, *Essential Malariology*, 89–95.

[59] Elise Pinckney, ed., *The Letterbook of Eliza Lucas Pinckney, 1739–1762* (Chapel Hill: University of North Carolina Press, 1972), 91; "The Manigault Family of South Carolina from 1685 to 1886," *Transactions of the Huguenot Society of South Carolina* 1 (1897), 70, 79–80.

transferred them to another plantation (unless they escaped). These moves sometimes worsened their health, because in moving to a new environment they could meet a type or strain of malarial parasite or some other pathogen to which they had no immunity, genetic or acquired.[60] Newly arrived and "unseasoned" Africans tended to have higher mortality rates than those born or long resident in the lowcountry. Moreover, many blacks whom the British returned to West Africa after the Revolution proved vulnerable to the fevers of that region, although they fared somewhat better than whites who went with them. In 1793, a group of freed slaves who had settled in Nova Scotia after the Revolution immigrated to the new British colony of Sierra Leone. Soon after their arrival, 800 of the 1,100 black settlers who had survived the voyage fell ill from "putrid fever," perhaps malaria or yellow fever or both, as well as dysentery. Boston King, a freed slave from South Carolina, recorded the death of his wife from the fever, which he also contracted. King survived, but many others in the little colony died: "[T]he people died so fast, that it was difficult to procure a burial for them." By the end of 1793, around 200 of the blacks from Nova Scotia were dead. One white settler wrote that he was surprised that the black settlers died in such large numbers. In fact, the blacks from Nova Scotia died at almost the same rates as the whites. A century later, British traveler Mary Kingsley claimed that when it came to malaria and yellow fever, the mortality of the descendants of freed blacks in Sierra Leone was almost as high as that of whites.[61]

Charleston's death records, which began in 1819, indicate – at first sight – that yellow fever largely spared the city's blacks. The records list 86 blacks who died of yellow fever between 1819 and 1859, whereas nearly 3,000 white deaths were ascribed to the fever. The proportion of black yellow fever deaths – less than 3 percent of the total – seems tiny given that during that time, blacks constituted about 50–55 percent of the population. But when one considers that the enormous majority of whites who died of yellow fever were listed as "strangers," and that few strangers were black in this period, the discrepancy does not seem quite so compelling. Moreover, when one looks in general at fever deaths of native Charlestonians over this period, the numbers for native whites and blacks are very similar: 603 whites and 640 blacks. It seems that natives, black or white, had a fairly equal chance of dying of fevers in antebellum Charleston. Moreover, the number of black deaths is

---

[60] Humphreys, *Malaria*, 18–20; Kiple, *Caribbean Slave*, 16–17; Wailoo, *Dying in the City of the Blues*, 55–56.

[61] Boston King, "Memoirs of the Life of Boston King, A Black Preacher," in *Face Zion Forward: First Writers of the Black Atlantic* ed. and intr. by Joanna Brooks and John Saillant (Boston: Northeastern University Press, 2002), 228–229; Alfred W. Crosby, *Ecological Imperialism: The Biological Expansion of Europe, 900–1900* (Cambridge: Cambridge University Press, 2004), 139; Adam Hochschild, *Bury the Chains: Prophets and Rebels in the Fight to Free an Empire's Slaves* (Boston and New York: Houghton Mifflin Co., 2005), 175, 209; A. B. C. Sibthorpe, *The History of Sierra Leone* (London: Frank Cass, 1970), 9–10; Sheldon Watts, *Epidemics and History: Disease, Power and Imperialism* (New Haven, CT and London: Yale University Press, 1997), 243.

probably understated. Perhaps the widespread belief in black immunity to yellow fever made the diagnosis unlikely; perhaps doctors just did not pay as close attention to black fever cases during an epidemic as to white ones; perhaps black deaths were less likely to be recorded than white deaths. Some doctors argued that blacks who died of yellow fever were actually mulattoes. People of mixed race were considered more susceptible to the disease because they were part white. The records reveal another intriguing development: The number of black deaths attributed to yellow fever rose sharply in the 1850s. Between 1819 and 1852, only thirty black deaths were attributed to that disease – less than one per year; between 1853 and 1859, the number jumped to fifty-six, or almost ten per year. After the epidemic of 1858, one doctor told the Medical Society of South Carolina that he was "struck by the fact that negroes had also suffered from yellow fever." Of course, more white natives also died from it in the 1850s than in any other decade of the nineteenth century.[62] Probably the number of nonimmunes among white and black natives had increased during the 1840s, when the disease had been largely absent. But the white population, being much more mobile than the black, would also be more likely to lack acquired immunity. The argument that some people of African descent possess a genetic resistance to yellow fever is widely but by no means universally accepted today.[63]

ROLE REVERSAL

After the Civil War, promoters of economic development in South Carolina asserted something that would have astonished their antebellum forebears: White mortality from fevers was in fact not much different from black mortality. *South Carolina, Resources and Population, Institutions and Industries* (1883) cited mortality statistics for 1857–1859 that showed "malarial influences" causing 5.93 percent of white mortality and 5.43 percent of black deaths – "a difference," the authors noted, "which amounts to nothing."

---

[62] City of Charleston Death Records, 1819–1859; Kenneth F. Kiple and Virginia H. Kiple, "Black Yellow Fever Immunities, Innate and Acquired, as Revealed in the American South," *Social Science History* 1 (1997), 424.

[63] For arguments for an African genetic resistance to yellow fever, see Henry Carter, *Yellow Fever; An Epidemiological and Historical Study of Its Place of Origin* (Baltimore, 1931) and Kiple and Kiple, "Black Yellow Fever Immunities," 419–436. J. R. McNeill thinks a genetic resistance probably exists but notes that the evidence is by no means conclusive. See McNeill, *Mosquito Empires: Ecology and War in the Greater Caribbean, 1640–1914* (Cambridge: Cambridge University Press, 2010), 44–46. Sheldon Watts questions the existence of genetic resistance in *Epidemics and History* (New Haven, CT and London: Yale University Press, 1997), 234, 241–243, and "Yellow Fever Immunities in West Africa and Beyond: A Reappraisal," *Journal of Social History* 34 (2001), 962. See also Kenneth F. Kiple, "Response to Sheldon Watts, "Yellow Fever Immunities in West Africa and Beyond: A Reappraisal," *Journal of Social History* 34 (2001), 969–974. Yellow fever has killed many Africans in recent decades. See Thomas P. Monath, "Yellow fever: victor, victoria? conqueror, conquest? Epidemics and research in the last forty years and prospects for the future," *American Journal of Tropical Hygiene* 45 (1991), 1–43.

By using statewide statistics, the authors masked a still high malarial mortality among lowcountry whites. They went farther. They "demonstrated" that overall black mortality in Charleston in recent years was about twice that of white mortality. The accuracy of their statistics is questionable. The point is that the authors used them to assure potential white immigrants that blacks, freed from the benevolent paternalism of slavery, were a declining or even doomed race, whereas whites could thrive in the state. The thrust of the book's sections devoted to climate and vital statistics was to encourage white immigration by demonstrating that South Carolina – even the lowcountry – was not an unhealthy place for whites to live and work, and that it would soon contain a white majority. Such claims stand in vivid contrast to those made by antebellum apologists for slavery who argued that blacks suffered little from disease in the lowcountry.[64]

An interesting change had taken place. The new goal of attracting investment and white immigrants to the state conflicted with the old claim that whites could not safely labor in the lowcountry fields during the hot months. Economic boosters claimed that since the Civil War, many white people had done exactly that. The key experiment had already taken place during the war. Many people on both sides predicted that soldiers would be unable to sustain operations in the lowcountry summers because the toll from disease would be intolerable. That did not prove to be the case. The war demonstrated that "large bodies of white men" could endure hard toil and exposure. The alleged success was partly due to the prophylactic use of quinine and "proper hygienic regulations." The danger to health in the region, its boosters concluded, had been exaggerated. Emancipation of the slaves had made an experiment in the use of white labor in the lowcountry necessary, and the results were surprisingly good:

The reverses of fortune, sustained as a result of the war, have forced many white families to reside the summer long where it was once thought fatal to do so, and the experiment has been successful, thus exploding the idea that white people could not enjoy health here during the summer months. Replies from twenty-three townships state without exception, that the inhabitants enjoy good health, and that a considerable portion of the field work is performed by whites – a great change since the war.[65]

A great change indeed. Once again – but for a different purpose – economic needs shaped perceptions of liability to disease. The happy, healthy black laborer gradually exits the scene, doomed by the demise of the paternalistic slavery that ensured his well-being. The healthy – if not quite happy – white laborer takes his place. One can be excused for seeing both as unconvincing characters.

[64] Harry Hammond, ed., *South Carolina, Resources and Population, Institutions and Industries* (Charleston, 1883), 417–419, 21–23, 54, 145; *Report of the Special Committee of the General Assembly of South Carolina on the Subject of Encouraging European Immigration* (Charleston, 1866), 3–8; Dan T. Carter, *When the War was Over: The Failure of Reconstruction in the South, 1865–1867* (Baton Rouge: University of Louisiana Press, 1985), 166–172.

[65] Hammond, *South Carolina, Resources and Population*, 22, 54.

PART II

COMBATING PESTILENCE

"Doctor, are you sure I'm suffering from pneumonia? I've heard once about a doctor treating someone with pneumonia and he finally died of typhus." "Don't worry, it won't happen to me," the doctor replied. "If I treat someone with pneumonia he will die of pneumonia."

Joke of unknown origin

He may rest satisfied that he will die neither of the dose nor the doctor, both which deaths are equally terrible, tho' the lot of many a poor man and unhappy woman.

Alexander Garden, 1761

I wish no person would send for me, for I know nothing of this disease, and am as ignorant as a child unborn – for let me do as I will, puke, purge or bleed still they all die.

Alexander Baron, 1794

8

"I Wish That I Had Studied Physick"

The God of verse and medic skill
Oft plies the Muses harmless quill,
Not still intent to write and kill.

James Kilpatrick/Kirkpatrick,
The Sea Piece, c. 1742

The object of [medicine] is not to accumulate wealth, but to promote the health
and happiness of the human race.

David Ramsay, 1800

MCDOCTORS

In the early 1740s, a young Scottish doctor named John Murray arrived in
Charleston. Soon he was writing home to report that he had achieved "incredible" success. South Carolina, he concluded, was "a fine place for a surgeon."[1]
The virulent-disease environment in itself was not much of an attraction, as
the lack of adequate medical care in the unhealthiest parts of the world today
attests. What made it a fine place was its combination of pestilence and prosperity. As another Scot, Adam Smith, observed in 1776, it is not demand but
effective demand that encourages people to supply a need or want. The great
wealth of the planters and merchants held the promise of a lucrative medical
marketplace, and a supply of Scottish medicos rushed to meet the demand.

Established medical practitioners in late colonial Charleston appear to have
earned a comfortable living. During epidemics they could make money "very
fast," according to his cousin, also named John Murray.[2] Another Scottish
doctor, Alexander Garden, who arrived in the early 1750s, was soon aver-
aging an income of 500 pounds a year. By the 1770s, he was making several

---

[1] John Murray to John Murray of Murraywhat, Nov. 6, 1747, Murraywhat Muniments, SRO/
GD219/284.
[2] John Murray of Murraywhat to Elizabeth Murray, Feb. 21, March 21, 1763, Murraywhat
Muniments, SRO/GD219/287.

times that much and was reputed the richest doctor in the province. A number of other doctors earned yearly incomes of 500 pounds or more.[3] Many doctors supplemented their incomes by opening shops where they mixed and sold drugs. One young immigrant, at least, envied their success. After his arrival in 1763, he wrote that he was concerned about his economic prospects, confessing, "I wish that I had studied physick."[4]

It is significant that the young man expressing these views was a Scot. The medical establishment of Charleston and the lowcountry during much of the eighteenth century was dominated by men of Scottish birth, parentage, and/ or training. This is not entirely surprising, considering that eighteenth-century Scotland was a virtual manufactory of medical men. Yet the extent of Scottish medical dominance and influence in Charleston is impressive. Seventeen of the twenty-eight doctors Joseph Waring identified as practicing for extended periods in Charleston between 1725 and 1780 had Scottish connections.[5] Most had been born in Scotland. The rest were Scottish-trained, and most of these had Scottish parents. In 1763, thirteen Charleston doctors agreed to a public petition to stop inoculating. Seven of the signers were born in Scotland, and one other probably was.[6]

Several of the Scottish doctors gained an international reputation. Alexander Garden was elected to the Royal Society in recognition of his work in natural history, and later became its vice-president. Swedish naturalist Linnaeus named the gardenia in his honor. Lionel Chalmers corresponded with England's Dr. John Fothergill and with his help published two medical treatises in London, one on fevers and another on the connection between weather and diseases in South Carolina. The latter work drew on meteorological records and metabolic experiments done by his older partner, John Lining, who corresponded with Benjamin Franklin and published in *The Transactions of the Royal Society*. Lining experimented with electricity and wrote an accurate early description of yellow fever published in Edinburgh in the 1750s. In 1749, John Moultrie, Jr. penned the first American description of yellow fever, his medical dissertation at Edinburgh University. James Kilpatrick, a.k.a. James Kirkpatrick, a pioneer of inoculation who practiced in South Carolina from the 1720s until 1742, authored and translated many books after moving to London in the latter year. He also became a prominent inoculator of wealthy Britons and French aristocrats.[7]

3 James E. Smith, *A Selection of the Correspondence of Linnaeus and Other Naturalists* 2 vols. (New York: Arno Press, 1978) 1: 552; Diane Sydenham, "Practitioner and Patient: the Practice of Medicine in Eighteenth-Century South Carolina," Ph.D. Diss., Johns Hopkins University, 1979, 141–150.

4 Alexander Camine to Alexander Ogilvie, March 21, 1763, Ogilvie-Forbes of Boyndlie Papers, Aberdeen University Special Collections.

5 Joseph I. Waring, *History of Medicine in South Carolina, 1675–1825* (Charleston: South Carolina Medical Association, 1964), 330.

6 *SCG*, June 18, 1763.

7 Waring, *Medicine in South Carolina, 1675–1825*, 268. Moultrie's Latin thesis of 1749 was later translated into French and German, but not English.

To a great extent, the large number of Scottish doctors in colonial Charleston was simply the result of effective demand there combined with an excess of supply in Scotland. During the eighteenth century, the four Scottish universities, especially Edinburgh, produced far greater numbers of medical men than did the two English ones, Oxford and Cambridge, and far more than the effective demand in Scotland.[8] To paraphrase Samuel Johnson, many an aspiring Scottish doctor took the high road to London, and some, such as brothers William and John Hunter, did extremely well there. But competition was fierce, and graduates of the English universities dominated the Royal Colleges of Physicians and Surgeons. As one Scot in London said of his brother in 1761, "if he inclines to continue [in medicine] he will find it a difficult matter to establish himself in this part of the world."[9] Others established themselves in the English provinces, became naval or army surgeons, or headed to the colonies. Under the circumstances, it was inevitable that many medical Scots would seek their fortune in the opportunities provided by the expanding British Empire, as Scottish merchants and soldiers often did.[10] Indeed, some Scots were attracted to medicine because it was a skill that could readily be transferred to other lands, and they trained knowing that they would likely be practicing far from home. In 1747, John Murray praised his cousin William's decision to study medicine because "physick is absolutely the best traveling business in the world." He offered his own success in Charleston as proof.[11]

Large numbers of Scots came to the Carolinas and Georgia throughout the colonial period. The Lords Proprietors, who governed Carolina from 1670 until 1719, encouraged Scottish immigration. In 1707, the Act of Union, which united England and Scotland into the United Kingdom of Great Britain, gave Scots greater access to opportunities in the colonies. As the number of Scots in British North America increased, so did the attractions of immigration. At the time of the first census in 1790, people of Scots or Scots-Irish origins made up about one-third of the population of South Carolina. The only state with a larger percentage of Scots was Georgia.[12]

This is not to say that the Scots left their homeland easily. Dr. John Murray confessed that when he left Scotland, he was unsure "whether grief or hope"

---

[8] Thomas Neville Bonner, *Becoming a Physician: Medical Education in Britain, France, Germany, and the United States, 1750–1945* (Baltimore: Johns Hopkins University Press, 1995), esp. 40–41; Lisa Rosner, *Medical Education in the Age of Improvement: Edinburgh Students and Apprentices, 1760–1820* (Edinburgh: Edinburgh University Press, 1991); Kenneth Ludmerer, *Learning to Heal: The Development of American Medical Education* (New York: Basic Books, 1996).

[9] John Murray of Murraywhat to Elizabeth Murray, Oct. 29, 1761, Murraywhat Muniments, SRO/GD219/287.

[10] Linda Colley, *Britons: Forging the Nation, 1707–1830* (New Haven, CT and London: Yale University Press, 1992).

[11] John Murray to John Murray of Murraywhat, Nov. 6, 1747, Murraywhat Muniments, SRO/GD219/284.

[12] Robert Weir, *Colonial South Carolina: A History* (Columbia: University of South Carolina Press, 1997), 205, 209.

was uppermost in his mind. His greatest desire, and that of many other Scots who followed the same path, was to return to his homeland a wealthy man. His cousin William Murray, who also came to Charleston to practice medicine, echoed this view. On arriving there, he declared that he was "resolved to make money at all events."[13] But the pursuit of wealth was not the only reason medical Scots came to the lowcountry. Alexander Garden was seeking a warmer climate for his health: He was suffering from a lung complaint, probably tuberculosis. Garden's lungs may have benefited, but he suffered severely from fevers. Garden was also attracted by the financial opportunities of South Carolina, and in that he was not to be disappointed.[14]

PRACTICING PHYSICK

In its early decades, the Carolina colony does not seem to have been a powerful magnet for doctors. The number of medical men who appear in the early colonial records was small, although some probably left no documentary trace. There is no evidence that any of them prospered in medicine, although some did amass wealth in land and slaves. The names of some of them show up in wills, land and court records, and records of the colonial council and assembly. They sometimes appear in the role of planters and political figures, but their work as doctors is largely lost. The most famous early doctor was Henry Woodward, who first came to Carolina in 1666 on an exploring expedition. But Woodward was known for his adventures with the Indians and capture by the Spanish rather than his doctoring. The first ship full of settlers, *The Carolina*, carried a surgeon named Will Scrivener, but he died the following year. Most early doctors left behind little more than their names in official records, often requesting or demanding payment for medical services. In 1692, Dr. John (Jean) Thomas sued for reimbursement for performing what may have been the colony's first autopsy. Some years later, Gideon Johnston wrote that Thomas was the only man in Charleston who deserved to be called a physician. Johnston's praise may have derived in part from the fact that Thomas had treated him for free. Like most Anglican ministers, Johnston complained frequently that medical costs were extremely high in proportion to his clerical salary.[15] During the first few decades of settlement in Carolina, doctors probably did not make great incomes from their trade. Robert Adams died a poor man in 1697, judging by the inventory of his will. He did not own a horse or have a pharmacy. It appears that his patients paid him primarily in rum and sugar, not money. His medical books were up-to-date, well-known

[13] John Murray to John Murray of Murraywhat, Nov. 6, 1747, Murraywhat Muniments, SRO/GD219/284; John Murray to John Murray of Murraywhat, June 10, 1753, Murraywhat Muniments, SRO/GD219/284; William Murray to John Murray of Murraywhat, Jan. 7, 1751, Murraywhat Muniments, SRO/GD219/288.

[14] Edmund Berkeley and Dorothy Smith Berkeley, *Dr. Alexander Garden of Charles Town* (Chapel Hill: The University of North Carolina Press, 1969), 26–27.

[15] Waring, *Medicine in South Carolina, 1670–1825*, 12–15; Klingberg, *Johnston*, 41, 55, 66–92.

texts, but they were written in English, not Latin, which indicates he had little formal schooling. He was probably a surgeon or apothecary trained by apprenticeship, which was true of most colonial practitioners before the late eighteenth century.[16]

Medical men often received reimbursement from the colonial government for services to the poor, sailors, and soldiers. In the late colonial period, doctors were paid for the treatment of military and naval personnel, criminals, Indians, Acadians, and French prisoners of war.[17] Care of the indigent sick provided a regular, if small, income for some physicians. South Carolina, like other British colonies, adopted the English Poor Law, which provided for the collection of a poor rate or tax to care for the indigent. The first formal act to provide for the poor in 1695 made the colony as a whole the unit of administration. In 1712, the assembly adopted the English Poor Law statutes in its entirety, and the unit of administration became the parish. Parishes sometimes paid doctors to provide medical care for the indigent. In most of the rural parishes, these payments were on an ad hoc basis. As early as 1733, St. Philip's Parish paid an annual stipend to a doctor to care for the sick poor of Charleston. In 1738, the parish established the town's first poorhouse, where many of the sick poor received medical care. In 1768, St. Philip's built a new poorhouse with an attached hospital. The cost of caring for the sick poor was a perennial concern of taxpayers because so many were transients and people who came to Charleston from other parishes to seek medical treatment.[18]

Charleston operated a number of medical institutions from the mid-eighteenth century on. The poorhouse hospital was intended for white indigents, but it occasionally received blacks. From at least the mid-eighteenth century, planters could send ailing slaves to private hospitals in Charleston. Drs. David Oliphant and Patrick Mackie advertised a "Hospital for Sick Negroes" in the *South Carolina Gazette* in 1749. Advertisements for privately operated slave hospitals appeared regularly in Charleston newspapers until the 1860s. In 1749, the assembly ordered the establishment of a hospital for sick sailors. After 1800, the federal government helped defray the costs of caring for sick seamen. In 1834, a federally funded Marine Hospital opened. In 1801, city council agreed to fund a public dispensary, later called the Shirras Dispensary. It was based on a plan

[16] St. Julien Ravenel Childs, "A South Carolina Physician, 1693–1697," *Journal of the History of Medicine* 26 (1971), 18–26.

[17] *Journal of the Commons House of Assembly of South Carolina, 1693*, ed. by A. S. Salley, Jr. (Columbia, 1907), 5; *Journal of the Commons House of Assembly of South Carolina for the session beginning Jan. 30, 1696, and ending March 17, 1696*, ed. by A. S. Salley, Jr. (Columbia, 1908), 27; *Journal of the Commons House of Assembly of South Carolina for the Two Sessions of 1698*, ed. by A. S. Salley, Jr. (Columbia, 1914), 26; *Journal of the Commons House of Assembly of South Carolina, 1703*, ed. by A. S. Salley, Jr. (Columbia, 1934), 41, 46, 50, 88–89, 104, 128.

[18] Barbara Bellows, *Benevolence Among Slaveholders: Assisting the Poor in Charleston, 1670–1860* (Baton Rouge: Louisiana University Press, 1993); Peter McCandless, *Moonlight, Magnolias, and Madness: Insanity in South Carolina from the Colonial Period to the Progressive Era* (Chapel Hill: University of North Carolina Press, 1996), 21–24, 31.

drawn up by the Medical Society and staffed by the society's members. The first general hospital, Roper Hospital, did not open until 1856.[19]

Before the twentieth century, most people, whether white or black, were treated at home by physicians, alternative healers, family members, neighbors, or themselves. Sick slaves were generally treated on the plantations where they resided, although they were sometimes sent away to be cared for by a physician at his home or at a slave hospital. In the nineteenth century, wealthy planters often contracted with a physician to care for sick slaves, and some planters established hospitals – or what they called hospitals – on their plantations. In the 1770s, Alexander Hewatt claimed that the slaves received better medical care than the poorest laborers of Europe. That may have been true, but the standard of comparison was not a high one, and in any case one might be better off without any medical care at all. It is also crucial to remember that slaves were commodities whose health was a matter of economic calculation. How much a master was willing to expend might depend as much upon his estimation of a slave's economic value as on humanistic considerations. Planters, overseers, and their wives often cared for sick slaves, using medicine chests and health guides of various kinds. A doctor might – or might not – be consulted with or called in to treat cases that seemed to be serious. The enslaved were not passive recipients of white-controlled medicine, however. They held on to African healing traditions, discussed in the following chapter.[20]

By the later colonial period, some established doctors were deriving comfortable incomes from medicine. But the road to establishing and maintaining a lucrative medical practice was strewn with obstacles. The possibility of profit attracted many practitioners, and competition for patients was often fierce. Average doctor-patient ratios in late colonial South Carolina were higher than in many states or the national average for the United States in the late twentieth century.[21] Epidemics and summer and fall fevers could keep them all busy, even too busy, but during relatively healthy periods, doctors might find themselves underemployed. In 1770, Lionel Chalmers wrote to Benjamin Rush that there were between 30 and 40 medical practitioners in a town of about 11,000 or 12,000 inhabitants, and most of them "have not much to do." People in the northern colonies assumed that the climate was always unhealthy, but in fact its diseases were "only periodical." They resulted from the effects of seasonal changes on people's constitutions. As in all places, everyday maladies gave the doctors "somewhat to do daily; tho' it may be of

[19] *SCG*, March 1, 1749, *The Courier*, June-December, 1804, April 12, 13, 1805, Aug. 4, 1807, May 18, 1812; *The Courier*, Aug. 23, 1806; Waring, *Medicine in South Carolina, 1670–1825*, 136; Waring, *Medicine in South Carolina, 1825–1900*, 14–21.

[20] Hewatt, *South Carolina and Georgia*, 2: 95; Waring, *Medicine in South Carolina, 1825–1900*, 97, 283; Sharla M. Fett, *Working Cures: Healing, Health, and Power on Southern Slave Plantations* (Chapel Hill: University of North Carolina Press, 2002), 111–192; James M. Clifton, ed., *Life and Labor on Argyle Island: Letters and Documents of a Savannah River Plantation, 1833–1867* (Savannah, GA: The Beehive Press, 1978).

[21] Sydenham, "Practitioners and Patients," 2–3, 23–29.

no great advantage, for several months together." Chalmers may have understated how busy the doctors were because Rush was contemplating moving to Charleston and he didn't want more competition. Rush didn't come, but he urged David Ramsay to go there a few years later.[22]

Establishing a viable practice could be difficult for newly arrived doctors without local connections or introductions from well-known physicians. As John Murray put it, "people here are very averse to employing newcomers."[23] When Chalmers arrived in 1737, he at first found it difficult to make a medical living. But his timing was fortunate, for him at least: Smallpox and yellow fever ravaged the town during the next two years, creating a high demand for medical services.[24] Some doctors never made what they considered a satisfactory living because they could not attract the wealthier clientele or collect their fees. Despite having an M.D. from Edinburgh University, Thomas Tudor Tucker was never able to secure enough wealthy patients to support his family in the style he expected, and he gave up medicine for politics. In 1801, he became Treasurer of the United States, a post he held until his death in 1828. At one point in his medical career, he wrote that he could barely keep himself out of jail, presumably for debt.[25]

A lack of patients was not the only reason for Tucker's financial problems. He also had difficulty collecting fees in a timely manner. Doctors desperate to collect fees often placed advertisements in the newspapers informing patients that they would sue for payment if it was not received by a certain time. Despite the region's wealth, people were sometimes hard-pressed to pay medical bills. This was especially true for newcomers and those who made a precarious living. Anglican missionaries complained constantly about their inability to pay medical expenses.[26] Even wealthy planters sometimes had difficulty paying their medical bills. This was particularly true during and after the Revolutionary War due to loss of trade, slaves, and rampant inflation. Eliza Pinckney was unable to pay Alexander Garden a bill of less than sixty pounds for medical services.[27] In the mid-1780s, Samuel Miller, fresh from studying medicine at Edinburgh, started a practice in St. Stephen's Parish along the Santee River. A few years later, he wrote to Edinburgh's William Cullen that the place had given him more business than he "could rightly manage," but

[22] Lionel Chalmers to Benjamin Rush, Library Co. of Philadelphia, Rush Mss. vol. 23, folio 28, quoted in Waring, *Medicine in South Carolina, 1675–1825*, 68.
[23] John Murray to John Murray of Murraywhat, June 10, 1753, Murraywhat Muniments, SRO/GD219/284.
[24] Waring, *Medicine in South Carolina, 1675–1825*, 188.
[25] Sydenham, "Practitioners and Patients," 132–133; Waring, *Medicine in South Carolina, 1675–1825*, 319–320.
[26] "Letters of Rev. Samuel Thomas," *South Carolina Historical and Genealogical Magazine* 4 (1903), letter 6, 281; Klingberg, *Johnston*; SPG Letter Books, Robert Maule, Jan. 23, 1714/15, A10: 79–80; SPG Letter Books, John Fordyce, March 16, 1741/42 B10: 148; William Orr, March 31, 1749, SPG Letter Books, B17: 172.
[27] Berkeley, *Alexander Garden*, 281.

his income did not reflect his exertions. The Revolution, he explained, had left many people "very much in debt."[28]

In 1755, some of the town's doctors founded the Faculty of Physic in the hope that by organizing they could increase their fees and secure prompter payment of them. John Moultrie, Sr. was president and William Murray secretary. Both were Scots. The announcement of the faculty's creation in the *South Carolina Gazette* was met with a frosty reception, followed by several letters and poems to the newspaper ridiculing the doctors as greedy and incompetent. It was hardly surprising. The horrendous toll of disease in the region created a demand for doctors but also highlighted their inadequacy. The doctors apparently got the message. The Faculty of Physic quickly disappeared from the scene.[29]

The doctors tried again with more success in 1789, when they formed the Medical Society of South Carolina. Incorporated by an act of the state legislature in 1793, it was effectively the medical society of Charleston. Most of its members practiced in the city or nearby. A statewide professional organization, the South Carolina Medical Association, was not established until 1848. One reason for establishing the Medical Society was the perennial problem of collecting fees. Another goal was to establish a system for licensing medical practitioners. This had been tried earlier. A bill to "regulate the practice of physic" through a licensing board had been considered and rejected by the South Carolina colonial assembly in 1744. Attempts to secure a licensing act failed again in 1765 and in 1793. In 1793, the Medical Society proposed to create a state College of Physicians and give it the power to license doctors. Opponents countered that such "monopolies" were antirepublican and a threat to private property and liberty. Skeptics added that it was absurd to give a medical monopoly to men who could not even agree about the causes and cure of diseases, pointing to the recent "medical uncertainty" of Philadelphia physicians addressing deadly yellow fever.[30]

South Carolina doctors finally achieved a licensing act in 1817. But it was a weak law and the legislature repealed it in 1838, bowing to Jacksonian antielitism and the rise of alternative medical systems such as Thomsonianism and homeopathy. The Thomsonians were followers of Samuel Thomson, a New Hampshire farmer, who developed a system of botanical medicine featuring

[28] Samuel Miller to William Cullen, Oct. 6, 1789, Letters to William Cullen, Cullen Mss., Royal College of Physicians, Edinburgh.

[29] *SCG*, May 2, June 12, 26, 1755; Sydenham, "Practitioners and Patients," 153, 163–173, 258; Waring, 65–67.

[30] *JCHA*, 5: 15–16, 19, Feb. 25, 1743/44; *JCHA*, Jan. 8, 1765–Aug. 9, 1765, ed. by A.S. Salley, Jr. (Columbia, 1949), 39, 46; *Stats.*, 6: 63–65, 597; *Columbian Herald*, Feb. 25, 28, 1788, Dec. 14, 1793; *MSM*, Nov. 30, 1793, 51–58; *Journals of the House of Representatives, 1792–1794* (Columbia: University of South Carolina Press, 1988), 363, 496–497; David Ramsay, *History of South Carolina* 2 vols. (Charleston, 1858), 2: 64; Waring, *Medicine in South Carolina, 1670–1825*, 109, 118–119; Waring, *Medicine in South Carolina, 1825–1900*, 102–106.

herbal purgatives and sweat baths. They and their imitators were highly successful in South Carolina during the 1820s and 1830s. Homeopathy, another alternative medical system, also found local supporters. The brainchild of German physician Samuel Hahnemann, homeopathy was based on two principles: the law of similars and the law of infinitesimals. The first claimed that the best way to combat a disease was to prescribe something that produced symptoms similar to the disease. The second law held that the smaller the dosages of the prescribed substance, the more effective it would be. Skeptics argued that such reasoning was absurd and that the dosages were so minute as to have no effect at all. But that was part of homeopathy's appeal. Planter James Henry Hammond put his finger on it: "If you hit right you make a speedy cure. If you miss, you do no harm." Hammond turned to homeopathy as a result of despair over the cost and failures of orthodox practitioners.[31]

Most doctors during the colonial period did not possess a medical degree. But an M.D. was no more essential to practice in British North America than in many parts of provincial Britain. Most of the medical practitioners for whom we have some biographical information had some formal university training, but few had an M.D. Many of them had previously served as naval surgeons.[32] Nevertheless, an M.D. brought benefit and prestige. Doctors who did not have one on arrival sometimes sought to earn one afterward. When William Murray went to Scotland in the early 1760s, his cousin John advised him that if he took "the Degree" and spent some time "with Dr. Hunter and Sons," it would give him "the vogue and a superiority over others."[33] Lionel Chalmers secured an M.D. from the University of St. Andrews in the 1750s with the help of Robert Whytt, professor of medicine at Edinburgh and a graduate of St. Andrews. William Bull of South Carolina became the first person born in British North America to receive a doctorate in medicine, from the University of Leyden in 1734. But Bull did not practice medicine, at least not for long. He soon became involved in the provincial government, rising to Speaker of the Assembly and Lieutenant Governor. John Moultrie, Jr. was the first native-born American to receive an M.D. from Edinburgh, in 1749. Like Bull, however, he soon gave up medicine for planting and politics. In 1763, Moultrie became Lieutenant Governor of British East Florida. During the late colonial period, more doctors began to arrive in Charleston with M.D. in hand. Most of them had graduated from Edinburgh University, twelve between 1768 and 1775 alone.[34]

Marriages to daughters of the local elite eased the path to wealth for some of the most successful eighteenth-century doctors. Kilpatrick married Elizabeth

[31] McCandless, *Moonlight, Magnolias, and Madness*, 201–203.
[32] Waring, *Medicine in South Carolina, 1675–1825*, 40, 268, 303; Berkeley, *Alexander Garden*, 15–19.
[33] John Murray to William Murray, Aug. 21, 1762, Murraywhat Muniments, SRO/GD219/285.
[34] Waring, *Medicine in South Carolina, 1675–1825*, 182–183, 188–189, 254–256, 269–270; Sydenham, "Practitioners and Patients," 42.

Hepworth, the daughter of the colony's secretary. Garden's wife, Elizabeth Perroneau, brought him 8,000 pounds and the means to buy a plantation. John Moultrie, Jr. married a wealthy widow, Dorothy Dry. Ramsay's third wife was Martha Laurens, the daughter of Henry Laurens, one of the wealthiest men in South Carolina. In the eighteenth century, most successful doctors bought plantations or gained them through marriage. In the nineteenth century, they often inherited them.[35]

Just as today, networking was important to the aspiring professional. Doctors were active in fraternal and civic organizations such as the St. Andrews Society, the Freemasons, the Charleston Library Society, and the St. Cecilia Society. Another common way for a doctor to get established was through a partnership with a senior colleague. In 1740, Chalmers formed a partnership with Lining that lasted until the latter retired in 1754. Garden entered into practice with David Oliphant in 1755. Many partnerships were formed and dissolved frequently.[36]

Some doctors enjoyed long and successful practices. Others turned to other types of work, left, or died after a short time.[37] Some sought advancement on a bigger stage. The most successful of these was James Kilpatrick. His rise to prominence began with the Charleston smallpox epidemic of 1738. The epidemic was a personal tragedy, as he lost a child to the disease. He also became embroiled in a bitter conflict with other Charleston doctors over the propriety and method of inoculation for smallpox. In the long run, however, the epidemic helped make his fortune and reputation.[38]

POX BRITANNIA

Some contemporary and historical works credit Kilpatrick with having revived inoculation in Britain after it had allegedly declined. In the 1950s, historian Genevieve Miller argued that this was a myth. Myth or not, his career provides a fascinating glimpse into the medical politics of inoculation in colonial America and its relationship to Britain's commercial empire. Kilpatrick is an elusive figure. Historians have called him Scottish, Irish, and English. Even his name is a problem. During his twenty-plus years in the colony, he was known as James Kilpatrick, sometimes spelled Killpatrick. Sometime after he went to London in the 1740s, he began to call himself James Kirkpatrick, and

---

[35] Waring, *Medicine in South Carolina, 1675–1825*, 271, 282; Berkeley, *Alexander Garden*, 65; Waring, *Medicine in South Carolina, 1825–1900*, medical biographies.

[36] *Gazette of the State of South Carolina*, May 12, 1777; SCG, March 1, 1749, April 27, 1752, Oct. 15, 1753; Oct. 20, 1758, Jan. 4, 1770, Jan. 3, 1771, May 23, 1771; Waring, *Medicine in South Carolina, 1675–1825*, 80, 82, 188–189, 192–197, 268–271, 328–329; John Murray to John Murray of Murraywhat, June 10, 1753, Murraywhat Muniments, SRO/GD219/284.

[37] Sydenham, "Practitioners and Patients,"133, 163; Waring, *Medicine in South Carolina, 1675–1825*, 318–320.

[38] Miller, *Adoption of Inoculation*, 25, 134–137; Charles Creighton, *A History of Epidemics in Britain* 2 vols. (Cambridge, 1894), 2: 489–494; Kilpatrick, *Essay on Inoculation*, 31.

most of his writings were published under that name.[39] An old theory of why he changed his name is that one that began with "kill" was unfortunate for a doctor. In fact, Kirkpatrick was his original name. He came from a Scots family implicated in the Jacobite Revolt of 1715 and probably changed his name to hide his identity. He was born, perhaps in Ireland, sometime between 1690 and 1702. He most likely attended Edinburgh University.[40]

By the 1730s – as Kilpatrick – he had become one of Charleston's established practitioners. He married well and bought a plantation. He wrote poetry and essays.[41] Like many an eighteenth-century Scot, he restyled himself as a British patriot, promoting Britain as the center of a benevolent mercantile empire in a long poem, *The Sea Piece*.[42] It was his work on inoculation that won him renown, however. After he came to London, he published a description of the Charleston smallpox epidemic of 1738 entitled *An Essay on Inoculation* (1743). In 1754 – as Kirkpatrick – he published a much longer work, *The Analysis of Inoculation*, a detailed discussion of the history, methods, and theories of inoculation. *The Analysis* was reprinted several times and translated into French, German, and Dutch, and it earned the praise of other advocates of inoculation.[43] Following its publication, prominent continental

[39] Donald Hopkins calls him John Kirkpatrick in *Princes and Peasants*, 58–59, 254.

[40] Two James Kirkpatricks matriculated at Edinburgh in the early eighteenth century. One attended the university between 1708 and 1711 and the other between 1717 and 1721. Letter from L.W. Sharp, Manuscripts Department, University of Edinburgh, June, 13, 1933, in James Kilpatrick file, WHL. *The Kirkpatricks of Closeburn* (Privately Printed, 1858), 59–60; Strachey Collection, Genealogical Papers, British Library, MSS EUR F127/478a, Box 1, Notes on Kilpatrick/Kirkpatrick, FF 142–193; William Dalrymple, *White Mughals: Love and Betrayal in Eighteenth Century India* (New York and London: Viking Penguin Books, 2004), 49; *Dictionnaire Historique de la Medicine Ancienne et Moderne*, T. iii, 1re Partie, 326; Genevieve Miller, *The Adoption of Inoculation for Smallpox in England and France* (Philadelphia: University of Pennsylvania Press, 1957), 25, 122, 134–161; Joseph I. Waring, "James Killpatrick and Smallpox Inoculation in Charlestown," *Annals of Medical History* 10 (1938): 306; Joseph I. Waring, "Doctors Afield: James Killpatrick," *The New England Journal of Medicine* 256 (1957): 266–267; David S. Shields, *Oracles of Empire* (Chicago: University of Chicago Press, 1990), 26–27; David S. Shields, "Dr. James Kirkpatrick, American Laureate of Mercantilism," in *The Meaning of South Carolina History: Essays in Honor of George C. Rogers, Jr.*, ed. by David R. Chesnutt and Clyde N. Wilson. (Columbia: University of South Carolina Press), 1991, 4; Richard Beale Davis, *Intellectual Life in the Colonial South* 3 vols. (Knoxville: University of Tennessee Press, 1978), 2: 925.

[41] Kilpatrick's arrival in Charleston is uncertain, but he was surely there by 1724, when he was appointed administrator of the estate of his uncle David Kilpatrick. Waring, *Medicine in South Carolina, 1670–1825*, 42–43; Waring, "James Killpatrick and Smallpox Inoculation in Charlestown," 1938, 304, 306–307; Shields, "Dr. James Kirkpatrick, American Laureate of Mercantilism," 39, 42; David S. Shields, *Civil Tongues and Polite Letters in British America*, (Chapel Hill: University of North Carolina Press, 1997) 293; "James Killpatrick," *American National Biography*, 667–678; SCG, July 16, 1741; Register of St Philip's Parish, May 4, 1727, SCHS.

[42] Shields, "Dr. James Kirkpatrick," 42; Shields, *Civil Tongues and Polite Letters in British America*, 293–295; Weir, *Colonial South Carolina*, 116–119; James Kirkpatrick, *The Sea-Piece: A Narrative, Philosophical, and Descriptive Poem in Five Cantos* (London, 1750).

[43] Daniel Cox, *A Letter from a Physician in Town to a Friend in the Country on Inoculation* (London, 1757), 30.

doctors began to consult Kirkpatrick and cite him as an expert on inoculation. In 1756 he was called to Paris to inoculate some French aristocrats.[44]

The experience Kilpatrick gained in the colonial periphery in Charleston became the basis for his success at the imperial center. He was a kind of medical nabob, as entrepreneurial as many of the merchants he admired, except that he returned to Britain with a skill, not a fortune. His subsequent success was an accidental benefit of what one might call the Pox Britannia, the spread of smallpox throughout the British Atlantic Empire. This microbial diaspora resulted from the trade he celebrated, which involved massive movements of people, willingly and unwillingly, around the Atlantic Basin. The upshot was virulent epidemics among a population rendered immunologically vulnerable by their relative isolation. For an ambitious doctor with an empirical mindset, which Kilpatrick was, the colonies provided an accidental laboratory for observing the effectiveness of inoculation. Because of their vulnerability to smallpox, colonials were more open to inoculation than their British cousins.

Knowledge of inoculation – or variation – spread to Britain and its American colonies after 1700. In Britain, it was promoted by a few doctors and famously by Lady Mary Wortley Montagu, who had learned about it in the Ottoman Empire. British pioneers were handicapped, however, by the fact that in London smallpox was largely a childhood disease, and most adults had already survived it. People did not take it lightly, but it did not produce the widespread terror it did in the colonies, nor would an epidemic cause London to grind to a standstill. Parents were understandably reluctant to offer their children for experiment. British innovators struggled to get a few convicts who had never had the disease to inoculate.[45] In the colonies, in contrast, most people were susceptible to smallpox due to the infrequency of epidemics. Many adults were willing to try the procedure in hopes that it might produce a mild case of the disease and future immunity. In North America, the first use of inoculation occurred in Boston. Its champion was Cotton Mather, who had learned about the Turkish practice from British sources. His slave Onesimus also told him that it was a common practice among his people in Africa. At Mather's urging, surgeon Zabdiel Boylston inoculated about 200 people in Boston in 1721 to 1722. Boylston's inoculations aroused violent opposition, but in time many people viewed the experiment as a success.[46]

[44] In 1796, a historian of inoculation in the British Isles, William Woodville, called the *Analysis* "the most comprehensive digest" on the topic. He also found it verbose, unclear, and often unhelpful. Kirkpatrick good-humoredly conceded his defects as a prose writer in the second edition of the *Analysis*, when he said he had heard that some wags had threatened to translate it into English. Woodville, *The History of the Inoculation of the Small-Pox in Great Britain* 2 vols. (London, 1796), 1: 305–306; Miller, *Inoculation*, 161, 210–211, 214–215, 220; Waring, "James Killpatrick," 305, 308; Creighton, *Epidemics in Britain*, 2: 491–492.

[45] Isobel Grundy, *Lady Mary Wortley Montagu: Comet of the Enlightenment* (London: Oxford University Press, 1999), 209–222; Miller, *Adoption of Inoculation*. Grundy and Miller disagree about the importance of Montagu's role in promoting inoculation.

[46] Miller, *The Adoption of Inoculation*; Hopkins, *Princes and Peasants*, 46–59, 246–247.

Methods of inoculation varied, but generally involved putting matter from the pustules of smallpox victims under the skin of the uninfected in hopes of producing a mild infection and immunity. The basic procedure was simple and quick, which presented a problem for medical professionals. If peasant women could do it, as they did in the Ottoman Empire, how could physicians claim that they needed to perform and supervise the operation, and how could they charge a substantial fee for it? They argued – perhaps sincerely – that it was necessary to prepare the patient for inoculation with a spare diet, bleeding, and purges over a period of two weeks or more. The drugs used for preparation included heavy metals such as mercury and antimony.[47] During the 1738 epidemic, one doctor complained in the *South Carolina Gazette* that some people were spreading the impression that inoculation simply meant placing some "pocky" pus into a small wound, something anyone could do. This mistaken notion was a potential threat to the community, and although he did not specifically say so, to medical incomes. Intelligent people knew that skillful preparation of the body for inoculation was necessary through a judicious use of medicines and diet, and a regimen tailored to the patient's age, sex, and constitution. These things could only be properly done by a physician, and only physicians should be allowed to inoculate. Kilpatrick made the same argument in the *Gazette*, although he added that preparation might be dispensed with in some cases.[48]

Doctors argued over many details such as where and how deep to make the incision or incisions. Kilpatrick advocated a gentler form of inoculation than was common among physicians at the time. Whereas many early inoculators insisted on making deep incisions into the skin, he argued that "the smallest violation of the surface of the skin, if it was stained with blood," was sufficient for effective inoculation. In this he anticipated the practice of the most successful inoculators of the late eighteenth century in Britain, the Sutton family and Thomas Dimsdale. Despite the hazards of preparation, added to the danger of the virus itself, contemporary statistics showed that inoculation was much less likely to kill or disfigure than would be a natural infection. Yet inoculation often aroused controversy and sometimes rabid hostility when it was introduced into a community.[49]

That was certainly true in Charleston. In 1738 its use also produced or exposed major divisions within Charleston's medical corps. Many people were familiar with the arguments against inoculation, because they had been publicized extensively in Britain and Massachusetts. The decision to adopt

---

[47] For examples of preparation for inoculation, see Thomas Frewen, *The Practice and Theory of Inoculation* (London, 1749), 18–19; James Burges, *An Account of the Preparation and Management Necessary to Inoculation* (London, 1754), 8–14, 19–21.

[48] *SCG*, June 15, 1738; Kilpatrick, *Essay on Inoculation*, 14–15, 41, 44, 51; Glynn, *Smallpox*, 76–77; Hopkins, *Princes and Peasants*, 60.

[49] *SCG*, June 8, 15, July 6, 1738; Burges, *Inoculation*, 4–5; Miller, *Adoption of Inoculation*, 24–25, 38, 40, 48–69, 100–171; Hopkins, *Princes and Peasants*, 46–59, 246–247; Glynn, *Smallpox*, 55–69, 75–76.

it was a difficult one. Despite lofty humanitarian sentiments, doctors had to attract patients to make a living, and they recognized that this situation could make or destroy their reputations. In 1738, they flung accusations at one another of inoculating primarily for profit, with little regard for the welfare of their patients or the community. The episode illustrates the tensions that inoculation aroused between professional medical ideals and the desire to advance wealth and standing in an increasingly commercialized empire. Kilpatrick's defense of inoculation in 1738 both revealed these tensions and inflamed them. His aim was to justify the initial resort to inoculation, which had been introduced by Arthur Mowbray, a naval surgeon stationed in Charleston, and his own use of the procedure. In the process he questioned the learning and competence of those who had at first opposed it. He suggested that they did so out of envy and then adopted it for fear of losing business. In effect, he implied that they were petty and greedy.[50] At the same time, he denied that he had any "mercantile interest" in the procedure. His claims infuriated other doctors.

One of them accused Mowbray – and by implication Kilpatrick – of making the epidemic worse through a "hasty" resort to inoculation. Use of the procedure had greatly increased the number of sick, filled the air more fully with the infection, and made the disease more virulent than it might have been. Inoculation also increased misery, he asserted, because the physicians could not properly attend to all their patients. Antagonism toward Mowbray was probably increased by his marginal position as a naval surgeon and his failure to consult with the town's "settled practitioners" before starting to inoculate. The writer contrasted what he called Mowbray's precipitate, profit-motivated action with the town doctors' more careful, professional course. They had refused to inoculate until they were sure of its propriety, "despising" the income they might gain from it. Once they began inoculating, they had done so with "equally happy success." As men of "established characters" they did not need to thrust themselves into "business."[51]

Kilpatrick also became involved in a bitter controversy with another prominent physician, Thomas Dale. For months, they carried on a pamphlet duel centered on the case of Mary Roche, an infant who had died of smallpox after being inoculated. The issue that divided the two men was not inoculation itself, which both employed. Nor was the conflict between them purely medical. It was part of a broader political, economic, and literary rivalry. Both men ran pharmacies. Both had political ambitions, and both viewed themselves as men of letters. Kilpatrick stated that he wrote against Dale to vindicate his literary as well as his medical reputation: "I could forgive his reflections on my [medical] capacity, since this at worst could only starve me.... But to assault my pen, my fame, and call my pretensions to wit and eloquence boyishness and affectation, these are solid, insupportable evils." Dale's writing, he countered, was an "accumulation of absurdity and incoherence ... a profusion of

[50] *SCG*, June 15, July 20, 1738.
[51] *SCG*, July [27], Aug. 10, 1738; Kilpatrick, *Essay on Inoculation*, 44.

filth and ribaldry" parading as "reason and argument, wit and raillery." Dale accused Kilpatrick of ignorance, malpractice, and "murder for experience" in his treatment of Roche. Kilpatrick charged Dale with similar failings in the Roche case and throughout the epidemic.[52]

Kilpatrick claimed that Dale could not even recognize smallpox the first time he saw it and that he misdiagnosed other cases. He also charged that Dale's approach to inoculation was careless and mercenary, driven by a desire to inoculate more patients than Mowbray. According to Kilpatrick, Dale had repeatedly inoculated where the procedure was questionable and without properly preparing patients for it. He had stated that preparation for inoculation was not needed. If the charge was true, Dale's method was surely an advantage to his patients, given the ordeal preparation could be. By the later eighteenth century, most inoculators were abandoning it. At the time, however, forgoing preparation was often denounced as commercial quackery. Kilpatrick declared that Dale could hardly have been more mercantile if he had put his patients onto scales and priced inoculation by the ton. His own motives, Kilpatrick insisted, were moral, professional, and humane. He had even sometimes recommended against the operation when asked to perform it, as in the Roche case.[53] Clearly, the doctors were anxious about the experiment with inoculation and how it would affect their status within the local medical hierarchy. They were on edge and ready to blame others if things went wrong. The counter-accusations of "mercantile" behavior reveal a tension between their desire to enhance their practices and incomes and a concern to appear as professionals and gentlemen. Their behavior, however, was anything but gentlemanly.

THE END OF SCOTTISH DOMINANCE

Scottish medical dominance in Charleston declined in the late eighteenth century. Lining died in 1760, John Moultrie, Sr., in 1771, Chalmers in 1777. The Revolution sent many others away. George Milligen, a vocal Loyalist, fled to Britain in 1775. Thirteen doctors, including the richest, Alexander Garden, were banished in 1783 as "obnoxious persons" for supporting the British cause. Most were Scots.[54] Their dominance of medicine in the colony had aroused ill will even before then. Some people resented the Scots for their alleged clannishness and penny pinching. The *South Carolina*

---

[52] James Killpatrick [sic], *A Full and Clear Reply to Doct. Thomas Dale* (Charles-Town, 1739), 3, 6–13, 28–32. This is the only one of the pamphlets extant, and Dale's version of the conflict must be largely extracted from it. For a discussion of the broader rivalry between Kilpatrick and Dale, see Shields, *Civil Tongues*, 293–295. For the publication notices of the Kilpatrick-Dale pamphlets, see Hennig Cohn, *The South Carolina Gazette* (Columbia: University of South Carolina Press, 1953), 163–164.

[53] Killpatrick, *Reply*, 31, 37, 38; Kilpatrick, *Essay*, 39–40, 44.

[54] Berkeley, *Alexander Garden*, 287–291; Waring, *Medicine in South Carolina, 1675–1825*, 107, 267, 345.

Gazette summed up much anti-Scottish prejudice when it claimed that their motto was "Scratch me countryman – and I'll scratch thee." In 1772 Richard Bohun Baker wrote Benjamin Rush, who was contemplating a move from Philadelphia to Charleston, urging him to come. Baker told Rush that Dr. Garden's health was declining, "and unless you come may get some Scotch man to succeed him." Politics played a major part in anti-Scottishness. In the early eighteenth century, Scots were often suspected of being closet Jacobites, or supporters of the exiled Stuart dynasty. In 1718, the St. James Goose Creek Parish requested the Society for the Propagation of the Gospel to send a minister to replace the recently deceased Francis Le Jau and requested that the replacement not be a "North Briton," as they put it. Governor James Glen promoted many Scots in his administration in the mid-1700s, which may have increased resentment of them. From the time of the premiership of Scot John Stuart, Lord Bute, in the early 1760s, many colonials (and English Whigs) claimed that Scots were the force behind unpopular measures such as the Stamp Act and the Coercion Acts.[55]

The impact of Scottish medical dominance receded slowly. Between the 1760s and 1790s, twenty-five South Carolinians received an M.D., most of them at Edinburgh.[56] Simultaneously, however, Americans began to study medicine at home. The University of Pennsylvania opened its medical college in 1765, and one of its first graduates was David Ramsay. It was soon joined by other schools in New England and New York. Southern states began to open medical schools in the early nineteenth century, partly out of fear that medical education was being monopolized by Northerners. In 1824, the Medical Society of South Carolina founded the Medical College of South Carolina. Georgia established its first medical college in 1828. After the 1820s, the great majority of lowcountry doctors trained in South Carolina or Georgia and the rest trained elsewhere in the United States. Wherever they went the training they received was inferior to that of the best European medical programs of the time. It was especially weak in many of the proprietary medical schools that mushroomed in the laissez-faire educational milieu of the antebellum era. These weaknesses were not confined to the lowcountry or the South but were generally true of nineteenth-century medical training in America. The turn away from Europe should not be exaggerated, especially in the South. Many elite Southerners continued to look to Europe for cultural models, and some antebellum doctors took additional training abroad, mainly in Paris, which had replaced Edinburgh as the premier center of Western medical learning. The Medical College of South Carolina sent fifty-one graduates to Paris before the Civil War, and almost half the Americans who went there

[55] Weir, *Colonial South Carolina*, 211, 220, 286; Churchwardens and Vestry of St. James Goose Creek, March 1, 1717/1718, SPG Letters, A:13, 142–144; Berkeley, *Alexander Garden*, 260; Colley, *Britons*, 101–145.

[56] Ramsay, *Improvements, Progress and State of Medicine*, 43; Waring, *Medicine in South Carolina, 1675–1825*, 336–338.

were Southerners. In contrast to this cosmopolitan approach, however, many Southern doctors became more insular. The status of medicine everywhere in the early nineteenth century was low. Perhaps in an attempt to raise it, some Southern doctors called for the creation of a distinctive Southern medicine based on attention to the local environment and populations. As we have seen, some doctors added medical authority to proslavery ideology and insisted that yellow fever was a locally generated disease. With some notable exceptions, the lowcountry medical outlook became increasingly parochial and defensive as the antebellum era proceeded.[57]

[57] Waring, *Medicine in South Carolina, 1675–1825*, 167–170, 242, and *Medicine in South Carolina, 1825–1900*, medical biographies; John Harley Warner, "The Idea of Southern Medical Distinctiveness: Medical Knowledge and Practice in the Old South," and "A Southern Medical Reform: The Meaning of the Antebellum Argument for Southern Medical Education," both in Ronald L. Numbers and Todd L. Savitt, eds., *Science and Medicine in the Old South* (Baton Rouge: Louisiana State University Press, 1989); Steven Stowe, *Doctoring the South: Southern Physicians and Everyday Medicine in the Mid-Nineteenth Century* (Chapel Hill: University of North Carolina Press, 2004). On the continued influence of European culture on the South during the antebellum period, see Michael O'Brien, *Conjectures of Order: Intellectual Life and the American South, 1810–1860* (Chapel Hill: University of North Carolina Press, 2004). On Americans going to France for training, see John Harley Warner, *Against the Spirit of System: The French Impulse in Nineteenth-Century Medicine* (Princeton, NJ: Princeton University Press, 1998).

9

"I Know Nothing of this Disease"

I have been greatly afflicted with nephritick pains and a stoppage of urine ... and there is little help to be had from any of the doctors of this place in so critical a disease, the best of them having originally been no more than barbers.

Gideon Johnston, 1710

[A] blessed state of health which the inhabitants of this town have enjoyed for some years past and which I hope will continue until all the doctors in the place die of old age.

Henry Laurens, 1770

Mr. Deas has got rid of his fever, but poor William's will not yet take leave of him. I have just been administering a dose of James's Powders, and I hope by the aid of arsenic to cure him in a day or two.

Anne Deas, 1814

DOCTORS DIFFER

In the decades leading up to the Civil War, some doctors in the slave states advocated a distinctive southern medicine, or what they sometimes called "states-rights medicine." They urged the creation of medical schools staffed by southern doctors, where students could learn to treat the distinctive diseases of the region and the "peculiarities" of black bodies and diseases. "Southern medicine" was more rhetorical than real, a reaction to the increase of sectional tension in the United States that produced secession. The healing arts as practiced in the southern states never differed hugely in practice from those in other parts of America or in the western world generally. Professional medical men ascribed to the same medical theories and principles, and employed the same kind of therapies, as their brethren elsewhere. Domestic medicine, or "kitchen physic," was also much the same as elsewhere, combining orthodox therapies and exotic, sometimes magical remedies. Alternative forms of medicine existed everywhere, from folk medicine to the medical sects of the nineteenth century. Yet the hot climate, ubiquity of "tropical" fevers, and large black population inevitably produced some differences in medical thinking and practice between North and South. These differences originated in part out of the epidemiological circumstances of the lowcountry, which were a product of climate, terrain, and rice cultivation using enslaved African labor. Even during colonial times, doctors stressed the need to tailor therapies to the different climate and constitutions of the lowcountry, a trend that later broadened out to produce calls for a medicine geared to southern environments, diseases, and bodies, both black and white.[1]

In one crucial respect, lowcountry doctors were no different from doctors anywhere. Before the twentieth century, they were largely helpless in the face of infectious diseases. In the midst of a yellow fever epidemic in Charleston in 1794, an anguished Alexander Baron wrote Benjamin Rush that he wished that "no person would send for me, for I know nothing of this disease, and am as ignorant as a child unborn – for let me do as I will puke, purge or bleed still they all die." A few years later, Dr. Frederick Dalcho concluded that the doctors' helplessness in the face of yellow fever was "either a reflection upon our talents, or a proof of the imbecility of our art."[2] Such confessions of utter impotence may have been unusual, but many doctors surely doubted their usefulness at times. That many of their patients doubted it as well is attested to by numerous literary and visual satires of the bumbling medico. In truth, doctors had little to offer beyond palliative care for many diseases. The value of such care should not be minimized, for it could reduce suffering and increase the chances of recovery. Unfortunately, many doctors insisted on subjecting patients to harsh and sometimes deadly remedies. During the period covered by this book, 1670–1860, academic medicine took on and threw off theories like suits of clothes, but physicians continued to treat patients in ways the ancients would have found familiar. Some of them adopted new medications and techniques. These were sometimes useful but often more drastic and potentially deadly than those of earlier times. Medicine in the lowcountry in that respect was not exceptional. Doctors there adopted the advances and followed the old routines.

At the time the Carolina colony was founded in 1670, orthodox western medicine was in the process of abandoning the humoral theories of Galen. Galenism had dominated medical thinking for centuries. The various systems that replaced it, however, employed many of the same kinds of therapies, with

---

[1] *Disease and Distinctiveness in the American South* ed. by Todd L. Savitt and James Harvey Young (Knoxville: University of Tennessee Press, 1988); *Science and Medicine in the Old South*, ed. by Ronald L. Numbers and Todd L. Savitt (Baton Rouge: Louisiana State University Press, 1989).

[2] Alexander Baron to Benjamin Rush, Oct. 11, 1794, Rush Mss. 2 (Library Company of Philadelphia), cited in Waring, *History of Medicine in South Carolina, 1670–1825*, 178; Frederick Dalcho, "An Oration Delivered before the Medical Society of South Carolina, December 24, 1805," *Philadelphia Medical Museum* 3 (1807), 131.

the addition of many new chemical remedies derived from Paracelsus and his followers. To justify their therapies, lowcountry doctors appealed to recognized authorities: Hippocrates, Thomas Sydenham, William Boerhaave, William Cullen, and Benjamin Rush were held in high esteem at different periods. Whom doctors followed largely depended on when and how they were trained. Some were receptive to experimentation, regardless of system. Hippocrates was almost always in vogue and always being "revived," a figure simultaneously classical and revolutionary. Sydenham, the "English Hippocrates," was nearly as iconic throughout the late seventeenth and eighteenth centuries. Boerhaave strongly influenced medical thinking among lowcountry doctors during the early and mid-eighteenth century. In the late eighteenth century, many South Carolina doctors studied under Cullen at Edinburgh. Rush, who trained under Cullen but rejected his theories, became a major influence in South Carolina between the 1790s and the 1830s. From then on to the Civil War, well-informed doctors looked to the "Parisian school" of medicine as a source of inspiration and more moderate supportive therapies. Yet old ideas and methods died slowly.[3]

Boerhaave ascribed disease to "morbific matter" in the blood and prescribed medicines to expel it. He put a lot of emphasis on expelling disease by sweating, purging, and vomiting. Patients were put into warm closed rooms and had blankets piled on them. They were dosed with sudorifics (perspiration-inducing medicines) such as spirits of niter, snakeroot, saffron, and camphor. Boerhaave recommended bleeding for pleurisies and acute rheumatism but rarely for other disorders. Whereas Boerhaave saw corruption of the body's fluids as the source of disease, Cullen located the source in the solids, particularly in spasmodic actions of the nerves. Cullen's followers made extensive use of emetics (vomit-inducing drugs) such as tartar emetic and other antimonials, or compounds of the heavy metal antimony to reduce the "spasms" of fever. Ramsay viewed Cullen's system as an improvement on Boerhaave's because it urged greater use of antimonial medicines, "which are much more powerful than the medicines which had been previously in common use."

Ramsay reserved the greatest praise, however, for the system developed by his mentor, Rush. Ramsay dubbed Rush "the American Sydenham" after "the English Hippocrates." Between the Revolution and the 1820s, Rush probably had more influence over medicine in South Carolina than any other physician, partly because of Ramsay's fervent advocacy and partly because so many of the state's doctors trained under him in Philadelphia. Rush decided in the 1790s that most disease was due to vascular inflammation or "arterial convulsions" that had to be combated by "depletion": heavy bleeding and purging with jalap, a powerful herbal cathartic, and calomel, a mercury compound.

---

[3] Roy Porter, *The Greatest Benefit to Mankind: A Medical History of Humanity* (New York: W.W. Norton, 1997); *The Medical Enlightenment of the Eighteenth Century*, ed. by Andrew Cunningham and Roger French (Cambridge and New York: Cambridge University Press, 1990).

One of the greatest benefits of Rush's system, Ramsay argued, was its simplicity. Cullen's classification of disease was extremely complex, with almost 1,400 diseases broken down into "orders, classes, and genera, in the manner of botanists ... requiring in some respects, different treatment." Rush had greatly simplified "this embarrassing, perplexing mode of acquiring knowledge of diseases." Students of medicine would forever be in Rush's debt, for the old European medical systems required "reading and memory, the new judgment and observation." Rush's simple system could be learned much more quickly than the old systems. In 1809, Ramsay claimed that calomel (chloride of mercury) and jalap (a strong herbal purgative) had become the favorite local remedies. At the same time, potent new medicines, such as digitalis and heavy metals and gases, were now in common use.

Ramsay argued that American practitioners of the colonial period had been therapeutically too timid, and that Rush's more active therapeutics was cause for celebration. To the patriotic Ramsay, the new medicine was a natural corollary to the political changes brought by independence: "The practice of physic has undergone a revolution in South Carolina, as well as the government of the state." The medical revolution was also necessitated by "a real change of the diseases of the country." Since 1792 – the year epidemic yellow fever returned to Charleston – local fevers had been "more inflammatory" and required "freer evacuations and more energetic prescriptions." The use of opium was an example of the new energetic approach. Colonial doctors had often used opium to combat coughing, but their dosages were generally too small, and they did not use it for other conditions to which it was now successfully applied. Many people once resisted taking opium because of the strong "prejudices" against it, and doctors had to disguise or conceal it. In former times, people had rarely taken opium without the advice of a physician, but "now, a phial of laudanum is to be found in almost every family." Ramsay admitted that some danger arose from the greater use of opium, for he added, "it is freely taken, not only without medical advice, but frequently in cases in which no prudent physician would advise it."

Ramsay also cautioned against the dangers of careless use of bleeding and calomel. The "depleting mercurial plan" had "done much mischief in the hands of persons who did not understand it." But he was hardly urging moderate use of these remedies. He sounds more like a vampire: "Bleeding should be repeated while the symptoms which first indicated it continue, should it be until four-fifths of the blood contained in the body are drawn away ... In fevers and other diseases, which run their course in a few days or hours, and which threaten immediate death, there can be no limits fixed to the quantity of blood which may be drawn at once, or in a short time."[4] Ramsay was merely

---

[4] David Ramsay, *History of South Carolina* 2 vols. (Charleston, 1858), 2: 65–66; David Ramsay, *A Review of the Improvements, Progress, and State of Medicine in the XVIIIth Century* (Charleston, 1800), 7–8, 18–19; David Ramsay, *An Eulogium upon Benjamin Rush, M. D.* (Philadelphia, 1813), vii, 20–27, 75.

following Rush's advice. During a Philadelphia yellow fever epidemic in 1794, Rush claimed that he took 144 ounces of blood from a patient in 12 bleedings in six days and gave him almost 150 grains of calomel during the same period, along with the powerful purgatives jalap and gamboge. The patient somehow survived to become proof of the virtues of Rush's theory and therapeutics.[5]

The colonial doctors Ramsay thought too timid probably included two of his former colleagues, Lionel Chalmers and Alexander Garden. Chalmers urged caution in bleeding. Heavy bleeding might be necessary in other places or on some occasions but in general, he argued, it "weakens the sick rather than gives lasting relief." Most people in health had just enough blood to maintain their health. It made little sense to take it from those already weakened by disease. When necessary, eight to ten ounces was the maximum amount a doctor should take from anyone's body. Chalmers also charged that many practitioners used vomiting too routinely in intermitting and remitting fevers. Experience convinced Chalmers that giving strong emetics in acute fevers – notably the newly fashionable emetic tartar (tartrate of antimony) – had led to "*epileptic* attacks, *stupors*, or *deliria*." He preferred to have the patient drink warm water when he saw them discharging much acrimonious bile upwards "until [the water] returns clear and tasteless." In contrast, Ramsay advised that patients should be vomited at the first indication of a fever.[6]

Garden also seemed timid by Ramsay's standards. He was well aware of his profession's deadly reputation. Of one of his patients he wrote that "he will die neither of the dose nor the doctor ... the lot of many poor man and unhappy woman." Garden counseled heavy reliance on nature, as in his advice about treating whooping cough, an occasional scourge of children: "I have only endeavoured to assist the little children in getting up the phlegm, clearing themselves from the oppression and stuffing about the stomach. When nature is left to herself she relieves them by vomiting and those who vomit easiest and soonest ... suffer less and recover soonest." The only medicine he gave them was an herbal expectorant made from squills "and only when nature seems to want it." The child's diet should be light and pleasant, emphasizing fruit and vegetables: "stewed black berries and milk makes an excellent light and cooling supper and they are fond of it." He sometimes applied a blister to the neck, but only when the symptoms persisted for more than five weeks. He declared that "all nostrums and specifics in this disease however much boasted of are nonsense." Garden's relatively gentle approach to therapeutics may partly explain why his services were in high demand.[7]

---

[5] *Letters of Benjamin Rush*, ed. by L. H. Butterfield 2 vols. (Princeton, NJ: Princeton University Press, 1951), 2: 752; Joseph I. Waring, "The Influence of Benjamin Rush on the Practice of Bleeding in South Carolina," *Bulletin of the History of Medicine* 3 (1961), 230–237.

[6] Lionel Chalmers, *Essay on Fevers* (London, 1768), 42–44, 49, 53–54, 79–82; Lionel Chalmers, *An Account of the Weather and Diseases of South Carolina* 2 vols. (London, 1776) 1: 177; David Ramsay, *A Dissertation on the Means of Preserving Health in Charleston, and the Adjacent Lowcountry* (Charleston, 1790), 17.

[7] Alexander Garden to Richard Bohun Baker, n.d., Baker-Grimke Papers, SCHS, 11/535/536.

That did not prevent Garden from being banished as an "obnoxious person" (a Loyalist) after the Revolution, and he went to London in 1783. Chalmers died in 1777. By the 1790s, Rush's drastic therapies – termed "heroic medicine" – became the vogue. (One inevitably wonders who the heroes were). Rush did not carry everyone with him by any means. Even at the height of enthusiasm for his therapies, some doctors urged caution in using them or rejected them altogether. Popular resistance to bleeding surely induced some doctors to moderate their practice from time to time. A satirical rhyme in the *South Carolina Gazette*, published before Rush had concocted his vascular theory, illustrates the point: "The people alarmed at such proceeding, resolve (tho' in fevers) not to be bleeding." In 1793, a Charleston physician argued that bleeding in fevers was not helpful in the lowcountry climate.[8] Another doctor, John Shecut, deprecated the overuse of bleeding and mercury. In 1819, he declared that in the treatment of yellow fever he had "long since sheathed my lancet." He had also rejected mercury, except in small doses, "because I have determined never to tremble for the consequences, resulting from its excessive use."[9] The consequences could certainly be frightful: They included loss of teeth, rotting of the jaw, paralysis, and death. An example was recorded by Alexander Robertson during the yellow fever epidemic of 1838: "Mr. Lewis is mending, but very slowly, poor old gentleman, he has had a cruel and severe bout of [yellow fever], he is so dreadfully salivated [from mercury] that he cannot speak but with the most excruciating pain; it will be, must be, some time before he gets over it." Nevertheless, Robertson did not question the wisdom of mercurial treatment. Lewis, he concluded, would "be better when he recovers than he has been for years." Alternatives to mercury were not necessarily an improvement. Matthew Irvine, who also rejected mercury and heavy bleeding for yellow fever, recommended sugar of lead instead.[10]

A more palatable, if not more effective, therapy was alcohol. When Alice Izard came down with a fever in 1814, her doctor advised her to drink wine, a common prescription, and one that Izard, like many, found remarkably helpful: "I felt better for it," she declared.[11] Military and naval surgeons considered a good supply of rum and wine as essential to the medical care of soldiers and sailors. Rum was considered to be a good preventive of fevers.[12] Wine was prescribed for a host of disorders. When Alexander Robertson was caring for a young girl severely ill with yellow fever in Charleston in 1838, the

---

[8] Waring, "Influence of Benjamin Rush," 231.

[9] John L. E. W. Shecut, *Shecut's Medical and Philosophical Essays*, (Charleston, 1819), 123–128.

[10] J. H. Easterby, ed., *The South Carolina Rice Plantation* (Columbia: University of South Carolina Press, 2004; 1945), 411; Matthew Irvine, *Irvine's Treatise on the Yellow Fever* (Charleston, 1820), 41.

[11] A. Izard to Mrs. Manigault, Aug. 24, 1814, Manigault FP, SCL.

[12] Alexander Leslie to Sir Guy Carleton, July 18, 1782, Great Britain, Historical Manuscripts Commission, *Report on American Manuscripts in the Royal Institution of Great Britain* 4 vols. (Boston: Gregg Press, 1972), 3: 24.

doctor recommended "old wine" for her and he "got her the oldest and best" he had. Unfortunately, it did not save her.[13]

"NEGRO STROLLERS AND OLD WOMEN"

Whatever medical system they professed, doctors stressed the need to adjust medical practice to the body of the patient and the climate, topography, and disorders of the region. They also believed that remedies for diseases often existed close to where the diseases were prevalent. Most doctors used botanical remedies that came from the local forests or other parts of America. Europeans learned the uses and preparation of many of these herbals from Native Americans. Indian healing was shamanistic, tied to religious beliefs, but healers also used numerous herbals. In 1680, colonial planter and official Maurice Matthews reported that he had learned much from local Indians about the medicinal uses of certain roots, barks, and leaves. A promotional pamphlet of the early 1680s ascribed an "exquisite knowledge" of botanical medicine to the Indians. The author referred to snakeroot as a cure for snake poison, malignant fevers, smallpox, and plague. Subsequently, doctors and other healers used different species of snakeroot as painkillers, emetics, sedatives, expectorants, diuretics, and sudorifics. They touted various types of snakeroot as cures for numerous disorders, including inflammation of the lungs, dropsy, rheumatism, yellow fever, and intermittent fevers. In the early 1700s Francis Le Jau reported that he had taken large doses of infused snakeroot with good results for a respiratory disorder. White Carolinians often used another Indian remedy, yaupon holly or cassine. In a pamphlet of 1695, John Peachie recommended drinking a tea made from it to cure smallpox. Nothing could or can cure smallpox, but people recommended yaupon tea for that disorder and others well into the nineteenth century.[14] In 1700, John Lawson was so impressed by Indian herbal remedies that he urged European medicine to adopt many of them. He urged intermarriage between whites and Native Americans because it would lead to "a true knowledge of all the Indian's skill in medicine and surgery." James Adair, an Indian trader, declared that all the Native American nations possessed "a great knowledge of specific virtues in simples: applying herbs and plants, on the most dangerous occasions, and seldom if ever, fail to effect a thorough cure." Naturalist Mark Catesby described Native American use of yaupon tea, sassafras, and especially pinkroot, used to combat the ubiquitous worm infestations.[15]

[13] Easterby, *South Carolina Rice Plantation*, 410–411.

[14] Maurice Matthews, "A Contemporary View of Carolina in 1680," *SCHM* 55 (1954), 157–158; Salley, *Narratives*, 144–145; "Seneka Rattle-Snake Root," *SCG*, Nov. 6, 1740; Klingberg, *Le Jau*, 103–106; John Peachie, *Some Observations Made upon the Herb Cassiny; Imported from Carolina: Showing its Admirable Virtues in Curing the Smallpox* (London, 1695); Virgil J. Vogel, *American Indian Medicine* (Norman: University of Oklahoma Press, 1990; 1970), 370–374.

[15] John Lawson, *A New Voyage to Carolina*, ed. by Hugh T. Lefler (Chapel Hill: University of North Carolina Press, 1967), 222–231; Mark Catesby, *The Natural History of Carolina*,

Several colonial physicians publicly promoted pinkroot's virtues as a vermifuge or antihelminthic (worm destroyer). John Moultrie Sr. and Alexander Garden sent specimens to Britain in the early 1750s. John Lining published the first medical description of pinkroot (or Indian pink) in an Edinburgh journal in 1754. Lining wrote that Indians had taught the English how to prepare it, and that all practitioners and planters had been using it for many years. They administered it in a powder or an infusion of the root made in boiling water. Lining claimed that Indian pink was less nauseous and safer than any other remedy he had used. He had recently given it to a negro child who voided thirty-nine large round worms in two days, ending the child's "worm fever." Garden also published descriptions of the pinkroot and how to prepare it for medicinal use. Chalmers and Ramsay declared that it was the best vermifuge in Carolina and perhaps in the world. Pinkroot was part of the official pharmacopeia of the United States from 1820 until 1926. Many varieties of snakeroot remained part of the pharmacopeia well into twentieth century.[16]

Lowcountry doctors also learned much about the medicinal properties of local plants from Africans. Because some Indians were enslaved, the two groups probably learned from one another. Many Africans arrived with considerable knowledge of herbals. Garden declared that African herbalists knew far more about plants than most local doctors. If it was not for what they learned "from the negro strollers and old women," Garden wrote sarcastically, "I doubt much if they would know a common dock from a cabbage stock."[17] Garden often criticized the botanical ignorance of local practitioners, perhaps unfairly, but he was an avid student of natural history who gained an international reputation for his accurate observations and descriptions. When he arrived in the early 1750s, the colony was gripped by hysteria over real or alleged slave poisonings. Doctors were often ascribing deaths in planters' families to poison administered by slaves. Initially, he concluded that some Africans knew of botanical poisons so lethal that even "the ablest practitioners in the province" had no effective antidotes. He soon changed his mind. Most alleged poisoning cases, he decided, were actually the result of doctors' mistakes in treating dysentery and other diseases. When the patients got worse, the doctors would blame poison. The family and friends "never blame the doctor's neglect or ignorance when they think that the case is poison, as they readily think that lies out of the power of medicine and thus the word *poison* ... has been as good a screen to ignorance here as that of *malignancy* was in Britain."

Florida, and the Bahama Islands (London, 1771), 1: xiv; James Adair, *Adair's History of the American Indians*, ed. by Samuel Cole Williams (New York: Promontory Press, 1930), 244–248, 364, 388; Vogel, *American Indian Medicine*, 51–58, 348–349.

[16] John Lining, "Of the Antihelminthic Virtues of the Root of the Indian Pink," *Essays and Observations, Physical and Literary* 1 (1754), 386–389; Chalmers, *Weather and Diseases of South Carolina*, 1: 67; Ramsay, *Preserving Health*, 4; Edmund Berkeley and Dorothy Smith Berkeley, *Dr. Alexander Garden of Charles Town* (Chapel Hill: University of North Carolina Press, 1969), 29–31.

[17] Alexander Garden to Charles Alston, Jan. 28, 1753, Edinburgh University, Special Collections, La. III.375/42–45. "Dock" here refers to a broadleaf weed.

Garden was often called on to deal with cases of obstinate dysentery that other doctors had called poisonous cases. He claimed that he had "often succeeded in curing the poor patient, who might have been actually poisoned by swallowing dubious antidotes." One of the antidotes that local doctors claimed to use was itself the prescription of a slave named Caesar. In 1749, he had given the provincial government his "secret recipe" for a poison antidote. In return, the assembly rewarded him with freedom, money, and the title of Dr. Caesar. When Garden arrived a few years later, he dismissed the antidote, claiming that the white doctor who had published it for the assembly was an incompetent botanist who had failed to describe accurately the plants required. Anyone using the recipe would be liable to make a mistake that might render the antidote useless or dangerous.[18]

If Garden was correct, medical mistakes in diagnosis and treatment had a high cost to more than their patients. In July 1749, a letter appeared in the *South Carolina Gazette* about a secret antidote for Indian and Negro poisons. The letter claimed that the Africans used a "strange and extraordinary" poison that had "no ill taste." It killed sometimes in hours, in other cases in months or years, apparently according to the poisoner's design. The symptoms of poisoning – as the writer described them – bore a striking similarity to diseases such as dysentery and consumption. The victims always died – without the secret remedy, of course. The letter may have helped ignite the hysteria. A few months after it appeared, the *Gazette* reported that "the horrid practice of poisoning white people, by the Negroes, has lately become so common, that within a few days past, several executions have taken place in different parts of the country, by burning, hanging, and gibbeting." In 1751, the assembly extended capital punishment to any "negro, mulatto, or mestizo" who aided a slave or slaves in poisoning or knew about a planned poisoning and did not reveal it to the authorities. The act made it a capital crime for any slave to teach knowledge of poisons to another slave; prohibited slaves from working for an apothecary; and banned them from administering medicine except under the direction of a white person. The exception was necessary; without it, it would have been illegal for slaves to act as healers on the plantations. The Virginia assembly had passed a similar act in 1748. Such legislation did not stop alleged or real poisonings, fears of poisoning, or executions of suspected slave poisoners. They continued to be a feature of southern life throughout the age of slavery.

The poisoning episode reveals a paradox in the mindset of the planters, who feared the very skills they most valued in some of their slaves. Nevertheless, the planter elite continued to draw on the knowledge or alleged knowledge of African healers. In 1754, the assembly rewarded another slave named Sampson for revealing his remedy for rattlesnake bites. Appropriately, it

---

[18] Alexander Garden to Charles Alston, Edinburgh, Jan. 28, 1753, Feb. 18, 1756, Edinburgh University, Special Collections, La. III.375/42–45; Berkeley, *Alexander Garden*, 31–32; *JCHA*, 9: 293, 303–304.

contained hart-snakeroot along with several other herbals.[19] On a more basic level, planters – especially in isolated areas – were highly dependent on the healing skills of their slaves. The primary caregivers on plantations were generally other slaves, often older women with knowledge of herbal medicine that the planters or overseers appointed to the task. In addition, an underground medical system also existed on many plantations in which slaves treated others with herbal and magical remedies. Planters often valued African medical knowledge and skills but also feared them. As the discussion over "slave poisoning" indicates, African healers possessed a power that could endanger the planters' control and even their existence.[20] On many plantations, slaves practiced a type of religio-magical medicine called root medicine , hoodoo, or conjure. These practices appealed to many blacks because they derived from and were an integral part of African religious and cultural practices. Africans explained many illnesses as the result of spells cast by conjurors. But they also employed conjurers or root doctors to take the spells off. To cast and remove spells, these practitioners – both men and women – used charms, incantations, and conjure packets containing all sorts of ingredients including herbs such as snakeroot, graveyard dust, bits of cloth, feathers, animal parts, whisky, and a fungus called "Devil's Snuff." The conjurers might also use purgatives or other medicines, much like orthodox white doctors. Planters sometimes ignored or winked at these practices and sometimes tried to stamp them out, without success. Whites sometimes consulted conjure doctors for their own disorders as well. Medicine in the lowcountry was a highly eclectic operation drawing on many different traditions.[21]

TAKING THE BARK

Perhaps the most effective remedy lowcountry doctors prescribed was introduced to Europeans by Native Americans, in this case in Peru. The Peruvian bark was introduced and used primarily as a specific for malarial fevers. It was also used for other conditions, with poorer and sometimes dangerous results. The bark was derived from the South American cinchona tree. Jesuit priests introduced it into European medicine in the mid-seventeenth century. British doctors were allegedly slow to adopt its use because it was often called Jesuits' Bark. Nevertheless, Robert Talbor promoted it in England in the late

---

[19] SCG, July 24, Oct. 30, 1749; *Stats.*, 7: 422–423; *JCHA*, 10: 211, 287, 292, 12: 335, 368, 13: 145; JCHA, computer file, 1757–1761, 154; Muhlenberg, *Journals*, Oct. 10, 1774; Sharla M. Fett, *Working Cures: Healing, Health, and Power on Southern Slave Plantations* (Chapel Hill: University of North Carolina Press, 2002), 159–166.

[20] Fett, *Working Cures*, 111–192; James M. Clifton, ed., *Life and Labor on Argyle Island: Letters and Documents of a Savannah River Plantation, 1833–1867* (Savannah, GA: The Beehive Press, 1978).

[21] Fett, *Working Cures*, 36–110; Charles Joyner, *Down by the Riverside: A South Carolina Slave Community* (Chicago: University of Illinois Press, 1984), 144–150; McCandless, *Moonlight, Magnolias, and Madness*, 204–205, 376 notes 60–61.

seventeenth century, and was knighted for his efforts. By the early eighteenth century, the bark was being widely used to combat malarial fevers.[22]

The bark was powdered and taken in decoctions of various kinds. Talbor provided several prescriptions for infusions of bark with wine and opium, and others added new recipes in the eighteenth century. One of the most famous was a tincture English doctor John Huxham included in his *Essay on Fevers* (1739). It is difficult to pinpoint when the bark was first used in the low-country, but it was widely prescribed by the late colonial period. Georgia official William Stephens took the bark for a fever in the summer of 1736. Apparently it worked, because he soon resumed his normal business. In 1741, Levi Durand, an Anglican minister in South Carolina, reported that he was "going at last to take the bark."[23] As with inoculation, doctors prepared the patient's body for receiving the bark by administering other treatments, such as vomits, purges, sweats, blisters, or bleeding. They stressed the importance of emptying the stomach and intestines and securing a remission of the fever before administering bark. James Lind provided detailed directions in his guide for Europeans living in hot climates. During the first hours of fever, the patient should be given a vomit and purgative or an enema. This was to be followed by an antimonial drink every six hours, particularly if the patient was perspiring. If this worked, the patient should have a remission or at least a mitigation of fever within twenty-four hours, "when the bark, if no symptom forbids its use, is immediately to be given." If the fever returned, it meant the patient had been given insufficient bark. Lind also cautioned against bleeding patients much in hot climates – a view that some lowcountry doctors shared.[24]

A major problem with the bark was that many patients could not tolerate its extreme bitterness. In the early 1760s, Garden prescribed it for the son of planter Richard Baker. The boy vomited it up. Garden told Baker that he must have "prepared the bark rather too strong for his stomach" and sent him a dose that he claimed would "check the fever and prepared so he will not vomit it up." Baker's daughter soon came down with a fever, and Garden advised omitting the bark for the time being and giving her hart-snake root tea. When fever struck Baker's wife, Garden sent a mild preparation that would "agree with her stomach" along with a more powerful decoction to take later. Garden hoped that the milder decoction along with some nourishment would prepare and strengthen her stomach to enable her to take the stronger dose of bark she needed. Baker may have had doubts about the use of the bark, because Garden added that the fevers had "been so obstinate to remove lately that

[22] Sir Robert Talbor, *The English Remedy; or Talbor's Wonderful Secret for Cureing Agues and Feavers* (London, 1682); Berkeley, *Alexander Garden*, 37, note 11.

[23] *Journal of William Stephens*, Appendix A, 251–258; Levi Durand, Feb. 3, 1741, SPG Letter Books, B10: 159; James Steuart to John Steuart of Dalgleish, Aug. 15, 1752, Steuart of Dalgleish Muniments, SRO/GD38/2/8/65.

[24] James Lind, *An Essay on Diseases Incident to Europeans in Hot Climates* (London, 1768), 167.

nothing but the bark in substance will overcome them." On another occasion, he prescribed bark with success when one of Baker's children came down with what he called worm fever. Garden claimed that worm fever sometimes included remissions or intermissions, and that bark rarely failed to check it. Many so-called worm fevers were in fact probably malaria.[25]

Many patients resisted taking the bark because of low tolerance; because they feared its side effects; or because they did not experience much improvement from taking it. Ramsay declared that many people "entertained great prejudices against" the bark, such as the belief that it collected in the bones and "disposed them to take cold." For all these reasons, physicians often disguised bark to get patients to take it, and they routinely used sugar, wine, or some other ingredient to moderate its bitterness. Chalmers recommended putting sugar into the bark tea but cautioned that too much would reduce its fever-reducing properties. He also suggested injecting the decoction via clysters into the rectum of the patient whose stomach could not tolerate it. Reducing the dosage was another common tactic, but he insisted that large doses were best because they would get rid of the fever more quickly. Chalmers also stressed the importance of continuing to take the bark for several weeks after the fever disappeared. Many patients stopped taking it too soon, and their fever returned. For patients who could not tolerate regular and sufficient doses of the bark, moving to a different climate might be the only solution. According to Alice Izard, members of the Deas family were unable to take the bark for fevers in the fall of 1815: "[B]ark does not agree with any of them."[26]

Producing decoctions of bark in dosages that would be effective, safe, and ingestible was a difficult task, complicated by the highly variable quality of the bark itself. It is likely that some sellers fraudulently sold other tree barks to those unfamiliar with the genuine product. Although experienced physicians could probably detect such frauds, many ordinary people might easily have been duped, and the resulting failures convince them the remedy was useless. Another problem was simply getting bark at all. During wartime – which was often between 1739 and 1815 – supplies from South America might be cut off. In the summer of 1776, with supplies cut off temporarily by the British navy, Henry Laurens reported that people were using dogwood bark as a substitute for Peruvian bark. Laurens claimed the substitution was successful. Others disagreed. In 1814, Alice Izard took dogwood bark instead of the Peruvian, which "my stomach would no longer bear." A friend had strongly recommended it, but it did Izard little good. Bark substitutes, she concluded, were "not to be depended on." She also reported that even Peruvian bark had

<hr/>

[25] HLP, 7: 125, Aug. 15, 1769; "Letters from Henry Laurens," SCHM 24 (1923), 11; Alexander Garden to Richard Bohun Baker, June 17, 19, 1761, and several other letters dated 1761 or undated, Baker-Grimke Papers, SCHS, 11/535–536.

[26] Ramsay, Improvements, Progress, and State of Medicine, 17; Ramsay, History of South Carolina, 2: 65–66; Chalmers, Weather and Diseases of South Carolina, 1: 150–156, 179, 182–183; Waring, Medicine in South Carolina, 1670–1825, 286; A. Izard to Mrs. Manigault, Oct. 19, 1815, Manigault FP, SCL.

not worked well of late. When Anne Deas found her son could not keep the bark down, she decided to try arsenic, and took it herself. Her husband could take neither. She also gave her children Dr. James's Powders, a concoction of antimony.[27]

During the Revolutionary War, the medical services of both armies in the South used large quantities of bark. They often ran out of it. While campaigning in Georgia in the summer of 1782, General Anthony Wayne reported that shortages of bark had led to the loss of some of his men. His superior, Nathanael Greene, reported that his army was also short of bark. As we have seen, hundreds of Greene's men died from malarial fevers that fall. High-ranking officers probably got what was available. One of Greene's staff, Colonel Lewis Morris, was able to take it regularly.[28]

Bark continued to be used into the early nineteenth century. In 1817, French chemists learned how to isolate the active alkali in cinchona bark, quinine, which made it possible to give precise and pure dosages. By the 1820s, some practitioners were prescribing quinine for malaria.[29] Even before then, however, doctors were noticing something ominous: Bark was less effective in curing malaria than it once had been and sometimes produced dangerous side effects. In 1808, Dr. Isaac Auld claimed that the bark was important but not as powerful a remedy as it once was. It often worked well in the milder cases, which had predominated in the recent past. Recently, however, autumnal fevers had become more resistant to the remedy: "Instead of expulsion by the bark, the fever derives additional strength from it and fatal termination has in this way been but too often the melancholy consequence." Patients with bilious fever who were treated with Peruvian bark were now "much to be pitied." Perhaps Auld was observing cases of "blackwater fever" – which may result from an allergic reaction to quinine. Yellow fever, which bark did not affect, is another possibility. Doctors often prescribed bark for yellow fever either because they believed it was just a higher grade of malarial fever or because of misdiagnosis. The failures of the bark in such cases undoubtedly contributed to the view that it was becoming less effective. Whatever Auld was seeing, he agreed with Ramsay that bilious fevers required stronger therapeutic measures than before: "[L]arge and repeated bleedings, assisted by active mercurial purges, and emetic and nauseating medicines." Blisters sometimes produced "astonishing effects." Auld's views were typical of many practitioners. This could not have been good news to fever sufferers.[30]

---

[27] *HLP*, 11: 255, Aug. 17, 1776; A. Izard to Mrs. Manigault, Sept. 28, 1814, Manigault FP, SCL; A. Izard to Mrs. Manigault, Oct. 5, 12, 19, 1815, A. I. Deas to Mrs. Manigault, Oct. 6, 1814, Sept. 29, 1815, Manigault FP, SCL.

[28] *The Papers of General Nathanael Greene* 11 vols., ed. by Dennis M. Conrad (Chapel Hill and London: The University of North Carolina Press, 2000) 11: 359–361, 486; "Letters of Col. Lewis Morris to Miss Ann Elliott," *SCHM* 40 (1939), 123–124. See also Chapter 5 of this book.

[29] Philip Curtin, *Disease and Empire* (Cambridge: Cambridge University Press, 1998), 23; "Medical Expenses," John Black Papers, SCL.

[30] Ramsay, *History of South Carolina* 2: appendix 1, 282, written by Isaac Auld.

CAN'T GET NO SATISFACTION

In 1843, a letter to the Charleston *Courier* proclaimed that "the practice of physic is little more than the making of experiments. Hence the frequent failures in medical practice ... and the longstanding suspicion that doctors *kill* sometimes." In 1861, James Henry Hammond charged that the prescriptions of regular medicine were lethal: "Observation ... and experience lead me to throw all physic to the dogs. Every drug in the apothecary shop is poison. I have seen hundreds die of doctors and scarcely a week goes by that I do not hear of a case."[31] The criticisms were not new or unusual, but public disdain for the medical profession was probably at its height in the antebellum period. In part, this may have been a reaction against heroic therapies, but criticism did not abate when doctors began to moderate their treatments in the 1840s. This only created a new problem for orthodox medicine: It jettisoned old therapies but had nothing much to offer in their place beyond careful nursing, tonics, and the course of nature. Doctors seemed more confused than ever about how to deal with disease. The public was not any kinder to uncertainty then than now, and the fact that so many antebellum doctors were poorly trained graduates of substandard proprietary medical schools did not inspire confidence. People complained that physicians' therapies were too drastic – or not drastic enough.[32]

Skepticism toward doctors' healing skills was a staple of public discussion throughout the colonial and early national periods. It derived from a long and honorable European tradition illustrated by the cartoons of Hogarth, Gillray, and Rowlandson.[33] It is important not to exaggerate it. Perhaps most patients were satisfied with their doctors. After all, they kept calling them back when they needed help. Just as today, some people concluded that they got little help, and often much suffering, in return for the money they spent on medical care. Gideon Johnston was convinced that he would not recover his health until he had returned to England and "good British physicians, air, and diet restore me to health." In 1749, William Orr, an Anglican missionary, complained that "notwithstanding all the advice and charges of physicians, I am but very little better."[34] After Henry Laurens took a prescribed vomit for an intermittent fever, he recorded that it had "strained my eyes very much and almost brought me to spectacles."[35]

[31] *The Courier*, April 5, 1843; Carol Bleser, *The Hammonds of Redcliffe* (New York: Oxford University Press, 1981), 101.

[32] Charles Rosenberg, "The Therapeutic Revolution," in *The Therapeutic Revolution*, ed. by Morris Vogel and Charles Rosenberg (Philadelphia: University of Pennsylvania Press, 1979), 5–20; John Harley Warner, *The Therapeutic Perspective: Medical Practice, Knowledge, and Identity in America, 1820–1885* (Cambridge, MA: Harvard University Press, 1986).

[33] Roy Porter, *Bodies Politic: Disease, Death, and Doctors in Britain, 1650–1900* (Ithaca, NY: Cornell University Press, 2001).

[34] Klingberg, *Johnston*, 90–92; William Orr, March 31, 1749, SPG Letter Books, B17: 172.

[35] *HLP*, 7: 131.

Some people entirely lost faith in their doctors. When the Deas family refused to call a doctor to treat their young son, Anne Deas wrote in explanation, "You will perhaps wonder ... that we have not sent for the doctor; the fact is that after our late misfortune we both had a horror of sending for him. He may be a good physician but he has not been a successful one with us, and we think him too fond of bleeding. He took blood twice from our beloved little William and ... it struck us that he must have bled him too much." Yet the domestic therapies many people employed were every bit as dangerous as those used by the regular doctors, partly because they were very much the same. As we have seen, Deas gave her son antimonial powders and arsenic. Many domestic prescriptions involved bleeding, drastic purges and vomits, and heavy metals, particularly mercuric compounds.[36]

Yellow fever provided doctors with the greatest challenge to their reputations. They could not cure it no matter what they tried. No one could. But that was true of nearly all microbial diseases before the twentieth century, and it remains true of yellow fever today. Doctors sometimes expressed frustration with their inability to cure or even allay the fever. Alexander Baron's confession that he could do nothing for his yellow fever patients became known in Charleston circles. William James Ball commented a few years later that "old Dr. Baron" had proclaimed that in a disease like yellow fever, "the greatest fool and the most skillful physician are equally unsuccessful." That Baron was not alone is indicated by Roger Pinckney's statement in 1817 that yellow fever "defies the skill of our best physicians, who declare themselves ignorant of a cure or how to check it."[37] In 1824, the Medical Society acknowledged the fact, at least indirectly. They refused to debate which therapies for yellow fever were most effective because such a deliberation "might lead to professional discussions of an unharmonious character." And embarrassing as well, one might add. Perhaps they recalled the professional mudslinging that accompanied the introduction of inoculation in 1738. The society had become more candid by the late 1850s. The members openly debated the merits of various treatments. The general agreement was that none of them worked. One doctor stated that he had tried every treatment that had ever been recommended and had found them all to be worthless. Another declared that no relation existed "between the disease and its treatment, or in fact any treatment yet used." A third was so disappointed with every medication that he had "abandoned all treatment and placed reliance on nursing and careful attention." In a way, that was progress.[38]

None of this stopped some people from claiming that they could cure yellow fever or any other disease. The advertising of cure-all remedies was a regular

[36] A. I. Deas, to Mrs. Manigault, Sept. 29, 1815, Oct. 6, 1814, Manigault FP, SCL.

[37] Waring, *History of Medicine in South Carolina, 1670–1825*, 178; William James Ball to his father, Dec. 18, 1805, Ball FP, SCHS; Roger Pinckney to his aunt, Oct. 2, 1817, Roger Pinckney Correspondence, SCHS.

[38] MSM, Nov. 1, 1824, 253, Sept. 1, 1858, 407.

feature of colonial newspapers from their beginnings. The earliest issues of the *South Carolina Gazette* included Dr. Varambaut's claim that he possessed a "remedy for the cure of all sorts of fevers." Another doctor promised to cure smallpox and worms and vowed to take no payment unless he achieved a thorough cure. Dr. John Lax, a self-proclaimed Indian doctor, peddled cures for the flux and "bleedings," presumably hemorrhages.[39] In 1759, Joseph Howard claimed that he had "performed several extraordinary cures" and informed the provincial assembly that he was willing to share his methods "for the benefit of the public" in return for a "suitable reward." The gullible legislators agreed to give Howard 3,000 pounds for revealing his secret recipes for the cure of the lame distemper, yaws, an old pox, canker, and "almost any corrupt blood." The prescriptions were duly printed in the *South Carolina Gazette* and in almanacs. The benefit to Howard was obvious. The benefit to the public was not. His cure contained nothing extraordinary, relying on purges and guaiacum, an old and useless remedy for syphilis.[40]

A frequently advertised disease preventive and remedy was tar water – a diluted decoction of pine tar. During the smallpox epidemic of 1738, the *Gazette's* editor, Lewis Timothy, promoted it as a means of preparing the body for the disease. Tar water was alleged to cleanse the body and bring about a mild case, even in people who had been in close contact with the infected. He added that a person who had drunk tar water was later inoculated twice and showed no symptoms, which proved it to be not only "a preservative but an antidote against the infection." It proved nothing of the sort. The person may have already had the smallpox as a child, which meant that he or she was immune. Timothy printed the recipe and instructions "for the benefit of the public."[41]

Most purveyors of medical nostrums had dubious if any medical credentials, but even regular physicians sometimes claimed astounding results for their therapies. No matter what therapy a physician used, some patients always survived, and the doctor could take credit for the "cure." During the yellow fever epidemic of 1817, Joshua B. Whitridge, a recent immigrant from Rhode Island, bragged to his father of "my reputed success in the cure of this direful malady." His reputation was gained, he claimed, by his ability to cure himself – a thing "unheard of in this country in such an alarming and fatal disease." During his illness, he had refused to see anyone, including other physicians. He considered them incompetent. While ill, he had referred patients to three other doctors "who suffered most of them to die." Before he had fully recovered, Whitridge resolved that he must use his discovery to aid others. Perhaps romantic interest spurred him from his sickbed. He had been moved by "a father in tears" to undertake the treatment of his daughter, "a most interesting young lady of 17." Once word spread that he had treated her with

---

success, "applications multiplied." He took on numerous cases, "restoring many wretched victims of disease to health." The secret of his success was hardly novel. It was bleeding and calomel, perhaps carried to an extreme: "[T]he extent [to] which I bled myself, the quantity of calomel I took, etc. etc. quite astonished the weak minds of the natives." Whitridge's melodramatic narrative, although written to his father, differs little in tone and substance from those of irregular practitioners whom orthodox physicians called quacks. He confessed that secretiveness about his methods undermined his credibility with some of his medical colleagues. They "took umbrage" at their exclusion from his sick room and later claimed that he had not actually had yellow fever. But Whitridge was no ordinary quack. He later served as president of the Medical Society and the Medical College of South Carolina.[42]

Yellow fever patients continued to die in large numbers whatever the treatment. The helplessness of professional doctors in this and many other disorders encouraged people to turn to alternative sources of help, as did lack of money or geographical isolation. People unable or unwilling to call on physicians had many options. They could employ domestic medicine or "kitchen physic" – that is, they could treat themselves or their families using folk remedies, recipes from almanacs and other publications, domestic medical manuals, or some combination of all of them. They could purchase drugs and proprietary medicines from pharmacies and merchants. From the 1730s, the columns of newspapers were filled with advertisements for medicines imported from Britain: Daffy's Elixir, Godfrey's Cordial, Dr. James's Powders, and countless other concoctions. The number of proprietary and patent medicines grew exponentially in the nineteenth century, most of them worthless or dangerous. Most contained alcohol and/or opium, often laced with heavy metals and acids.[43]

Apothecary shops sold medicines and ready-made medicine chests for plantations. People could also buy domestic medical manuals that began to proliferate in the late seventeenth century.[44] The domestic manuals, along with almanacs and home remedy books, contained cures for everything imaginable: from yaws to yellow fever, ague to asthma, rheumatism to rabies, whooping cough to worms, measles to malaria. *The South Carolina Almanac for*

[42] Joshua B. Whitridge to William Whitridge, Sept. 8–10, 19–21, 1817, Whitridge Papers, SCHS; Waring, *Medicine in South Carolina, 1670–1825*, 325.
[43] *SCG*, Oct. 19, 1747, Jan. 19, 1751, Oct. 20, 1758, March 29, Oct. 11–18, 1760, May 14–21, Nov. 5, 1763, Jan. 7, Feb. 9, 23, 1765, Nov. 3, 1766, Aug. 22, 1768, June 25, July 9, Aug. 20, 1772, July 26, 1773; *South Carolina Gazette and Country Journal*, Aug. 11, 1772; *The Courier*, June 25, 1804; McCandless, *Moonlight, Magnolias and Madness*, 203–209.
[44] Early settlers could have brought Nicholas Culpeper's *English Physician* and his *Complete Herbal* (1652, 1653); John Archer's *Every Man His Own Doctor* (1671); and *Kitchin-Physick: or, Advice to the Poor* (1676). In the late colonial period, John Wesley's *Primitive Physick* (1747) and William Buchan's *Domestic Medicine* (1769) became popular favorites. The first manual published in America was in 1734, John Tennent's *Every Man His Own Doctor; or, The Poor Planter's Physician*. Many other American manuals followed in the nineteenth century.

1758 contained a selection from William Salmon's *New London Dispensary* (1676) describing the medicinal uses of various garden herbs. Almanacs contained prescriptions for countering many common diseases, notably fever and ague.[45] Recipes for the cure of dysentery were common. Most included ipecac, an emetic derived from the rhizome and roots of the ipecacuanha plant. Ipecac was often given with opium in the form of Dover's Powders, a concoction imported from England. Gideon Johnston wrote that he and his wife Harriet had used ipecac and laudanum (a tincture of opium) with some success against the flux, but nothing could free them entirely from its grip.[46] Many doctors advised taking bark with ipecac – a reminder that people often suffered from malaria and dysentery together, and that malaria can produce severe diarrhea.[47]

People often kept home remedy books in which they wrote or pasted recipes for medicines. The recipes often came from domestic manuals and almanacs. The recipe books contain many prescriptions for common scourges such as intermittents, agues, fevers, fluxes, colic, pleurisies, and worms. The Deas family's commonplace book from 1749 contains an Indian cure for the "spleen (probably the enlarged spleen caused by malaria), which had originally been published in John Lawson's *A New Voyage to Carolina* (1709): "They cure the spleen by burning with a reed. They lay the patient on his back, putting a hollow cane in the fire till 'tis very hot and on fire at one end, then they lay a bit of thin leather on the patient's belly between the pit of the stomach and the navel, pressing the hot reed on the leather, burning the patient so that in many the print of the cane never wears out. This is also used for the belly-ache sometimes."[48] Dr. Philip Porcher's account book for the 1780s lists many similar recipes and ingredients. One, Van Swieten's Liquor, sounds much better than its main ingredient, corrosive sublimate of mercury. It was used to treat syphilis and perhaps yaws.[49]

A detailed example of "kitchen physick" exists in a series of letters written by planter William Dry. He was managing the estate of missionary Richard Ludlam who had willed it to the Society for the Propagation of the Gospel on

[45] John Tobler, *The South Carolina Almanac for 1758* (Germantown, 1757); *The South Carolina and Georgia Almanac for the Year of Our Lord 1793* (Charleston, 1792); *Palladium of Knowledge: or, the Carolina and Georgia Almanac* (Charleston, 1796).

[46] Klingberg, *Johnston*, pp. 50–60.

[47] *Bountheau's Town and Country Almanac for Carolina and Georgia for 1805* (Charleston, 1804?); James Lind, *An Essay on Diseases Incident to Europeans in Hot Climates* (London, 1768), 248–250; Richard Towne, *A Treatise on the Diseases Most Frequent in the West Indies* (London, 1726); William Hilary, *Observations on the Changes of the Air and the Concomitant Epidemical Diseases in the Island of Barbados* (London, 1759); Benjamin Moseley, *A Treatise on Tropical Diseases* (London, 1792); Robert Jackson, *An Outline of the History and Cure of Fever* (London, 1798).

[48] Harriott Horry's Recipe Book, 1770, Pinckney Family Papers, SCHS, 38/19/2; Deas Commonplace Book, 1749, SCHS, 34/100; John Lawson, *A New Voyage to Carolina*, ed. by Hugh T. Lefler (Chapel Hill: University of North Carolina Press, 1967), 228–229.

[49] Philip Porcher Account Book, 1770–1800, typescript, SCL, 107–108.

his death in 1728. That winter, Dry treated several of Ludlam's slaves for a "pestilential pleuritick fever" (probably pneumonia or influenza). When two of them became ill with severe colds, he gave them snakeroot to sweat them, followed by a vomit to alleviate stomach pains. The next day he bled one of them and put them both in a hot house to sweat. A few days later, six slaves developed an inflammation of the lungs and one died. Dry lost two of his own slaves at this time from the same disorder. At this point, he decided to call in a doctor, because the disorder had become "very mortal amongst both whites and blacks." Dry also treated a slave boy named Mark for an intermittent fever and "moving pains," which he thought might be pneumonia. He bled him and the next day, Mark vomited two or three worms and a great deal of bile. Dry then gave him a vomit with sulfuric acid, which he thought ineffective. Mark's fever worsened and he became very low-spirited. He complained of great pain in the stomach and shoulder. Dry cupped him (with heated glasses) to raise blisters and gave him "a composing draft of Squire's grand elixir." When Mark failed to improve, he asked a local doctor to visit the boy, but the doctor refused, claiming that the problem was simply worms. Dry carried on alone. Within a few days, he boasted, he had cured Mark "without any doctor's assistance (tho' I looked upon him as past recovery) and that without putting the Honorable Society to any charge." He was hopeful that he could sell the rejuvenated youth for a good price. Dry did not do all the healing himself. He paid 8 pounds for "nursing, physicking, and bleeding" for the sick slaves. Perhaps he hired someone like Rebecca Pollard, who advertised her services as a nurse or midwife in the *South Carolina Gazette* in 1742. Pollard announced that she "had nursed many people through the smallpox" and added, perhaps unnecessarily, that "she was not dead."[50]

The doctor's reluctance to visit Mark was probably not unusual. Doctors did sometimes visit plantations to treat their inhabitants personally, but such trips were time-consuming and sometimes impossible. Instead, doctors often sent written advice and prescriptions. In 1761, Richard Bohun Baker consulted Garden about an enslaved woman who was probably suffering from a severe respiratory disorder. Garden sent detailed instructions for her treatment, along with several prescriptions. He complimented Baker on the accuracy of his description of the case and added a bit of caution: "I'm in hopes if the above course be carefully followed that it may be of service to the wench, but I should not advise you to think much of the want of success, for her case is very dangerous, especially as she is a new negro."[51] Garden's letters illustrate that healing was often a collaborative effort between a doctor and a member of the family. When Baker's son was ill of a fever in the fall of 1762, Garden

[50] St. Julien Ravenel Childs, "Kitchen Physick" Medical and Surgical Care of Slaves on an Eighteenth Century Rice Plantation," *Mississippi Valley Historical* Review 20 (1934), 549–553; *SCG*, March 27, 1742.

[51] Alexander Garden to Richard Bohun Baker, May 30, 1761, Baker-Grimke Papers, SCHS, 11/535–536.

was uncertain how to proceed because he considered Baker's description too vague. He sent Baker some powders to counteract the fever and recommended giving the boy a little wine if the fever subsided. Apparently Baker had bled the boy, for Garden added that he might take "a little more blood" if the state of the pulse and strength indicated it, "but this I will leave to your own discretion."[52]

As this episode shows, people on plantations and farms had to be prepared to perform many medical tasks. In the summer and fall of 1817, fevers, including yellow fever, were ravaging Barnwell District. When Sarah Ayer came down with "burning fevers and chills," her father, Lewis, was away from home and sick with fever himself. Her mother, Rebecca, gave Sarah a puke of hippo, and she improved. A few days later, she relapsed. Rebecca sent for the doctor, but he was away visiting other sick patients. By the time he came several days later, Sarah was better but still very weak. He complimented Rebecca on her treatment and directed her to continue it.[53] The outcome in this case may have been a happy one, but immense uncertainty and confusion reigned in the world of healing, be it professional, domestic, or alternative. The prospect could be frightening. In August 1817, The Charleston *Courier* published a letter recommending a tea of Seneka Snake Root and salts for yellow fever. The next day, a letter appeared in the paper protesting that the recipe was wrong and that taken in the way described, "death perhaps would soon be the fatal result."[54] A fatal death was a result to be feared, from yellow fever or its treatment. Confused and confronting a lack of effective medical remedies, many people looked for ways to avert disease through appeals to Providence and changes in behavior. Some simply counseled stoic resignation.

[52] Alexander Garden to Richard Bohun Baker, Oct.? 1762, Baker-Grimke Papers, SCHS, 11/535–536; Accounts of Henry Ravenel with Dr. William Keith (1755–1756) and Dr. Hugh Rose (1777) for medicines and medical treatments, Henry Ravenel Papers, SCHS, 43/07/09.

[53] Rebecca Ayer to Lewis Malone Ayer, Aug. 9, 1817, Sept. 7, 1817, Louis Malone Ayer Papers, SCL.

[54] *The Courier*, Aug. 11, 12, 1817.

10

Providence, Prudence, and Patience

Infidelity, profaneness, heresy, blasphemy, and the most offensive breaches of common morality, have scarce ever appeared with more insolence in that province, and tho' for these things the Lord does yearly visit, sending pestilential diseases among men and beasts, which yearly sweep away numbers of both, yet none regard those things.

Levi Durand, 1747

I did perceive that the fever and agues were generally gotten by carelessness in their clothing, or intemperance.... What I write is not to encourage any to depend upon natural causes, but prudently to use them with an eye to God, the Great Lord of the universe and dispenser of human affairs.

John Archdale, 1707

PROVIDENCE

In late November 1774, a delighted George Ogilvie wrote from Myrtle Grove plantation that his overseer's three-year-old son was "running about in his shirt rejoicing that the frost has killed the mosquitoes." Only the day before, the mosquitoes had been as thick as during the summer. Several earlier frosts had not "been severe enough to destroy these Devils in miniature." Neither Ogilvie nor anyone else at the time realized that mosquitoes were more than a source of annoyance and red, sometimes agonizingly itchy bumps.[1] But many people noticed that frost killed more than mosquitoes. If hard enough, it ended the seasonal reign of fever. Many people looked forward to "Dr. Frost" with pleasure. He might arrive later in some years than expected, but unlike the local doctors, his prescriptions were always effective. But frost was a force of nature and – nearly everyone agreed – the work of Providence.

[1] George Ogilvie to Margaret Ogilvie, Nov. 22, 1774, Ogilvie-Forbes of Boyndlie Papers, University of Aberdeen Archives.

Faced with medical treatments that were often of little help, many people combated disease through a combination of piety, prudence, and patience. They would have agreed with the Rev. Robert Maule who, after thanking God for his recovery from a severe bout of illness, declared, "I wholly resign myself up to the disposal of the Divine Providence."[2] Another minister, Michael Smith, lost his wife, one of his children, and two servants to fever a few months after coming to the lowcountry in the 1750s, but noted that it had "pleased God" to give him and other family members "the strength to get over the seasoning."[3] The Rev. William Hutson repeatedly thanked God for sparing him and his family during the "sickly season" of 1757. When his wife Mary later became ill, he castigated himself for despairing and not submitting patiently to God's will: "But, alas! I found my heart hard, very hard and stupid.... 'tis amazing that God should allow such an unworthy creature so large a shard of mercy." When his wife died, he reminded himself that he should be thankful that God had ever granted him a wife possessed of such "piety, prudence and good sense."[4]

These men were clergymen, but laypeople expressed similar thoughts. A Swiss immigrant who arrived in the 1730s and suffered numerous illnesses recorded that his "doctor in these perilous times was our Lord God, for I did not take medicine from men, but trusted to divine care." When doctors first used inoculation in Charleston, some people objected to it as interference with Providence. God had sent the smallpox, they proclaimed, and He would decide whether or not someone should be inflicted with it. For man to interfere would only anger God and make things worse. An opponent of inoculation protested that it was "the prerogative of God to preserve whom he will from that very distemper." Lewis Timothy, editor of the *Gazette*, claimed that inoculation spread the disease more than would have been the case if people had trusted Providence.[5]

Trusting Providence could be consoling. When Henrietta Heyward lost her son in 1819, her friend Mary Barnwell urged her to see it as an example of divine benevolence: "[H]owever dark and mysterious the dispensations of Providence are to you and I at present let us endeavour ... to trust that eventually these severe and trying afflictions may be sent for our benefit." God sent them "to lessen our interest in the world." The repeated losses of loved ones, Mary insisted, helped us "reflect on God's plan of salvation."[6] When a

[2] Robert Maule, March 6, 1708/9, SPG Letter Books, A4: 472; Klingberg, *Le Jau*, 182.

[3] Memorial of Rev. Michael Smith [1755?], SPG Letter Books, B5: 55.

[4] "A Faithful Ambassador: The Diary of William Hutson, Pastor of the Independent Meeting in Charleston, 1757–1761," ed. by Daniel J. Tortora, *SCHM* 107 (2006), 299–305; Anne Hart to Oliver Hart, May 14, 1785, Oliver Hart Papers SCL.

[5] R. W. Kelsey, "Swiss Settlers in South Carolina," *SCHM* 23 (1922), 89; *SCG*, Aug. 3, 1738; George Fenwick Jones, ed., *Detailed Reports on the Salzburger Emigrants Who Settled in America*. (Athens: University of Georgia Press, 1993), 17: 121.

[6] Mary Barnwell to Henrietta Manigault Heyward, Sept. 2, 1819, Heyward-Ferguson FP, COCSC.

young girl came down with yellow fever in the Charleston house of Alexander Robertson in late October 1838, near the end of the fever season, he wrote her aunt that for "poor Charlotte to be taken ill at this 11th hour when we were indulging the fond hope that all danger was over shews us the inscrutable ways of Providence, to whom we must at all times trust and confide." When the girl died, Robertson decided it was inevitable, for they had taken every precaution, keeping her confined in the house from the early part of August. God would have called her away "had she been anywhere, for taking all circumstances attending her case, we cannot come to any other conclusion."[7]

Providence could be vengeful. Often people simply said – as Governor Robert Johnson did after a yellow fever epidemic in 1732 – that God was "pleased" to afflict the community with pestilence, without examining His reasons for doing so. But many people explained epidemics as divine chastisement for collective sins. The Rev. Hugh Adams feared that the yellow fever epidemic of 1699 was the first of a series of "terrible impending judgments ... hovering over Carolina to be rained down in snares, fire and brimstone and a horrible tempest, as the portion of our cup for the yet tolerated and practiced abominations, and Sodom like sins of this land." The "destroying Angel" had "slaughtered ... furiously with his revenging Sword of Pestilence."[8] Quaker John Archdale explained the epidemic of 1706 as a sign of "the immediate Hand of God." The Lord was displeased with the recent "unchristian broils" in the colony, by which Archdale meant the nasty fight over the establishment of the Anglican Church. God had brought the settlers to "a land that flows with milk and honey," and now He had "brought a pestilential fever amongst" them. They needed to reflect that only "His infinite mercy" had spared them from worse.[9] Anglican Governor Nathaniel Johnson saw the events of 1706 a bit differently. In his view, God had rescued the Carolinians from their human and pestilential foes. The French and Spanish had attacked Charleston during the epidemic, but it had "pleased God not only to deliver us from the raging of the sickness, but also from the violence and malice of our public enemies by giving us victory over them."[10]

Anglicans and Dissenters might differ in their views of God's aims, but both saw His hand in epidemics. Gideon Johnston declared the epidemics of 1711 and 1712 "a kind of judgment upon the place (for they are a very sinful people)." His colleague Francis Le Jau blamed the diseases on the "irreligion and lewdness" of the people to which he added mistreatment of Indians and "barbarous usage of the poor slaves." As evidence, he cited a recent law decreeing castration for male slaves who ran away and cutting off of the ears for female runaways. Le Jau claimed that the law violated God's decrees. He added that

---

[7] Easterby, *South Carolina Rice Plantation*, 410–411.

[8] JCHA, Dec. 7, 1732, SCDAH; Extract of a letter from Hugh Adams to Samuel Sewell, Feb. 23, 1700, in Diary of Samuel Sewell, April 22, 1700, Massachusetts Historical Society, *Collections* 5th series, 6: 11–12.

[9] Salley, *Narratives*, 304, 308.

[10] JCHA, March 6, 1706/07, 3.

the reason slaves ran away was "immoderate labor and want of victuals and rest." He mentioned a master who punished slaves for "small faults" by chaining them for twenty-four hours in a "hellish machine," a "coffin where they are almost crushed to death" by a heavy lid pressing on their stomach. Le Jau also condemned the traders' habit of promoting wars among the Indians and then purchasing war captives as slaves. He hoped that God's visitations would turn their minds to "better things than worldly advantages," but they were slow to learn the error of their ways. Nine years after coming to the colony, he noted that he had seen many "frequent and dreadful visitations upon this place" but little "disposition to repentance."[11]

Later observers agreed, although the sins they condemned might differ. On a visit to Charleston in 1738, evangelical George Whitefield noted that "God's judgments have been lately amongst them by the spreading of the small-pox. I hope they will learn righteousness." The people seemed to be "wholly devoted to pleasure." Yellow fever, slave rebellion, a major fire, and an earthquake soon followed, giving Whitefield more fuel for his fiery sermons. When he returned to Charleston in 1740, he compared its misfortunes to those of Sodom and Gomorrah. He and his disciple Hugh Bryan also blamed the Anglican clergy's lack of evangelistic fervor and overattention to ritual for recent epidemics and other disasters.[12] Local Anglican ministers took up the refrain. Levi Durand of Christ Church cited "infidelity, profaneness, heresy, blasphemy, and the most offensive breaches of common morality" as the cause of recent epidemics, "for these things the Lord does yearly visit, sending pestilential diseases among men and beasts." No doubt gritting his teeth, Durand reminded himself that "he should endeavour to content himself with that province God had allotted him in one of the dark corners of the world even tho' amidst a perverse and crooked generation."[13]

To many religious folk, Charleston was a particular focus of divine displeasure. Salzburger leader Johann Bolzius wrote during a trip there in 1742, "I long to get out of this sinful city," as if he feared an imminent calamity.[14] Given recent disasters, the feeling was understandable. When smallpox exploded across the region in 1760, a Salzburger in Ebenezer, Georgia, commented that God was once again "chastising the Carolinians." He mocked their trust in inoculation and "a powder prepared with mercury." They recklessly ignored the Scripture-proven means of cure and prevention, "repentance and conversion."[15] Methodist leader Francis Asbury came to Charleston in

---

[11] Klingberg, *Johnston*, 99; Klingberg, *Le Jau*, 108–109, 153–154.
[12] *George Whitefield's Journals, 1737–1741* (Gainesville, FL: Scholars' Facsimiles & Reprints, 1969), 159–160; *The Fulham Papers in the Lambeth Palace Library; American Colonial Section Calendar and Indexes*, compiled by William W. Manross (Oxford: Clarendon Press, 1965), no. 150.
[13] Levi Durand, April 23, 1747, SPG Journals, 10: 287.
[14] George Fenwick Jones, "Johann Martin Boltzius' Trip to Charleston, October 1742," *SCHM* 82 (1981), 101.
[15] SCG, June 1, 15, July 13, August 3, 1738.

1795 to find that many of his friends in the city had recently "gone in eternity" in a recent yellow fever epidemic. The cause was obvious: "the unparalleled wickedness of the people." Those who came to the Methodist meetings were mainly women and Africans, along with some strangers. The "white and worldly" – mostly men – vexed him with their ignorance of God and their addiction to plays, balls, racing, and swearing. And yet, he marveled, these "sinners wonder that they have been afflicted." After a stay of two months, Asbury "left this seat of wickedness" with mixed feelings of "grief and joy." After his next visit, he referred to the city as the place of "the rich, rice and slaves; the last is awful to me." When Asbury came to Charleston in the fall of 1803, he found that several members of the Methodist society had perished of yellow fever. The news seemed to energize him: "[W]ho knows what God will yet do for wicked Charleston?" God's work was already having an effect: "[S]ome appeared to be in distress." The city, he added, was becoming "a paradise to me, and to some others." Clearly, the society had attracted some penitents courtesy of the divinely sent fever.[16] The idea that Charleston was a special object of divine wrath lasted well into the nineteenth century; indeed it still has advocates in the upper parts of the state, to judge by letters to its newspapers. So closely did yellow fever become associated with Charleston that upcountry statesman John C. Calhoun called it "a curse for their intemperance and debaucheries."[17] In 1838, The Charleston *Courier* more temperately referred to an epidemic as an affliction with "which an all-wise Providence has been pleased to chasten us."[18]

If God's anger brought pestilence, the natural response was to placate Him with prayer, repentance, and sacrifice. During epidemics, government leaders often proclaimed a day of repentance, urging people to fast and pray for God's mercy. The message was not only that the epidemic was in some sense divine punishment for the community's sins, but that what God had produced He could take away – if people were truly penitent. During the yellow fever epidemic of 1732, Governor Robert Johnson called for a day of fasting and prayer "to avert the present calamity." The *Gazette* reported that it was faithfully observed throughout the province. Such proclamations were routine during epidemics. On fast days, people flocked to their churches, where they would listen to jeremiads, sermons that traced communal misfortunes to divine displeasure with their behavior. On such a day in April 1760, proclaimed to combat the combined disasters of smallpox and war with the Cherokee, William Hutson suitably preached on the text of Jeremiah 5:9: "Shall I not visit for these things? saith the LORD: and shall not my soul be avenged on such a nation as this?" During the next few weeks, Hutson repeatedly returned to

[16] *The Journal of the Reverend Francis Asbury, 1771–1815* 3 vols. (New York, 1821), 2: 213–216, 241, 244, 278, 3: 120–122.

[17] Robert L. Meriwether, ed., *The Papers of John C. Calhoun 1801–1807* (Columbia: University of South Carolina Press, 1959), 28.

[18] *The Courier*, Oct. 23, 1838.

the theme of repentance. Days of "humiliation and prayer" continued to be proclaimed during nineteenth-century epidemics.[19]

People sometimes invoked Providence as a model whose lead humans would be wise to follow. In 1820, Joseph Johnson told the Medical Society that Charleston was spared from yellow fever that year because Providence had "kindly" arranged for "our drains to be cleansed of their fermenting contents" at the right time through copious rains. The city could achieve the same result artificially by flushing out the drains every few days in the absence of sufficient rainfall: "[W]ashing the drains, paving the streets, and filling wet cellars are within the power of Man."[20]

On a more individual level, people often blamed the sins of the victims for their illness: It was the result of imprudent or impious behavior, or perhaps a combination of the two. Some people blamed their own indiscretions. After a long bout of fevers, Le Jau recorded that "it has pleased Almighty God because of my sins to visit me with a tedious fit of sickness." People also blamed themselves for the sufferings of others.[21] Anne Deas was uncertain if her son's death from fever in 1815 was a divine punishment or a sign of divine favor: "[I]t is in vain to weary oneself with conjectures – it was God's will to take my beloved boy, and we must endeavor to bow with submission to his will. I sometimes think I must have been very bad to require such severe chastisement as I have met with. I derive consolation from believing that God loves those whom he chasteneth."[22]

Some people sought consolation in a stoical resignation. When an acquaintance died of yellow fever in 1748, Henry Laurens rationalized his death as man's fate: "Poor Capt. Gould just now quitted this troublesome stage of life. He died of a yellow fever which I fear will carry off many more. But why fear? We are born to die!"[23] A century later, Frederick Augustus Porcher put a cheery Panglossian spin on fever deaths: "The truth is, that disease, fevers particularly, come from God; to what end, we know not precisely, but a good one, we may be certain. If there were no fevers provided for us, we would be deprived of one of the means for quitting this world, and it is worse than useless to speculate upon the causes." Porcher conceded that fevers killed many children, but coolly – or callously – admonished his community: "Regard not their death. That is the debt of nature."[24]

[19] *SCG*, Aug. 5, 1732, June 29, 1738, April 7–12, 1760; Journal of His Majesty's Council of South Carolina, Jan. 29, 1728/29; "Diary of William Hutson," 87–88; Joshua B. Whitridge to Dr. William Whitridge, Rhode Island, Sept. 10, 1817, Whitridge Papers, SCHS; *The Courier*, Sept. 3, 11, 1817, Oct. 9, 1824, Oct. 31, 1827; *Charleston Mercury*, Sept. 10, 1824.

[20] MSM, Sept. 1, 1820.

[21] Klingberg, *Le Jau*, 34–37.

[22] A. I. Deas to Mrs. Manigault, Sept. 29, 1815, Manigault FP, SCL.

[23] *HLP*, 1: 171.

[24] Frederick Augustus Porcher, *Historical and Social Sketch of Craven County, South Carolina*, first published in *Southern Quarterly Review*, April 1852, reprinted in *A Contribution to the History of the Huguenots in South Carolina* by Thomas Gaillard, M.D. (New York, 1887; reprinted Columbia, SC: The R. L. Bryan Company, 1972), 159–165.

Porcher's views were probably unusual. He was a professor at the College of Charleston. Most folk were more likely to resort to prayer and charms than stoic philosophy. This was true even among the elite. In 1794, Elizabeth Drayton sent Susannah Carnes a charm for combating ague and fever. It appears to have been in circulation for several generations, for her mother had been told that it should be worn next to the skin. The charm consisted of a piece of paper with the following words: "When Jesus saw the place where his body was to be crucified, his body did shake, and the Jews asked Him, hast thou an ague? Jesus answered and said: whosoever shall be troubled with fever or ague, let him keep this in memory or writing, and he shall never be troubled with fever and ague more. So help me God, so be it."[25] As in most cultures, people often employed a mixture of natural and supernatural remedies supplied by reputed "witches," wise women, or African root and conjure doctors. One aspiring physician lamented the widespread resort to such superstitious practices, which of course could reduce his earning potential. He ascribed any improvement among those who used amulets and charms to their psychological influence on simple minds, or what today would be called the placebo effect.[26] Of course, the effect could apply to any therapy.

PRUDENCE

Recipes for good health routinely mixed piety with prudence. John Archdale advised prospective colonists to live temperately and prudently and acknowledge the divine power. They should not rely wholly on "natural causes" but use them "with an eye to God."[27] Peter Purry, Swiss promoter of the 1730s settlement of Purrysburg, blamed the colony's reputation for sickliness on the immoral and ignorant. Those who knew how "to regulate themselves suitably to the country" and observed the proper precautions had "as good health there as they would in other places." Purry conceded that "sudden changes of weather" helped cause fevers, but so did consuming too much punch and wine, eating unripe fruit (a remarkably common source of illness in the eyes of contemporaries), and unspecified "debauches." Careless, "sensual persons" took too many stimulants, exposed their bodies to extremes of heat and cold, and then blamed the country instead of themselves for the sickness that followed. If they lived regularly, avoided damp air, kept their breasts warm, and covered themselves well at night, especially in the summer, people would enjoy health as good as people anywhere. Many doctors agreed. Lionel

[25] Elizabeth Drayton to Susannah Carnes, March 4, 1794, SCHS, 43/884.
[26] Charles Joyner, *Down by the Riverside: A South Carolina Slave Community* (Chicago: University of Illinois Press, 1984), 144–150; Margaret Washington Creel, *A Peculiar People: Slave Religion and Community Among the Gullahs* (New York: New York University Press, 1988), 56–58; J.A. Moore, *On Intermittent Fever*, Medical Theses, WHL; Joshua Gordon "Witchcraft Book," 1784, SCL. I owe the Moore reference to David Brown.
[27] Salley, *Narratives*, 290.

Chalmers declared that local diseases were often precipitated by "some indiscretion or other in those who suffer."[28]

Advice as to what constituted the details of prudent behavior was often contradictory. Chalmers recommended a diet heavy in meat to avoid summer fevers. In contrast, Ramsay declared that eating too much animal food, especially in summer, was dangerous: Its tendency to putrefaction helped produce putrid diseases. If one insisted on meat, salted meat, being less liable to putrefaction, was preferable to fresh meat in summer. In the days before refrigeration, this was sensible advice but not likely to prevent the seasonal fevers. Another example of contradiction is advice about bathing. Ramsay urged regular cold bathing because it braced the system, which heat relaxed, against fevers.[29] A set of instructions for keeping soldiers healthy in the papers of General Benjamin Lincoln contains the recommendation that they keep their bodies clean by bathing often. However, in the summer of 1782, another general, Nathanael Greene, prohibited his soldiers from bathing in the Ashley River because his medical advisers claimed that it had "been found to increase the number of sick." Bathing in a sluggish river in a malaria-infested spot was certainly not prudent, although it is difficult to see how any soldier who spent the fever season camped in the area could have avoided infection. The records indicate most did not. The best advice commanders received was to avoid low, marshy areas and stagnant water, and camp in high, dry, windy locations. Unfortunately, that was difficult in the lowcountry.[30]

Other types of prudent action were of limited use. Chalmers declared that people who lived "in well-aired houses" and avoided "excesses or fatigues of any sort" were safer from fevers than people who lived "in small, damp houses," drank too much water, and ate "a low or less nourishing diet." He might have added that it is best not to be poor or enslaved.[31] Ramsay recommended cheerfulness as a major aid to preserving health, because an excess of bile was a major source of illness. He didn't explain how to stay cheerful.[32] John Shecut advised people to avoid "excessive labor" and "convivial assemblies" where one might overindulge in food and drink.[33] This advice was

---

[28] *Proposals by Mr. Peter Purry*, in B. R. Carroll, *Historical Collections of South Carolina* 2 vols. (New York, 1836) 2: 135–136; Lionel Chalmers to Benjamin Rush, Library Co. of Philadelphia, Rush Mss., vol. 23, folio 28, quoted in Waring, *Medicine in South Carolina, 1675–1825*, 68.

[29] David Ramsay, *A Dissertation on the Means of Preserving Health in Charleston, and the Adjacent Lowcountry* (Charleston, 1790), 6–26, 32.

[30] "Letters of Thomas Pinckney, 1775–1780," *SCHM* 58 (1957), 156; "Observations on the Means of Preserving the Health of Soldiers in the Camp," Benjamin Lincoln Papers, Boston Public Library, Reel 3-I; David B. Mattern, *Benjamin Lincoln and the American Revolution* (Columbia: University of South Carolina Press, 1995), 58; *NGP*, 11: 449.

[31] Lionel Chalmers, *An Account of the Weather and Diseases of South Carolina* 2 vols. (London, 1776) 1: 169.

[32] Ramsay, *Preserving Health*, 6–26, 32.

[33] J. L. E. W. Shecut, *Shecut's Medical and Philosophical Essays* (Charleston, 1819), 109, 168, 171.

not much help to the great majority of the population, who could not avoid excessive labor and were seldom invited to convivial assemblies.

Many doctors and others ascribed fevers to imprudent alcohol consumption, especially after the Revolution. In the 1780s, John Smyth blamed "the great intemperance" of the planters "and the excesses of every kind they are involved in" for deadly fevers and a surplus of wealthy widows. Women lived longer, he claimed, because they led more temperate lives.[34] A Hessian soldier charged that men hastened "their death by misusing alcoholic beverages, in which they seek relief and strength against the enervating effects of the hot climate."[35] Ramsay declared that spirits inflamed the blood and added fuel to the fire of an already hot climate. "The practice of drinking daily drams," he avowed, "has slain its thousands."[36] Samuel Henry Dickson, a teetotaler, agreed and explained that when it came to yellow fever, "for the intemperate there is almost no hope."[37]

Some types of drinking were perceived as more dangerous than others. John Moultrie, Jr. argued that "guzzling" copious amounts of spirits, combined with hard labor in the sun and exposure to the night air, made white laborers and seamen especially liable to yellow fever. They suffered more than the elite, who also drank abundantly but primarily "a strongly acid gentleman's drink called *Punch*." Moultrie claimed that it helped prevent fevers because it reduced the "alkalesence of the fluids" and promoted their expulsion through sweat and urination. Nevertheless, he agreed that the more temperate the life people led, the less susceptible to fevers they would be.[38] Conflicting advice about alcohol consumption was common. John Shecut claimed that Charleston natives who lived regular lives were generally safe from yellow fever, but if they were intemperate they might turn a remittent fever (malaria) into a full-blown case of yellow fever. Elsewhere, he argued that the intemperate and irregular were not more liable to an attack of yellow fever than their opposites. Experience had taught him that "the most delicate, temperate, and regular of both sexes" were equally susceptible.[39] To drink or not to drink, that was the question. Most seem to have drunk.

To further confuse matters, alcohol, as we have seen, was a common medication. Most prescriptions contained it and many recipes for healthy living

[34] J. F. D. Smyth, *A Tour in the United States of America* 2 vols. (London, 1784), 2: 53–54.

[35] Johann Conrad Döhla, *A Hessian Diary of the American Revolution*, ed. and trans. Bruce E. Burgoyne (Norman: Oklahoma University Press, 1990), 127. I owe this reference to Elizabeth Fenn.

[36] David Ramsay, *Preserving Health*, 6–26, 32.

[37] Henry L. Pinckney, *Report, Relative to the Proceedings for the Relief of the Sick Poor, during the Late Epidemic* (Charleston, 1838), quoted in Fraser, *Charleston! Charleston!*, 217; Samuel Henry Dickson, *Essays on Pathology and Therapeutics* (Charleston, 1845); M. Foster Farley, *An Account of the Stranger's Fever in Charleston South Carolina, 1699–1876* (Washington, DC: University Press of America, 1978), 114–120.

[38] Joseph I. Waring, "John Moultrie, Jr., M.D., Lieutenant Governor of East Florida, His Thesis on Yellow Fever," *Journal of the Florida Medical Association* 54 (Aug. 1967), 775.

[39] *The Courier*, July 9, 1803. The British doctors were Benjamin Moseley, Robert Jackson, and Colin Chisholm; Shecut, *Medical and Philosophical Essays*, 109, 168, 171.

proclaimed the prophylactic virtues of moderate alcohol consumption. John De Brahm maintained that only a "prudent and moderate use of spirits" could counteract the corrosive, fever-inducing "slime" that arose from stagnant waters and coated the stomachs of the inhabitants. Ardent "wholesome" spirits would "dulcify all corroding matters, otherwise apt to coagulate the humidities, relax the tonum, and cause putrefaction." (De Brahm surpassed the most erudite doctor in the obfuscation of his medical language.)[40] During the Revolutionary War, Col. Thomas Pinckney wrote home while on campaign in Georgia that his family need not fear for his health "as long as the rum holds out." Benjamin Lincoln, who later became Pinckney's commanding officer, noted that many people believed that drinking rum was an effective preservative of health in a hot climate. Lincoln's papers include a recipe for preserving soldiers' health in hot weather that recommends the use of alcohol in moderation. More useful was the advice to give the men "an infusion of bark in spirits" every morning and evening when they were on duty. Lincoln received a personal prescription from a doctor on how to avoid fevers. It included a mixture of Huxham's Tincture and Madeira wine at lunch. Huxham's tincture was a concoction of bark, rum, snakeroot, and spices. At dinner and other times, Lincoln was to take "quantum sufficient" of rum, spring water, lemon or lime juice and sugar. What "quantum sufficient" was awaits explanation, but prophylactic consumption of rum in the colonial lowcountry was high.[41]

When Benjamin West arrived from Massachusetts in the 1770s, locals advised him to drink grog [rum and water] if he wanted to stay healthy. But he considered Carolinians to be intemperate and chose a life of abstinence: "They tell me I can't possibly live in Carolina unless I drink grog, but I will try the experiment." He ate nothing but rice gruel for breakfast and supper for five months. At dinner he ate "sparingly and of the plainest food." He drank no spirits except on one occasion when he mixed wine with some salt water. He avoided the hot sun but walked about two miles just before sunset – a questionable strategy given the biting habits of mosquitoes.[42] Drinking rum as a fever prophylactic seems to have moderated after the Revolution. In the 1790s, David Ramsay noted a recent decline in punch drinking, which he believed – probably correctly – had reduced the incidence of dry belly ache. He urged moderate drinking of porter ale and wine. The latter was "highly antiseptic" and prevented and cured putrid diseases. Drinking a lot of strong tea, however, was "pernicious."[43]

Blaming disease on imprudent or irregular habits was routine. This was especially true if the people in question were immigrants, black, or poor

[40] John G. W. De Brahm, *Report of the General Survey in the Southern District of North America* ed. with an introduction by Louis De Vorsey, Jr. (Columbia: University of South Carolina Press, 1971), 79.

[41] Dr. Browne to Benjamin Lincoln, Oct. 14, 1778, Benjamin Lincoln Papers, Boston Public Library, reel 2.

[42] *Life in the South, 1778–1779: The Letters of Benjamin West*, ed. by James S. Schoff (Ann Arbor, MI: The William L. Clements Library, 1963), 23–25, 35.

[43] Ramsay, *Preserving Health*, 6–26, 32.

and lived in crowded and disreputable quarters. Doctors and planters often attributed the illnesses and deaths of the enslaved to their own carelessness. A student at the Medical College of South Carolina echoed this view when he cautioned planters not to build airtight houses for slaves because "their known negligence of habit, and natural laziness would cause them to live ignorantly in a foul atmosphere." Yellow fever epidemics often began in the crowded alleys near the Charleston waterfront and docks, where many poor whites lived in squalor. In the 1820s, Thomas Y. Simons hinted that an epidemic was due in part to a combination of urban and human filth: "The first cases were exhibited in a narrow dirty alley, occupied by debauched females, and sailors, and from thence it extended among the shipping, then generally attacking strangers and latterly children."[44] In 1838, Mayor Henry Laurens Pinckney explained the high mortality from yellow fever among poor whites as due to intemperance and "vicious and destructive habits." The city council called these places "hotbeds of infection" that should be regulated more closely.[45]

"Imprudent exposure" was a commonly alleged source of fevers. Many people warned against going outside in the fogs and dews of the morning and evening. This was good advice given the heavy activity of mosquitoes around dawn and dusk, but that was not the reasoning. Lincoln's doctor advised him not to expose himself to the night air of Carolina or ride out in the morning until the sun had dispelled the noxious, fever-inducing vapors.[46] Ramsay warned against walking on dew-covered grass. Wet feet, he insisted, were a source of fevers. Drafts were as well. Ramsay advised sleepers to keep their windows closed to avoid drafts. He conceded that the air of a closed room would soon become foul and suggested keeping the bedroom door open to an adjoining room with open windows. He also advocated wearing flannel in bed and elsewhere. Many people recommended wearing flannel next to the skin during the fever season, especially in the vicinity of rice fields or stagnant waters. Hot sun, chill air, and sudden changes of temperature were all dangerous.[47]

Moving about too much was also dangerous, because it might expose the body to rapid changes in temperature, moisture, and type of air. Chalmers argued that many fevers resulted from "shifting the climate; either by going into the country, or the contrary."[48] To Alice Izard, prudence meant staying in one place during the sickly months. She wrote of one family member that he

---

[44] F. Perry Pope, *A Dissertation on the Professional Management of Negro Slaves, 1837*, Medical Theses, WHL. Thomas Y. Simons, "Observations on the Yellow Fever, as it occurs in Charleston, South Carolina," *Carolina Journal of Medicine, Science, and Agriculture* 1 (1825), 2–3.

[45] Pinckney, *Relief of the Sick Poor*, quoted in Fraser, *Charleston! Charleston!*, 217; M. Foster Farley, *An Account of the Stranger's Fever in Charleston South Carolina, 1699–1876* (Washington, DC: University Press of America, 1978), 114–120.

[46] Dr. Browne to Benjamin Lincoln, Oct. 14, 1778, Benjamin Lincoln Papers.

[47] Ramsay, *Preserving Health*, 6–26, 32; *The Courier*, July 9, 1803.

[48] Chalmers, *Weather and Diseases*, 1: 169.

"recovered his health so well last summer, and his wife and children were so much better while they remained at their own place, that it would have been prudent for him to have remained there, could he have contented himself with a quiet life, but that he cannot do." Families sometimes shut themselves up in houses to wait out the fever season. During the yellow fever epidemic of 1838, the family of Rawlins Lowndes did this and escaped, but a young neighbor who did the same perished.[49]

Admonitions to sit still came into conflict, however, with another common strategy for preventing fever that we will examine more closely later. Around the 1750s, many planters began to think it imprudent to remain on their estates during the fever season. Failure to remove was not merely dangerous, it might be socially unacceptable. In 1769, Eliza Lucas Pinckney begged her son-in-law, Daniel Horry, to bring his family to town by the end of June, not just because they might become ill, but also because "people in general think it wrong ... I know (from what was formerly said) you would be blamed: and prudence dictates to us to defeat malice and envy as much as we can by giving them as little room as possible to display their malevolence."[50] What began as a disease prophylactic was becoming a social convention, perhaps even a sign of one's superior status, for most people white or black could not avail themselves of the prescription.

Despite the dangers, many planters continued to visit or even live on their plantations during the sickly months, often after removing their families. Charles Cotton declared that for such men, economic interest predominated over health, and they "regularly compound for a severe fever during the warm season."[51] This was true even of the wealthiest planters. In 1785, Henry Laurens wrote a friend that in spite of the danger of fever, he had to visit his plantation and stay for a couple of weeks. His son feared his father had endangered his health that summer by going to the country.[52] John Ball's family worried about his frequent warm weather visits to his plantations. Ball was acutely aware of the danger. He wrote his son, then at Harvard University, that the dangers he was exposed to "in this sickly climate by going up and down in order to attend to my business, and see my family, will probably shorten my life, or even cut me off ere you return."[53] In the 1820s, another planter, Gabriel Manigault, wrote that he had nearly died from an attack of country fever. Some of his friends had blamed a trip to his plantation, but "doctors differ," he noted.[54]

[49] Easterby, *South Carolina Rice Plantation*, 410; A. Izard to Mrs. Manigault, April 27, 1815, Manigault FP, SCL; Susan Blanding to Elizabeth Carter, Sept. 29, 1808, William Blanding Papers, SCL.
[50] "Letters of Eliza Pinckney, 1768–1782," *SCHM* 76 (1975), 143.
[51] "Letters of Charles Caleb Cotton," *SCHM*, 51 (1950), 132–144, 217.
[52] "Letters from Henry Laurens," *SCHM* 24 (1923), 9, 11.
[53] John Ball, Sr. to John Ball, Jr., Aug. 15, 1799, Jane Ball to John Ball, Jr., Sept. 4, 1798, Ball FP, SCHS, 11/516/10.
[54] Gabriel Manigault to Charles I. Manigault, Sept. 15, 1819, Manigault FP, SCL; Joyce Chaplin, *Anxious Pursuit: Agricultural Innovation and Modernity in the Lower South, 1730–1815* (Chapel Hill: University of North Carolina Press, 1993), 97.

Many people considered such behavior reckless among a class that had overseers to run their plantations. When Frederick Law Olmsted visited the lowcountry in the mid-1850s, he heard several cautionary and possibly apocryphal tales about the dangers of the rice country in the warm season. One told how a group of six ladies and gentlemen took a day trip from Charleston to a rice plantation on a nearby island. An accident to their boat prevented their return before nightfall. They shut themselves up in the house, sat around fires all night, and observed every prudent means of warding off the deadly miasma. In spite of their precautions, all of them contracted fever and four of them died within a week. If the story was true, the high and quick mortality makes yellow fever a more likely cause than malaria. The other story concerned two brothers who owned a plantation, where they lived during the winter. When summer approached, one was careful to leave for another residence, but the other stayed too long and caught a fatal fever.[55] Hetty Heyward told her mother in September 1817 that she was "perfectly astonished" to hear that her sisters were going to Pinckney's Island near Hilton Head. Heyward's reaction was a bit uncharitable: "I hope they won't get sick, but I think they deserve to have the fever and ague the whole winter." Heyward also condemned another form of risky behavior: returning to the fever districts before the frost. She rhetorically asked her mother "I suppose you don't expect to see Brother William before the middle of November as it certainly will be imprudent in their venturing back before that time." In another letter, she confessed that she was anxious about her husband Nathaniel, because she felt he had gone to his plantation too early, at the end of October. She had heard that several planters who had gone to their plantations the week before had come down with fever. Because they had not yet had a frost, she observed, the danger was as great as it had been all summer. People were mistaken to follow "the plan of going to the country on a certain day whether there is a frost or not." Similarly, a writer discussing fever cases in Pineville in 1808 blamed them on planters who imprudently visited their plantations during the warm months.[56]

Conversely, many people considered it the height of imprudence to go to Charleston when yellow fever was in town. In the case of malignant epidemics, the best advice had always been to "flee from the infected." During the yellow fever epidemic of 1739, Anglican Commissary Alexander Garden called on the missionaries serving rural parishes to come to Charleston to help the sick. Aiding the sick was one of the duties of Christian ministers, and most of the time they probably fulfilled it, but in this case most of them stayed away for fear of becoming victims themselves. Their fear was justified, even if their behavior was un-Christian. The one minister who answered Garden's appeal, Robert Small of Christ Church Parish, died within a week.[57] During the yellow

[55] Frederick Law Olmsted, *A Journey in the Seaboard Slave States* (New York, 1856), 419.
[56] Hetty Heyward to Mother, Sept. 13, Nov. 8, 1817, Heyward and Ferguson FP, COCSC; David Ramsay, *History of South Carolina* 2 vols. (Charleston, 1858; first ed., 1809), 2: 293–294.
[57] George W. Williams, ed. "Letters to the Bishop of London from the Commissaries in South Carolina," *SCHM* 78 (1977), 214.

fever epidemic of 1817, Charles Kershaw warned Charlotte Allston not to send her son from their Waccamaw plantation to the city to catch a ship to New York, but to have him land a few miles away at Sullivan's Island: "I would not have him visit Charleston on any consideration, for he would as certain take the strangers' fever as he now exists." If he went to the island and became infected anyway, "we could console ourselves with having done every thing that was prudent, but if he was to land in Charleston ... we might continually reflect what little care we took."[58]

One could exercise considerable care and still become ill as a result of a minor deviation from prudent behavior. During the same epidemic of 1817, Dr. Joshua Whitridge followed what he considered a prudent mode of life. Like most doctors at the time, he viewed corrupt air as the "predisposing cause" of yellow fever. Living in Charleston, he believed his system was predisposed by the fatigue of treating patients and saturation with the corrupting mephitic or marsh gases. To prevent infection, he needed to avoid any "exciting cause." But the evening before the illness struck, he recklessly went to a friend's for a bit of socializing and exposed himself to a draft. He caught a chill, which was "the exciting cause of my disease." That night he experienced chills and fever. He went out the next morning on his rounds, but was forced to return in the early afternoon, completely exhausted. After fruitlessly trying to make up medicines, he collapsed in his bed, from which he did not rise for twelve days.[59]

PATIENCE

Another strategy for coping with fevers was, quite simply, patience: waiting and hoping that they or their causes would eventually disappear. People quickly learned that the onset of cold weather would bring an end to the fevers. One observer claimed that the short winter of South Carolina was the only advantage it had over Jamaica: The occasional frost restored people's health and rid them for a time of the "abominable insects" that devoured them.[60] Lionel Chalmers phrased the well-known fact in a series of questions: "Why, when the weather becomes fifteen or twenty degrees colder ... [do] the sick oftentimes recover, who were it not for that change, must assuredly have died? Whence may it be, that the pestilential disease which we call yellow fever, shall put off its malignant disposition by degrees as the cool season advances, and be no more seen when the air is forty or a few more degrees colder than our blood?" Chalmers and other doctors explained the change as the result of cold bracing the bodily fibers. Whereas hot weather relaxed the fibers and thinned the blood, cooler temperatures strengthened the body by contracting the fibers and "condensing the blood."[61]

[58] Easterby, *South Carolina Rice Plantation*, 364.
[59] Joshua B. Whitridge to William Whitridge, Sept 21, 1817, J.B. Whitridge Papers, SCHS.
[60] Mary Inglis Hering to Mrs. Henry Middleton, Jan. 8, 1800, SCHS, 43/0034.
[61] Chalmers, *Weather and Diseases*, 2: 60–61.

Whatever they thought of such reasoning, people quickly learned that cold weather reduced their miseries. Every year, sufferers and their families waited out the sickly season in expectation of the frosts that would bring it to an end. Unlike northerners, who dreaded the onset of winter, people living in·the lowcountry positively longed for it as a kind of spring. As one observer put it, winter "is vulgarly called the great physician of the country, as by its force it clears the air of the putrid autumnal effluvia" and brings relief to sufferers of "obstinate intermittents."[62] In September 1776, Richard Hutson predicted that "cold weather will be more efficacious than pounds of bark in checking the fevers, and bracing our relaxed fibers."[63] Recovering from a severe bout of malaria in August 1782, Patriot Colonel Lewis Morris looked "forward with anxious expectation for the return of the frost, when my languid constitution and all who have suffered by the climate, will revive and return to their natural state." By late October, his longing was rewarded: "The *Good Doctor* [frost] has been generous in his attentions to us. This army already experiences the happy effects of his prescriptions."[64] They were lucky. In some years, frosts came much later, if at all.

Before the end of the nineteenth century, people did not know that the onset of cold weather brought relief by killing off the insect vectors of fever. Observers sometimes noted that the mosquito season and fever season coincided, but none suggested that the one might be the cause of the other before the nineteenth century. Lord Adam Gordon, a British officer stationed in South Carolina in the 1760s, came close to making the leap. He observed that the great quantity of stagnated water in the rice fields and swamps during the summer increased the number of insects and produced "fall fevers and agues, dry gripes and other disorders."[65]

Promoters of immigration tended to minimize the mosquito problem, much as they minimized the problem of disease. In the 1730s, Jean-Pierre Purry declared that few insects in Carolina were troublesome except what "they call muscatoes; and there is scarce any of these except in low grounds, or near the Rivers." That little problem was easily remedied "by opening the windows about sun-setting, and shutting them again a little before the close of the twilight." The mosquitoes would invariably leave the house around that time. In case some of them were boorish enough to remain, putting gauze curtains around one's bed would keep them off.[66] After reading this, it is easy

[62] Harry J. Carman, ed., *American Husbandry* (Port Washington, NY: Kennikat Press, Inc., 1964; originally published in London, 1775), 264–275.

[63] Hutson to John Godfrey, Sept. 26, 1776, Richard Hutson Papers, SCHS.

[64] "Letters of Col. Lewis Morris to Miss Ann Elliott," *SCHM* 40 (1939), 124, 41 (1940) 4; A. Izard to Mrs. Manigault, Oct. 19, 1815, Manigault FP, SCL; David R. Williams, to James Chesnut, Society Hill, Oct. 7, 1820, Williams – Chesnut – Manning FP, SCL.

[65] "Journal of Lord Adam Gordon," in Newton D. Mereness ed., *Travels in the American Colonies* (New York: The Macmillan Co., 1916), 399.

[66] *Proposals by Mr. Peter Purry*, 2: 136.

to sympathize with Purry's Swiss critics who called his description of South Carolina mendacious.

Others wrote more realistically of the mosquito problem. Alexander Hewatt observed how difficult it was for people to defend themselves against swarming millions of "pestiferous" mosquitoes. People sought various ways of warding them off, but complete escape was nearly impossible. Many people used gauze pavilions or nets.[67] Soldiers on marches and in camps were highly vulnerable to mosquitoes. When Thomas Pinckney was ordered to Sullivan's Island in July 1776 to help guard Charleston against the British, he asked his sister to procure a mosquito net for him, as he had heard that the mosquitoes were numerous there. Later he told her he had lost much sleep due to the "mosquitoes which have quartered themselves on this unfortunate island (as their Brother Blood Suckers of Great Britain would fain do on the whole continent)."[68] Pinckney's comparison was understandable, but he erred in describing the mosquitoes and British as common enemies. As we have seen, the mosquitoes proved to be one of the revolutionaries' greatest allies.

[67] Hewatt, *South Carolina and Georgia*, 1: 88; A. I. Deas to Mrs. Manigault, Oct. 8, 1813, Manigault FP, SCL; Shecut, *Medical and Philosophical Essays*, (Charleston, 1819), 99; George Ogilvie to Margaret Ogilvie, Nov. 22, 1774, Ogilvie-Forbes of Boyndlie Papers, University of Aberdeen Archives.

[68] "Letters of Thomas Pinckney, 1775–1780," *SCHM* 58 (1957), 72–74.

Buying the Smallpox

Spoiler of Beauty! For this once forbear,
To print thy Vengeance on this blooming Fair,
O spare these brilliant Eyes, that Angel's Face,
Nor Heaven's fair Portrait with thy Spots disgrace.
Wisely determin'd to prevent the Foe,
Nor wait unguarded to sustain the Blow,
*Bravely resolved the doubtful war to wage,
She mocks thy Fury, and eludes thy Rage;
In perfect Lustre soon again she'll shine,
+With H____ and A____ in the Train divine:
They too, escaped the Danger of thy Harms,
In pristine Beauty glow, and wonted charms.
Thus a slight Hurt upon the Trojan Plain,
Venus received from Diomede – in vain!
The Wound soon clos'd again, no Scar remain'd,
And Queen of Beauty still the Goddess reign'd.

* Inoculated
+ Two Ladies recently inoculated, now in perfect Health
  "Address to the Small-Pox," *South Carolina Gazette*,
                                            April 19, 1760

"FEW OF THEM HAVE HAD IT"

Dr. Thomas Morritt, master of the Charleston free school, found himself with little to do. An outbreak of smallpox in 1723 had stripped his school of all but a few pupils. Rural people were afraid to send their children into town.[1] Their fear was understandable, given the deaths and disfigurements smallpox caused. Moreover, no effective treatment existed – then or now. In 1772, the family of Alexander Chesney landed in Charleston on their way to the backcountry. On the voyage from Ireland, some passengers had come down with smallpox. On arrival, the ship and passengers were put into quarantine at Sullivan's Island

---

[1] "Thomas Morritt and the Free School in Charleston," *SCHM* 32 (1931), 39.

for seven weeks, and then disembarked several miles north of the city, before making their way inland. Chesney observed that there was "no disorder the Americans are so afraid of as the smallpox ... as few of them have had it."[2]

The Americans' fear of smallpox was indeed strong, and it was justified. In densely populated parts of Europe, smallpox was endemic. It was primarily a childhood disease, because survival normally confers immunity. But in more sparsely populated areas of Europe and in the Americas, it remained an episodic epidemic disorder that could threaten a large part or all of the population. Epidemics in such places were often spaced fifteen-to-twenty or more years apart, which allowed the number of susceptible people to grow. As a result, smallpox attacked many adults and could virtually prostrate a community for months. Smallpox could bring commerce to a standstill for an even longer period, creating huge economic problems for a busy port like Charleston, heavily dependent as it was on the flow of goods and people to and from the region.

Smallpox is an acute, highly contagious, viral disease. It killed and disfigured untold millions of people globally before the World Health Organization declared it eradicated in 1977. The characteristic symptoms include fever; external and sometimes internal eruptions with pustules (the "pox"); sloughing and scarring of skin; and internal and external hemorrhaging. During the sixteenth century, a virulent form of smallpox (*variola major*) seems to have developed and spread around the globe. With the decline of plague in Western Europe in the late seventeenth century, smallpox became perhaps the world's most feared epidemic disease because it killed up to 25 percent or more of the infected, blinded some survivors, and scarred many with facial pock marks.[3]

Smallpox arrived in the lowcountry via ship from Europe, Africa, and the Caribbean, and by sea or land from other parts of North America. Major epidemics struck Charleston and its hinterland several times between 1697 and the 1860s, with the worst coming before 1800. During epidemics, ships avoided the place and so did people from the surrounding country, imperiling not only local commerce but food supplies and defense in time of war. In 1711, when Britain was at war with France and Spain, the assembly discussed the need to find some method to prevent the introduction of smallpox lest it "cause the country people to desert the town."[4] Most smallpox epidemics occurred

[2] *The Journal of Alexander Chesney, a South Carolina Loyalist in the Revolution and After*, ed. E. Alfred Jones; *The Ohio State University Bulletin*, (1921) 26: 2–3; SCG, Aug. 20,1772.
[3] Donald R. Hopkins, *Princes and Peasants: Smallpox in History* (Chicago: University of Chicago Press, 1983); Ian and Jennifer Glynn, *The Life and Death of Smallpox* (New York: Cambridge University Press, 2004), 37–39; Genevieve Miller, *The Adoption of Inoculation for Smallpox in England and France* (Philadelphia: University of Pennsylvania Press, 1957); Ann G. Carmichael and Arthur M. Silverstein, "Smallpox in Europe Before the Seventeenth Century: Virulent Killer or Benign Disease?" *Journal of the History of Medicine* (1987) 42: 148–168; Frank Fenner, D. A. Henderson, et al., *Smallpox and Its Eradication* (Geneva: World Health Organization, 1988).
[4] JCHA, Oct. 26, 1711, SCDAH.

during wars: in 1697–1698, 1711–1712, 1738–1739, 1759–1760, 1763, and 1779–1781. Quarantine and the isolation of infected persons was one method the colony adopted to keep the disease at bay. It was an old and well-established tradition, if always controversial. It also contained its own danger. If successful for many years, quarantine created the potential for a devastating epidemic by allowing the proportion of susceptible people to increase.

During the 1730s, the inhabitants began to use a new method of prevention mentioned in earlier chapters: inoculation. It was sometimes called "buying" or "purchasing" the smallpox – in contrast to natural infection. After 1800, inoculation gradually gave way to vaccination, which British doctor Edward Jenner began to promote in the late 1790s. This procedure involved "buying" a related and much milder disease, often called cowpox. The disease was actually horse-pox, a now extinct infection that farm workers sometimes got and spread from horses to cows. Milkmaids – and some who weren't maids – often contracted it from milking infected cows. Jenner noticed that such people never seemed to get smallpox. A few other doctors had observed the same effect and used the procedure locally before Jenner. But he promoted it far more effectively and got the credit, a knighthood, and a huge reward from Parliament. Jenner's method involved placing material from the cowpox pustules under the skin in the same manner as inoculation. Vaccination – from the Latin *vacca* (cow) – was safer than inoculation, and many physicians in Europe and the Americas quickly adopted it.[5] Both reduced the ravages of smallpox, and both aroused opposition, especially inoculation, the main focus of this chapter.

Arguments against inoculation shifted considerably over time. Opponents mounted three main arguments, ones that would have been familiar to contemporaries in Britain and its colonies. The first was discussed in the previous chapter: that inoculation was an interference with Providence, with God's power to decide whether to inflict a disease on someone or not. The second argument was medical and focused on its danger to individuals: It killed or disfigured people who might have escaped the natural disease altogether. This argument sometimes divided medical men themselves, especially in 1738. The third argument was both medical and economic: Inoculation could spread the disease and prolong an epidemic, bringing both physical and economic suffering to a community.[6] The arguments against inoculation gradually shifted in a way that reflected changes in religious, medical, and political thinking. In 1738, opponents used all three arguments, but placed the most emphasis on the religious objections and the danger to inoculated individuals. In the 1760s, opponents no longer focused much on these arguments. Instead, they

---

[5] Waring, *Medicine in South Carolina, 1670–1825*, 132–133, 155–156, 229, 294–297, 309; Hopkins, *Princes and Peasants*, 8–9, 77–78.

[6] Genevieve Miller, *Adoption of Inoculation*, 100–133; Elizabeth Fenn, *Pox Americana: The Great Smallpox Epidemic of 1775–82* (New York: Hill and Wang, 2001), 36–39; Hopkins, *Princes and Peasants*, 46–51, 59–59, 246–247.

emphasized the threat of *uncontrolled* inoculation to the medical, economic, and even political welfare of the broader community. During the Revolution, inoculation aroused little if any opposition, but conditions were far more chaotic.

Opponents had little success against inoculation at the height of a smallpox epidemic. Fear of the disease trumped the arguments against the procedure, and people willing to inoculate for a fee were never wanting. When the epidemic began to wane, however, opposition arguments carried more weight. At this point, the strongest argument against inoculation was that it was keeping the disease alive or might even revive it. Opposition on these grounds was more economic than medical. The presence of smallpox brought about a virtual cessation of the commerce by land and sea that Charleston depended and thrived upon. Exchanges of goods, labor, and services within the local economy declined as people susceptible to the disease avoided the town. A town as dependent on the global economy as Charleston could not tolerate such a situation for long. No one had more to lose from this situation than the merchant and planter elite. During the epidemic of 1763, however, those opposed to the continuation of inoculation in Charleston mounted a new, essentially political objection. They denounced it in broader political terms that a few years later would be used to condemn the actions of the British government. They argued that allowing doctors to continue to inoculate against the will of the community was a violation of "natural justice" and the "general welfare." The word "continue" is critical in this context, and "opponents" should be understood in situational rather than absolute terms. Many of those who sought to bring an end to inoculation, especially in the 1760s, had already used it to protect their families and sometimes their slaves. At some point, however, they became convinced that to continue inoculation threatened the basis of their prosperity. In each epidemic, the opponents were able to halt inoculation in Charleston.

MASS INOCULATION

On May 4, 1738, the *South Carolina Gazette* reported that some slaves who had recently arrived on board the ship *London Frigate* from West Africa had come down with smallpox. The slaves had already been sold, but the Governor's Council ordered their masters to return them to the ship, which was quarantined off Fort Johnson. Attempts to contain the epidemic failed and by midsummer it had spread widely in the town and surrounding country.[7] It infected more than 2,000 people in Charleston alone, about one-third of the population. It killed between 300 and 400 there before moving inland and destroying about half of the Catawba Nation and perhaps one-third of the

[7] SCG, May 4, 11, 1738, James Kilpatrick, *An Essay on Inoculation* (London, 1743), 31; Walter B. Edgar, ed., *The Letterbook of Robert Pringle*, 2 vols. (Columbia: University of South Carolina Press, 1972), 1: 18, 20, 25–26, 44, 52.

Cherokee. As we have seen, it also led to perhaps the largest mass inoculation to that point in British North America. James Kilpatrick later estimated
the number inoculated at between 800 and 1,000 and claimed that this was
more than anywhere in the British Empire or Europe, except in the Ottoman
Empire, during such a short period of time. This may not be true. Another
source claimed that as many as 3,000 people were inoculated in Barbados
the same year.[8] But thanks to Kilpatrick's writings, South Carolina's inoculations became widely known in Britain and Europe. He placed the death rate
from inoculation in Charleston in 1738 at about 1 percent of those inoculated.
The *Gazette* – whose printer, Lewis Timothy, was no friend of inoculation –
claimed the death rate was about 3 percent. In contrast, the death rate for
the natural disease was around 15–20 percent of the infected and sometimes
much higher.[9]

Inoculation was discussed in South Carolina before 1738. When a few
smallpox cases occurred in 1732, an article in the *South Carolina Gazette*
explained the procedure for its readers. The author noted that numerous
observations had shown it to be effective and usually safe for the inoculated
individuals, but recommended against its use because of the danger of spreading the disease throughout the community.[10] In 1738, inoculation began soon
after the first cases of smallpox were confirmed. On May 21, naval surgeon
Arthur Mowbray inoculated three young girls who came through the process
without much difficulty. The fact that the first to undergo inoculation were
adolescent girls is significant: a pock-marked face reduced a woman's value in
the marriage market.[11] As we have seen, James Kilpatrick defended Mowbray's
action in a series of articles in the *Gazette*. He began by asking for tolerance
on both sides. In the midst of such a terrible epidemic, everyone wanted to
do what was best to protect their families. The most compelling motive for
inoculation, he argued, was not profit but fear. No one would risk inoculation
unless smallpox was actually present in the community. The high fatality rate
and disfigurement the disease caused created demand for the procedure. "Did
any of the people of Charlestown inoculate last year," he asked, "for fear the
small-pox should be brought from Guinea amongst them this [year]?"[12]

[8] Kilpatrick, *Essay on Inoculation*, 31; James Kirkpatrick, *Analysis of Inoculation* (London,
    1754); SCG, Oct. 5, 1738; Larry Stewart, "The Edge of Utility: Slaves and Smallpox in the
    Early Eighteenth Century," *Medical History* 29 (1985), 70; Richard B. Sheridan, *Doctors and
    Slaves: A Medical and Demographic History of Slavery in the British West Indies, 1680–
    1834* (Cambridge: Cambridge University Press, 1985), 252.
[9] In Boston in 1721–1722, more than 200 were inoculated and 6 died. In 1730, 400 were inoc-
    ulated, with 12 deaths. Around 130 persons were inoculated in Philadelphia in 1736–1737,
    and 1 died. John B. Blake, "Smallpox Inoculation in Colonial Boston," *Journal of the History
    of Medicine and Allied Sciences*, 8 (1953), 286–287; Blake, "The Inoculation Controversy
    in Boston, 1721–22"; Duffy, *Epidemics In Colonial America* 26–36; Kilpatrick, *Essay on
    Inoculation*, 11, 34; SCG, Oct. 5, 1738.
[10] SCG, April 15–22, 1732.
[11] SCG, July 20, 1738, Feb. 2, 1747; Kilpatrick, *Essay on Inoculation*, 44.
[12] SCG, Aug. 31, 1738.

Kilpatrick's advocacy of inoculation then and later creates a potential problem for anyone seeking to understand its use in 1738. He wrote the only detailed account of the episode and he had an incentive to present the results in the most favorable light possible. However, many Carolinians later agreed that inoculation in 1738 had been highly successful. Kilpatrick claimed that he had refrained from inoculating at first for fear he would be accused of spreading the disease and only began after one of his children died of natural smallpox.[13] His fears of public hostility were well founded. Immediately after inoculation began, some people blamed the inoculators for spreading the disease. Lewis Timothy declared that the number of cases might have been smaller if people had trusted to Providence and taken prudent measures to prepare their bodies in case of infection – presumably with tar water, the remedy Timothy was then promoting in his newspaper. But some people, "being fond of having" smallpox, had selfishly chosen to be inoculated, to the great peril of the community. In mid-June, the newspaper reported that the disease had become more epidemic since inoculations had begun, and that several deaths had occurred among those who had been inoculated. Timothy implicitly questioned the motive as well as the method of the inoculators. If they wanted to show that they sought the general good and not just an increased income, they needed to keep an accurate account of deaths by inoculation and by natural smallpox. By this means they could show whether "purchasing" artificial smallpox was preferable to resigning oneself to the will of God. Other opponents of inoculation aired their views in the *Gazette*, reiterating and expounding on Timothy's arguments.[14] Kilpatrick rejected the argument. Reason, he argued, dictated that men had a duty to use all natural and moral means to preserve life and then put their trust in God. Inoculation was no more inconsistent with this duty than employing a physician and no more harmful than many standard medical remedies. Using religious arguments to prohibit it was a violation of sound theology. Inoculation was no more a violation of God's prerogative than staying away from the infected.[15]

In the end, opponents of inoculation prevailed. At the end of August, the colonial council declared that allowing country people to come to Charleston to be inoculated would keep smallpox circulating there. The council's concern was probably more economic than medical, because the epidemic had stifled trade for months. In September, the provincial assembly passed an act prohibiting inoculation for one year within two miles of Charleston, with violators subject to a fine of 500 pounds. The primary declared justification of the act was military. War was looming between Britain and Spain, the so-called War of Jenkins' Ear. The assembly was concerned that the continued presence of the disease in the town through inoculation would deter country people from coming to

[13] Edgar, *Letterbook of Robert Pringle*, 1: 20, 26, 44, 52; Kilpatrick, *Essay*, 28, 42, 44–45; Kirkpatrick, *Analysis*, 111, 134.

[14] SCG, June 1, 15; 1738; see also, June 29, July, 13, Aug., 3, 1738.

[15] SCG, June, 8, 15, July 6, Aug. 10, 17, 24, 31, 1738.

Charleston's aid in case of a Spanish attack. The rationale conflicted oddly with the council's claim that inoculation was attracting country people to town.[16]

The geographic and chronological limits on the prohibition indicate that the ruling elite had not rejected inoculation itself, but rather its continuation in Charleston. Indeed, many elite families had their children inoculated in Britain or the North during the following decades. Locally, families sometimes held "inoculation parties" at a house, where several young people would be inoculated at a time, and could spend the time together to relieve the tedium and isolation of a process that could last several weeks.[17] Most people probably chose to forego the procedure because of the danger, expense, inconvenience, and public hostility it might arouse. When smallpox returned in the 1760s, however, it produced a sudden and enormous demand for inoculation.

"INOCULATION MAD"

Between 1738 and 1760, Charleston was free from epidemic smallpox, but the threat was never absent for long. Ships, especially slave ships, often arrived with smallpox cases on board. Quarantine of ships found to have smallpox cases and isolation of the infected at the pest house on Sullivan's Island kept the disease out of the town. Or perhaps the town was just lucky.[18] But like a fort with guns pointing only in one direction, quarantine of ships could not protect against another danger: that smallpox might arrive by land. In 1749, a Chickasaw embassy was coming to Charleston when reports arrived that smallpox had broken out in their country (mainly in Mississippi and Alabama). A panicked colonial assembly debated how they could turn them back without offending them. In 1755, a correspondent of the *Gazette* pointed out that there was no law to prevent the introduction of contagious diseases by travelers from Georgia or North Carolina. Smallpox had been present in Georgia for some time, and if someone brought the infection from there, he declared, "all our precautions by sea" would be worthless. The writer suggested that the assembly should adopt the German practice of requiring travelers to carry certificates of health.[19] Nothing came of this suggestion, but the fear that

[16] Journals of His Majesty's Council, Aug. 30, 1738, SCDAH; Journals of the Upper House of Assembly of South Carolina, Sept. 12, 1738, SCDAH; *Stats.*, 3: 513

[17] Edgar, *Letterbook of Robert Pringle* 1: 26, 44; "Peter Manigault's Letters," ed. by Mabel L. Webber, *SCHM*, 31 (1930), 175; 32 (1931), 176; Peter Manigault to Ann Manigault, Oct. 10, 1750, July 13, 1751, Manigault Papers, SCHS, 11/275/6, 8; "Letters Concerning Peter Manigault," *SCHM* 21 (1920),43; Gabriel Manigault to Ann Manigault, Sept. 28, 1774, Manigault FP, SCL; *HLP*, 7: 482–483; 8: 16, 75, 127–128, 325, 624; 10: 139, 264; *The Letterbook of Eliza Pinckney, 1739–62*, ed. by Elise Pinckney (Chapel Hill: University of North Carolina Press, 1972), 75, 109, 131–134, 143–145, 160–161; Kirkpatrick, *Analysis of Inoculation*, 2d edition, 1761, 148; 276–280; Harriott H. Ravenel, *Eliza Pinckney* (New York: Scribners, 1925), 141–143.

[18] Council Journals, July 1, 31, Sept. 16, 1745, SCDAH; *JCHA*, March 10, 1752; *HLP*, 1: 250–251, 2: 43, 64, 179, 546; *SCG*, May 21, 1759; Henry Bouquet Collection, British Library, Add. 21631, June 23, 1757.

[19] *JCHA*, 9: 293, 298, 304–306; *SCG*, March 13–20, 1755.

smallpox might arrive by land remained. In 1758, the *Gazette* noted that it was spreading in the backcountry around Augusta, Georgia. The following May (1759), the newspaper reported that the smallpox had broken out among "the Chickasaw and some other Indians." The editor, however, assured readers that the disease was mild in form, and that the governor, William Henry Lyttleton, had issued "the necessary orders" to prevent its spread to South Carolina. A few weeks later, the newspaper reported that the smallpox had retreated from Augusta and had subsided among the Chickasaw.[20]

Celebration was premature. Within a few months, a devastating smallpox epidemic spread throughout the colony. As some people had feared, it came from the interior. In November 1759, Governor Lyttleton led a military expedition from Charleston to the Cherokee town of Keowee, in northwestern South Carolina. His goal was to punish a group of warriors who had killed some backcountry settlers. Virulent smallpox was raging through the interior and had already killed about one-half of the Catawba Nation. When the colonial army reached Keowee in early December, the disease had broken out among the Cherokee. To keep it from spreading to his men, many of whom were already battling measles, Lyttleton forbade them to enter the town or for the Cherokee to enter the army's camp without his authority. He also demanded that the Indians burn the houses and clothes of those who had been infected with smallpox and remove the ill to a location several miles away. They complied, and agreed to his terms, which included the surrender of two of the alleged murderers and a promise to deliver the others. With the spread of measles and the fear of smallpox, Lyttleton's army began to disintegrate. Some soldiers fled and many others threatened to do so. Lyttleton decided that he could not wait for the arrival of the other twenty-two alleged murderers. He demanded and received hostages and prepared to remove his army. About two days later, smallpox broke out in the army's camp.[21]

While the army straggled back in disorder, amid hunger and disease, the governor returned to Charleston and a hero's welcome, to the astonishment of several locals. Not only were the returning soldiers spreading smallpox throughout the colony, but open war had broken out with the Cherokee. As Alexander Garden put it a few weeks later, "[o]ur governor returned from the Cherokee country in January, as we then thought crowned with laurels; but alas, bringing pestilence along with him, and having war at his heels. The soldiers that came down with him brought a most fatal and malignant smallpox." In early January, the disease broke out at one of John Drayton's plantations near Charleston.[22]

[20] *SCG*, June 30, 1758, May 21, 1759, June 30, 1759; "A Faithful Ambassador: The Diary of William Hutson, Pastor of the Independent Meeting in Charleston, 1757–1761," ed. by Daniel J. Tortora, *SCHM* 108 (2007), 82–86.

[21] *SCG*, Dec. 29, 1758–Jan. 12, 1759; Milligen-Johnston, *Short Description*, 84–85.

[22] *SCG*, Dec. 15, 22–29, Dec. 29–Jan. 5, Jan. 8–12, 1759; Milligen-Johnston, *Short Description*, 84–85; James E. Smith, *A Selection of the Correspondence of Linnaeus and Other Naturalists* 2 vols. (New York: Arno Press, 1978) 1: 552; George Fenwick Jones, ed., *Detailed Reports on the Salzburger Immigrants Who Settled in America* (Athens: University of Georgia Press,

At first, some Charlestonians viewed the disease as a potential ally against the Cherokee. On January 19, the *Gazette* reported that smallpox had "destroyed a great many" of them at Keowee, and the uninfected had fled into the woods, "where many of them must perish as the Catawba did." At the same time, the paper noted that smallpox had broken out in Charleston, but in only one house, which was immediately put under quarantine. The newspaper was confident that the authorities had taken "every other precaution necessary" to keep the disease from spreading.²³ Garden harbored no such illusions. A few days after the governor's return, he wrote to John Ellis in London: "We are just now on the eve of having the smallpox. We have not had it for [22 years], so that there must be more than two thirds of the people to have it."²⁴

By early February, Garden's prediction was proving accurate. The disease was spreading rapidly.²⁵ Factor Robert Raper predicted disaster: "[V]ery few of this country have had [the smallpox], therefore I am afraid it will make a great havoc among them." People who could began to flee. On February 10, William Hutson, minister of the Independent (Congregational) Church, recorded that the disease "flew about the place so fast that I thought my duty by and with the advice of friends to remove my family to James Island." He was concerned about his wife, who was close to delivering a child. The move did not save her; she died several days later.²⁶ The rapid spread of the epidemic, along with daily reports of Cherokee attacks on the backcountry settlers, produced a sense of gloom. The people, Raper reported, were "low spirited." Eliza Pinckney noted: "A great cloud seems at present to hang over this province."²⁷ Garden's description of the situation was almost apocalyptic. In his view, the governor's ambition and folly had precipitated an appalling crisis in which the colony was threatened by three powerful opponents at once: the Cherokee, the smallpox, and – at least potentially – the slaves.²⁸

The epidemic severely disrupted the local economy. Many people fled to the country, and business and other contacts between Charleston and surrounding

---

1993), 17: 117; William Simpson to John Drayton, Drayton Hall, Jan. 14, 1760, ALS, SCL. On the Cherokee War, see Tom Hatley, *The Dividing Paths: Cherokee and South Carolinians through the Era of Revolution* (New York and Oxford: Oxford University Press, 1993); John Oliphant, *Peace and War on the Cherokee Frontier, 1756–1763* (Baton Rouge: Louisiana State University Press, 2001); David H. Corcoran, *The Cherokee Frontier: Conflict and Survival, 1740–62* (Norman: University of Oklahoma Press, 1962).

²³ *SCG*, Jan. 19, Jan. 26, 1760. See also, Suzanne Krebsbach, "The Great Charlestown Smallpox Epidemic of 1760," *SCHM* 97 (1996), 30–37.

²⁴ James E. Smith, *A Selection of the Correspondence of Linnaeus and Other Naturalists* 2 vols. (New York: Arno Press, 1978) 1: 552.

²⁵ *SCG*, Feb. 9, 1760, Feb. 16, 1760.

²⁶ Robert Raper to John Colleton, Feb. 9, 1760, Robert Raper Letterbook, 1759–1770, SCHS, 34/511; "Diary of William Hutson," 82.

²⁷ Robert Raper to John Colleton, Feb. 9, 1760, Raper Letterbook, SCHS, 34/511; Pinckney, *Letterbook*, 147–148.

²⁸ Smith, *Correspondence of Linnaeus*, 1: 473–475; *SCG*, Jan. 19, Jan. 26, Feb. 9, 16, 1760; Robert Raper to John Colleton, Feb. 9, 1760, Raper Letterbook, SCHS, 34/511.

districts were greatly restricted.[29] Colonel Archibald Montgomery, who arrived in April 1760 to command a British expedition against the Cherokee, confirmed the chaotic conditions: "This place has been in great distress with the smallpox, few people have escaped it, many died, and the people in the country, afraid of the disorder spreading amongst their Negroes, are unwilling to have any communication with the town or the people that come from it." Montgomery prudently kept his Highlanders away from Charleston. He disembarked them seven miles north of the city, and then marched them to Moncks Corner, about thirty miles to the northwest.[30]

Mass inoculation began almost immediately after the outbreak of the disease. On February 2, a letter to the *Gazette* advocated inoculation, citing its success in 1738. He had probably read Kilpatrick's essay on the epidemic because he cited the latter's statistics on inoculation exactly. He had also been one of those inoculated in that year and "passed thro' the disease, in the mildest manner, under the care of one of them; and the smooth faces of hundreds of other people, will shew that they did likewise."[31] Members of the elite who had accepted inoculation in 1738 were quick to employ it in 1760, but most other citizens were demanding it, too. On February 11, Robert Pringle had seven family members and relations inoculated. During the next few days, five of his house slaves were inoculated, and two more on April 1.[32] On February 14, another supporter of inoculation, Ann Manigault, wrote in her journal that she had had her entire family inoculated, which probably included her house slaves. Eliza Pinckney claimed that the people had gone "inoculation mad." They "rushed into it with such precipitation that I think it impossible they could have had either a proper preparation or attendance." The doctors had no choice but to meet the demand: "[T]he people would not be said nay."[33]

The demand for inoculation overwhelmed the doctors. Garden reported that "many more people were inoculated than could be attended by the practitioners of physic." He estimated that between 2,400 and 2,800 people were inoculated in less than two weeks, in a town of perhaps 10,000 residents. The total number of inoculations was variously reported at 3,000 to more than 3,500.[34] Lionel Chalmers estimated that more than 6,000 people had been infected, about 2,500 naturally and more than 3,500 by inoculation. Deaths

[29] Pinckney, *Letterbook*, 147–148; Robert Raper to John Colleton, April 3, May 22, 1760, Raper Letterbook, SCHS, 34/511; Smith, *Correspondence of Linnaeus*, 1: 473–475; *Pennsylvania Gazette*, March 6, 1760; "Diary of William Hutson," 84.

[30] Archibald Montgomery to Lord Amherst, April 12, 1760, James Grant to Lord Amherst, April 17, 1760, WO 34/47.

[31] *SCG*, Feb. 2, 1760.

[32] "Entries in the old Bible of Robert Pringle," *SCHM* 21 (1921), 25–33; "Extracts from the Journal of Mrs. Ann Manigault," *SCHM* 20 (1919), 134; *SCG*, March 7, 1760.

[33] Pinckney, *Letterbook*, 147–148.

[34] *SCG*, Feb. 16, 1760; Smith, *Correspondence of Linnaeus*, 1: 473–475; Samuel Urlsperger, ed., *Detailed Reports on the Salzburger Immigrants*, tr. George Fenwick Jones et. al. (Athens: University of Georgia Press, 1981), 17: 137–138.

numbered 940, or about 16 percent of infections and close to 10 percent of the population. How many people died in the colony as a whole is unknown, but it must have been several thousand, including Native Americans, rural whites, and rural blacks. Of those infected naturally in Charleston, 848 died – about one in three. Of those inoculated, ninety-two died – about one in thirty-eight. Other sources claimed deaths from inoculation totaled 140 or 160, but Chalmers thought that exaggerated. Accurate accounting was difficult. The disease had spread so rapidly that it was impossible to say how many of the inoculated had contracted natural smallpox before being inoculated. Chalmers conceded that the percentage of deaths from inoculation was higher than usual due to the great number of inoculations in such a short time. In the panic, proper medical and dietary preparation of patients was impossible. He had taken only four days to prepare his patients, a much shorter time than most inoculating physicians of the day advised. Other circumstances worsened the situation. Some practitioners had never seen or practiced inoculation. The doctors were not able to select subjects for the procedure but had to operate on all who asked. Moreover, many people did not wait for the doctors, and "inoculated their own and other families." During one two-week period, Chalmers inoculated more than 550 and attended more than 200 others who had become infected naturally.[35]

In contrast to 1738, no one in 1760 publicly opposed inoculation on either religious or medical grounds. Indeed, at the height of the epidemic, no one publicly denounced inoculation for any reason. The *Gazette*, which had opposed inoculation in 1738, supported it this time. The newspaper printed "Hints on Inoculation from Dr. Kilpatrick," and "Plain Instructions for Inoculation in the Smallpox" by William Heberden, a prominent English physician. Heberden's instructions were designed to enable anyone to "perform the operation and conduct the patient through the distemper." Unfortunately, Heberden did not mention the need to isolate inoculated patients to prevent them from spreading the infection. Lack of this precaution was often a problem.[36]

From the beginning, some observers worried justifiably about the effects of inoculating thousands of people simultaneously. It was not just the fear that inoculation would spread the disease, for its spread seemed inevitable. The biggest concern was that many of the inoculated would lack needed care because of their sheer numbers. The burden of inoculating and attending to more than

---

[35] Milligen-Johnston, *Short Description*, 84–85; SCG, Dec. 22,1759–April 19,1760; Waring, *Medicine in South Carolina, 1670–1825*, 74–76; Ramsay, *History of South Carolina*, 2: 44; Suzanne Krebsbach, "The Great Charlestown Smallpox Epidemic of 1760," *SCHM* 97 (1996), 37. James Kirkpatrick printed Chalmers's description and statistics in *Analysis of Inoculation*, 2d ed., 1761, 319–321. Ramsay cited the bill of mortality and Chalmers's statistics.

[36] Heberden printed large numbers of his instructions at his own expense and sent them to Benjamin Franklin for distribution in America. *SCG*, April 26, 1760; George Andrews, *South Carolina Almanack and Register for 1760* (Charleston, 1760) also contained instructions for inoculation; Glynn, *Smallpox*, 71.

500 people, Garden lamented, exceeded his strength.[37] Chalmers wrote that the scarcity of nurses, "who were not to be procured in a sufficient number" even at high prices, greatly hindered proper care of the infected. Many of the ill also suffered from a lack of basic necessities because country people who normally supplied them were avoiding the town.[38] The lack of basic care was particularly lethal to the poor, slaves, and Acadian detainees. As we have seen, the Acadians had been dispersed throughout the colony in 1756. By the time of the epidemic, many of them had drifted back to Charleston, destitute and dependent on the charity of those who viewed them as enemy sympathizers and papists. About one-third of the more than 300 Acadians in Charleston died in the epidemic. The South Carolina colonial assembly blamed "improper care" for their high mortality.[39] Even the elite were not immune to the problem of inadequate attention. In the chaos, infant Martha Laurens was nearly buried by mistake. She was thought to have died, but after being laid near an open window to be prepared for burial, the fresh air revived her.[40]

It is impossible to know how many slaves were inoculated, but some certainly were. Their fate naturally depended on their owners. Inoculation of slaves who lived in Charleston seems to have been common. Plantation slaves were sometimes inoculated, but masters balked at the economic consequences of inoculating all of them. It was not only the cost of the inoculations, though that would be substantial. If all the slaves were inoculated at once, the labor force would be incapacitated for several weeks, and it would be impossible to provide adequate nursing and care. The problem of expense was lessened in the late eighteenth century as inoculators began to reduce the lengthy and elaborate preparation. In the 1770s, doctors in the West Indies reported that they had successfully inoculated many slaves, with little or no preparation, except for some purging. One doctor made it clear that a major incentive for reducing the extent of preparation was economic rather than medical: the "scanty allowance" masters were willing to provide for it. How far the idea of reducing the amount of preparation had penetrated Carolina in 1760 is not clear. A few years later, Garden argued that elaborate preparation was unnecessary, but that patients should be given a cool vegetable diet for about ten days prior to inoculation, and a mercurial purge or vomit the day before.[41]

[37] Smith, *Correspondence of Linnaeus*, 1: 473–475, 481, 492–493.

[38] *SCG*, Feb. 16, 1760; Kirkpatrick, *Analysis of Inoculation*, 2d ed. 1761, 320.

[39] Ruth Allison Hudnut and Hayes Baker-Crothers, "Acadian Transients in South Carolina," *The American Historical Review* 43 (1938), 500–513; Marguerite B. Hamer, "The Fate of the Exiled Acadians in South Carolina," *The Journal of Southern History* 4 (1938), 199–208; Chapman J. Milling, *Exile without an End* (Columbia, SC: Bostick and Thornley, Inc., 1943).

[40] David Ramsay, *Memoirs of the Life of Martha Lauren Ramsay* (Boston, 1812), 11–12.

[41] John Quier, et al., *Letters and Essays on the Small Pox and Inoculation* (London, 1778), 22, 107–108; Edmund Berkeley and Dorothy Smith Berkeley, *Dr. Alexander Garden of Charles Town* (Chapel Hill: University of North Carolina Press, 1969), 140.

Planters who did not have any immune slaves on their plantations faced a dilemma. They needed to send slaves to Charleston for supplies, but the slaves could bring back the infection if not immune from inoculation or natural smallpox. One solution was to inoculate a few of them so they could travel off the plantations, and hope the rest did not get the disease. Estate manager Robert Raper had several of John Colleton's slaves inoculated so they could take the plantation boat to town. Raper wanted to inoculate all of them at the plantations of James Michie but did not get permission, to his evident frustration. Smallpox had broken out on a nearby plantation, and Raper believed that Michie's slaves would soon be infected. As it turned out, he was wrong: They escaped the disease.[42] Given the lack of caregivers, inoculating them may have produced greater mortality than doing nothing. Eliza Pinckney reported that "the poor blacks have died very fast even by inoculation," an outcome she attributed to inadequate nursing.[43]

By mid-April, some citizens began to oppose the continuance of inoculation. They were not so much opposed to inoculation itself, however, as to inoculation within Charleston.[44] They presented medical arguments, but their primary objection was economic. Opponents presented their case in a petition to the provincial assembly on April 18. The epidemic in the town, they claimed, was almost over. Nearly every inhabitant of Charleston who was susceptible to smallpox at the beginning of the epidemic had now had it through inoculation or by natural infection. The problem now was that many country people (often slaves brought by their masters) were coming to Charleston to be inoculated or treated for the disease. The presence of smallpox in the town was being unnecessarily prolonged by these actions, with drastic effects on trade and increased economic hardship for the inhabitants. Many were already suffering severely from the scarcity and high prices of food and other necessities. As long as the disease was present in the town, commerce would be crippled. Inoculation was responsible for its continued presence; thus inoculation within Charleston had to stop.[45]

The provincial assembly acted immediately. The act's preamble even restated the arguments in the petition almost verbatim. The legislation differed little from that of 1738. It prohibited inoculation within two miles of Charleston for one year. The only innovation was the appointment of a commission to enforce the law and to report on cases of smallpox until the town and its environs were clear of the disease.[46] Shortly after the act went into effect, Robert Raper predicted that the town would be free of smallpox within a month. It did not happen that quickly. The commissioners did not declare Charleston

[42] Robert Raper to James Stringham, Feb. 22, 1760, Raper to James Michie, April 17, June 17, 1760, Raper to John Colleton, May 22, Aug. 30, 1760, Raper Letterbook, SCHS, 34/511.

[43] Pinckney, *Letterbook*, 147–148, 153; *SCG*, March 22, 1760.

[44] Ramsay, *History of South Carolina*, 2: 44.

[45] *JCHA*, April 18, 1760, 504; *SCG*, April 19, 1760, 507.

[46] *Stats.*, 1760, 4: 106; Jones, *Detailed Reports on the Salzburger Immigrants*, 17: 233.

smallpox-free until early December. Either the disease continued to spread naturally, or someone continued to inoculate in violation of the ban.[47]

THE INOCULATION BUSINESS VERSUS COMMERCE

Three years later, smallpox struck again. As in 1738 and 1760, inoculation was widely adopted in Charleston and aroused opposition. As in 1760, religious objections to inoculation were not a major public issue. The 1763 epidemic differed in some ways from the earlier epidemics, however. First, it was much less virulent; few people died, from either natural or inoculated smallpox. The *Gazette* summed up the situation in May: "The smallpox continues favorable; nobody dies of it, and inoculation still prevails." Garden claimed that only 2 of about 800 patients he inoculated died.[48] It must have been a mild strain of the virus in this case. Also, most of the settled population was immune from the infections and inoculations of 1760. Large numbers of newcomers were pouring into the backcountry, however, and many of them were susceptible. As a result, the people inoculated in Charleston in 1763 often came from the country. Another way in which the 1763 epidemic differed from earlier ones was that local doctors approached inoculation in a more organized, business-like fashion. They established and advertised smallpox hospitals for inoculation and treatment.

The epidemic broke out in late December 1762 and spread quickly. By New Year's Day, Ann Manigault reported that many people were coming to Charleston from the country to be inoculated. Soon, the only people coming to town were those seeking inoculation. Rural residents were reluctant even to accept letters from town for fear of infection. Henry Laurens reported in early January that many townspeople were fleeing their homes. The disease broke out in so many places at once that Laurens doubted it could be stopped unless all susceptible people left town. Following his own advice, he sent several of his susceptible slaves to his plantation at Mepkin and went there himself when one of them came down with the disease.[49]

Several physicians and others opened "hospitals" for inoculation and the care of smallpox, generally in their own or others' houses. This practice became common in Britain and America in the late eighteenth century. Although some of the hospitals took in white patients, their main clientele was slaves. In early April, Dr. William Loocock opened a smallpox hospital at his house for the care of "town and country Negroes." To inspire confidence, he offered to insure the patients. Several other doctors and at least one woman,

[47] Raper to James Michie, June 17, 1760, Raper to John Colleton, August 30, 1760; *SCG*, Aug. 9, Sept. 6, Nov. 8, Dec. 6, 1760, Raper Letterbook, SCHS, 34/511.

[48] *SCG*, May 21, 28, 1763. I have not found any estimate of the mortality in 1763, but it appears to have been low. Dr. William Loocock claimed that he had inoculated 463 patients and lost only 4. *SCG*, May 28, 1763.

[49] "Extracts from the Journal of Mrs. Ann Manigault, 1754–1781," *SCHM* 20 (1919), 204; *HLP*, 3: 206, 216, 208, 237; Glynn, *Smallpox*, 151–152.

Elizabeth Girardeau, opened inoculation hospitals in or near Charleston during the following weeks, with charges varying between 10 and 15 pounds per inoculation. To some planters, the cost may have been justified, from an economic if not a humanitarian point of view. Replacing a dead slave would cost many times the price of inoculation. On the negative side, inoculation would mean loss of the slave's labor for several weeks and possibly forever.[50]

More than 2,000 people were inoculated between January and July.[51] Inoculation in 1763 aroused little hostility at first, compared to 1738 or even 1760. This may be partly due to familiarity with the procedure and acceptance of its advantages over taking smallpox naturally. Yet, as in the earlier epidemics, a move to stop inoculation arose – in this case, abetted by the mildness of the epidemic. If the smallpox was not deadly, some asked, why was it necessary to inoculate at all? Once again, however, the main rationale for ending inoculation was economic. In late April, Henry Laurens complained that the continuation of inoculation was turning Charleston into one large smallpox hospital, to the "detriment of the inhabitants." Because nearly all the town's inhabitants were probably immune to smallpox by the time Laurens wrote, the detriment he meant must have been primarily economic. He repeatedly complained about the difficulty of getting supplies and labor from town, and collecting money he was owed. The persistence of smallpox, he fumed, had become an excuse for people not to pay their debts. Laurens was not opposed to inoculation when it was in his interest. On June 2, more than a month *after* he singled out inoculation as the cause of the continuing woes of the town, he compared his house to a smallpox hospital, with nine people inoculated and two more about to be. Apparently, Laurens did not see the inconsistency in condemning a procedure he was using himself. To be fair, perhaps he saw his use of it as necessitated by the doctors' continuation of it.[52]

In mid-June, a number of citizens signed a petition to the "gentlemen of the practice of physic" asking them to cease inoculation after July 1. In 1738 and 1760, those who wanted to stop inoculation had gone to the assembly. However, as the petitioners of 1763 noted, they could not do that on this occasion because the assembly was not in session. Interestingly, in a society that often placed individual (white) liberty above all other values, they justified their appeal to the doctors on the grounds of natural justice and the general welfare: "[I]t is an invariable principle, that the desires and interests of individuals, especially non-residents, should be postponed to those of the community." The community they had in mind, however, was the white citizenry of Charleston. The nonresidents were country people, mostly blacks, coming or

[50] *SCG*, April 2, May 21, June 11, 25, 1763; Miller, *Inoculation*, pp. 165–166; Robert Raper to John Colleton, July 8, 1763, Robert Raper Letterbook, SCHS, 34/511.

[51] *SCG*, May 21, 1763; Smith, *Correspondence of Linnaeus*, 1: 316, 517; Lionel Chalmers to Robert Whytt, May 2, 17[63], Edinburgh University Special Collections, Dc.4.98/1, ff. 230–231; John Murray of Murraywhat to Elizabeth Murray, Feb. 21, March 31, 1763, Murraywhat Muniments, SRO/GD219/287.

[52] *HLP*, 3: 216, 273, 363, 420, 467–469, 7: 479, 8: 16, note 5.

brought to town to be inoculated. Allowing this to continue endangered the community's health because the bodies of the inoculated produced "vitiated air." The petitioners did not argue that the vitiated air would spread small-pox in the town. They could not reasonably make that claim, because most Charleston residents were now immune to that disease from inoculation or natural infection. Instead, drawing on a contemporary medical theory that one disease could mutate into another, they argued that the smallpox-corrupted air might cause other "malignant and alarming diseases." On several occa-sions in the past, smallpox epidemics had been followed by epidemics of yellow fever or other diseases. Another danger was that fear of smallpox in town was keeping many planters in the country, where the advancing heat would soon expose them to fevers. Inoculation was bringing the wrong sort of people to Charleston and preventing the right sort from coming. The petitioners added that continuing inoculation also threatened the livelihoods of the townspeople. A lack of needed goods had inflated prices. Many people who had fled to the country endured a double blow: the loss of their regular income and increased living expenses. The petitioners appealed to the doctors' "known humanity and disinterestedness" to bow to the wishes of the community.[53]

A large group of them agreed, with conditions. First, they did not promise to stop inoculating, only to refrain from it within one mile of Charleston. Second, they would adhere to the agreement only if the residents did so as well. In effect, the doctors were reminding the petitioners that the demand for inoculation had come from the community that now wanted to outlaw it. Implicit, too, was the warning that the doctors would not allow the profit-able business of inoculation to be carried on by anyone outside their ranks.[54] The response did not placate everyone. A letter to the *Gazette* applauded the agreement but doubted the doctors' commitment. The correspondent argued that anyone who inoculated henceforth should be treated as an enemy to the "welfare and prosperity of the community." For a few people to endanger the broader society in their own interest was "contrary to justice and equity." The writer apparently did not see the irony of making that statement in a community that had a slave majority. He hinted that the doctors might need to be restrained by law: "[W]henever there is a power of legislation, history and experience shew it to be the result of common policy, to lay restraints on individuals, in such instances."[55] Another correspondent had no faith in the physicians' promises at all. He was irate that the people had to "seek redress of their grievances" by supplicating "the men who are engaged, by interest, to reject their applications." Why, he asked, cannot we appeal to the legisla-ture, "a right purchased with the blood of our ancestors; is it abolished? By whose authority? To be more plain, where are our [Representatives]?"[56] The

---

[53] *SCG*, June 18, 1763.
[54] *SCG*, June 25, July 2, 1763.
[55] *SCG*, June 25, 1763.
[56] *SCG*, July 2, 1763.

controversy died away by early July, but it took longer to clear the town of smallpox than had been expected. At the end of August, the disease was still present in two houses. The *Gazette* suggested that someone was still inoculating contrary to the agreement. The episode probably increased resentment of the doctors, who were mostly Scots, and may help explain why so many of them supported the British government in the Revolution.[57]

In 1764, the South Carolina colonial assembly legislated once again on the problem of inoculation. The act they passed was similar in most respects to those of 1738 and 1760, except that it was to be in force for three years. But it introduced a new approach. Instead of banning inoculation, it tried to control it. It prohibited inoculation throughout the province without the permission of the governor and the assembly, or the council if the assembly was not in session. Those who had received permission could continue inoculating until the governor and council ordered them to stop it.[58] The aim of this clause was apparently to permit a flexible response to inoculation. It allowed it under certain controlled circumstances but also provided a mechanism to stop it if it seemed to be causing harm to the "welfare and prosperity" of the community. The new inoculation law appears to have satisfied enough of the elite to end the controversy over the procedure. The law was never tested. When epidemic smallpox returned during the Revolutionary War chaos made the law irrelevant.[59]

CHAOTIC INOCULATING: 1780–1781

In late May 1780, just after Charleston surrendered to the British, Colonel Alexander Innes reported that in his vicinity smallpox had "spread so universally that almost every family is inoculated."[60] Smallpox had broken out in New England in 1775. Between 1779 and 1781, it spread throughout the southeast. According to General William Moultrie, it appeared in Charleston in November 1779. He claimed that its presence frustrated attempts to attract the help of militia from the surrounding regions. Unlike regular Continental soldiers, who were routinely inoculated by this time, few of the militia had such protection. The commanding general in Charleston, Benjamin Lincoln, denied that smallpox was present there as late as February 29, 1780. But Lincoln was desperate to get reinforcements and undoubtedly downplayed the

---

[57] *SCG*, Aug. 6, 20, 27, 1763.
[58] *Stats.*, 4: 182.
[59] Ramsay, *History of South Carolina*, 2: 44–5.
[60] Alexander Innes to [John Andre], May 21, 1780, Henry Clinton Papers, 1730–1795, William L. Clements Library, University of Michigan, Ann Arbor. I owe this reference to Elizabeth Fenn; Fenn, *Pox Americana*, 110–128; Waring, *Medicine in South Carolina, 1670–1825*, 100; Sylvia Frey, *The British Soldier in America: A Social History of Military Life in the Revolutionary Period* (Austin: University of Texas Press, 1981), 43–44; Ravenel, *Eliza Pinckney*, 288–290.

danger.[61] When the city surrendered on May 12, an epidemic was underway. The British immediately began to inoculate their susceptible soldiers. David Ramsay claimed that "a general inoculation took place" in Charleston after the surrender, but sources disagree about how general it was. Meanwhile, Sir Henry Clinton had paroled hundreds of rebel militiamen, some of whom no doubt spread the disease as they returned home. Fighting in the hinterland during the next few months also helped spread the disease.

Suddenly everyone was seeking inoculators or information on how to inoculate. In June 1780, Harriott Horry went to Charleston to consult Alexander Garden on inoculation and sent a copy of his instructions to her friend, Mrs. Motte. In July, Elizabeth Pinckney wrote that smallpox was present on every plantation within fifteen miles of her home, and that a doctor from the "Northward" had inoculated more than 1,000 people, both black and white. Thomas Charlton, a physician-planter who lived in Camden, inoculated many of the soldiers of both armies after the battle there in August. In the fall of 1780, smallpox infected many patriot prisoners in Charleston, and Lincoln requested that the British allow the prisoners to be inoculated.[62]

How many people were inoculated and how many died in the epidemic of 1779–1781 is unknown. The totals of both must have been in the thousands. Thousands of blacks died of smallpox and camp fevers after the fall of Charleston. The greatest mortality was among slaves who fled their plantations to the British lines in search of freedom but often found microbes to which they had no immunity. Boston King, one of the runaway slaves, recalled that he and other slaves with smallpox were isolated from the British camp to avoid infecting the soldiers. They received little attendance, although King was given critical aid by a British soldier and later taken with about twenty-five others to a hospital. David George, another runaway, claimed that he survived smallpox only because some people gave him a little rice.

Some blacks were immune to smallpox from earlier inoculations or previous epidemics, but many, especially the young, were vulnerable. The same was true of many whites. Probably few rural people had been inoculated since the early 1760s, to judge by the urgent demand for inoculators across the Carolinas in 1779 and 1780. In August 1780, smallpox broke out on the plantation of Keating Simons. He claimed that "four fifths of the whole of my family of blacks and whites" had never had the disease naturally or by inoculation. A few months later, William Burrows recorded that he had lost more than thirty of his slaves to smallpox and camp fevers and expected to lose

---

[61] William Moultrie, *Memoirs of the American Revolution* 2 vols. (New York, 1802) 2: 43–44, 48–49, 55–56; David Ramsay, *The History of the Revolution of South Carolina* 2 vols. (Trenton, 1785), 2: 46; *Pennsylvania Gazette*, April 5, 1780.

[62] Ramsay, *History of South Carolina*, 2: 44; Fenn, *Pox Americana*, 110–128, 268–269; Ravenel, *Eliza Pinckney*, 289; *HLP*, 10: 285n; Eliza Pinckney to [?], Sept. 25, 1780, Charles Cotesworth Pinckney Family Papers, Library of Congress, Washington, DC, 1st ser., box 5. I owe the last reference to Elizabeth Fenn.

seven more. Securing the services of an inoculator in the chaotic conditions of war was understandably difficult. Planters sometimes inoculated slaves themselves.[63]

After the Revolutionary War, the South Carolina General Assembly decided that inoculation had proved a greater boon than danger, or perhaps that it was impossible to stop. It repealed the laws restricting the procedure. Legal or not, inoculation continued to arouse opposition in some communities. When smallpox broke out in the Wateree region in 1793, Henry Rugeley wanted to have his children inoculated but was afraid to anger his neighbors because the disease had not yet appeared in their neighborhood. He did not want "to be the first that brings it." He had his family inoculated that May but came to repent it. He lost "a fine Negro girl" and spent several months nursing two severely ill sons back to health. He blamed the doctor for giving them mercury.[64] In spite of these problems, David Ramsay declared in 1800 that inoculation had largely eliminated the danger from smallpox. Within a few years, however, inoculation was obsolete. In 1802, Ramsay himself became one of the first doctors in South Carolina to use Edward Jenner's new method for preventing smallpox: vaccination.[65]

VACCINATION

"They died under circumstances horrible to see, and painful to relate. Covered with confluent sores, they could neither stand, sit, nor lie, without exquisite pain. Their bodies, and their bedclothes, were stiffened with foetid discharges from every part of their skin. The whole emitted a stench intolerable to bystanders. Humanity was put to the rack." In these words, David Ramsay described the effects of a smallpox epidemic in 1802. Horrible as it sounds, this epidemic was relatively mild. Deaths totalled only twenty-four in

---

[63] Boston King, "Memoirs of the Life of Boston King, a Black Preacher," in *Face Zion Forward: First Writers of the Black Atlantic*, ed. and intro. by Joanna Brooks and John Saillant (Boston: Northeastern University Press, 2002), 212; "An Account of the Life of David George," in Brooks and Saillant, eds., *Face Zion Forward*, 182; *SCG*, Dec. 26, 1774, Jan. 30, Sept. 19, Oct. 24, 1775; Josiah Smith, "Diary, 1780–1781," *SCHM* 33 (1932), 21; Josiah Smith Letterbook, 1771–1784, SHC, 405–406, 412, 416, 418, 426, 431; William Ancrum to James Edward Colleton, July 14, 1780, in Harold Easterby, ed., *Wadboo Barony: Its Fate as Told in the Colleton Family Papers, 1773–1793* (Columbia: University of South Carolina Press, 1952), 4, 6; William Burrows to [?] Feb. 27, 1781, PRO/30/11/105; Keating Simons to Cornwallis, Aug. 11, 1780, PRO/30/11/63/36–37.

[64] Henry Rugeley to Elizabeth Rugeley, March 10, 1793, Henry Rugeley to Matthew Rugeley, Jan. 11, 1794, Rugeley Papers, Bedfordshire Record Office, Bedford, England, X311/146, X311/148.

[65] David Ramsay to Henry Laurens, June 3, 1794, *Letters of Edward Jenner* ed. by Genevieve Miller (Baltimore: Johns Hopkins University Press, 1983), 117; David Ramsay, *A Review of the Improvements, Progress and State of Medicine in the XVIIIth Century* (Charleston, 1800), 41; Ramsay, *History of South Carolina*, 2: 44–45.

the city – a tiny toll, compared to most eighteenth-century epidemics. Many of the infected "suffered little," according to Ramsay.[66]

The 1802 epidemic was nevertheless significant. It saw the first use of Jennerian vaccination for smallpox into South Carolina. In 1798, Jenner had published several pamphlets describing his experiments using cowpox as a preventive of smallpox.[67] Jenner's account quickly aroused the interest and support of medical men in the United States. In January 1800, David Ramsay discussed Jenner's success in England and the introduction of vaccination into America by Benjamin Waterhouse. The following year, John Vaughan, secretary of the American Philosophical Society in Philadelphia, sent a batch of vaccine and instructions to Charleston's Dr. Philip Tidyman.[68] Vaughan soon sent vaccine to Ramsay as well. Waterhouse also sent vaccine to Charleston. Ramsay later claimed to have introduced vaccination to South Carolina in 1802, but several other local doctors also used the procedure that year. In a letter written during the epidemic, he reported that vaccination had already become widely accepted in Charleston: "I scarcely know any persons of consequence who are unbelievers in vaccination." He added that the Medical Society of South Carolina had begun vaccinating charity patients at the newly opened dispensary.[69] A few years later, Ramsay predicted that "a general and simultaneous vaccination" would quickly bring about the extermination of the disease.[70] The dream of universal extermination of smallpox did not become a reality until 1977 and then through selective rather than general vaccination. It is doubtful that Ramsay or anyone else at the time foresaw all the difficulties a global eradication program would have to overcome.[71]

Ramsay did see several immediate obstacles. Ironically, one was the need for doctors to discredit inoculation – not an easy thing to do when they had been advocating and practicing it for decades. During the epidemic of 1802 and after, the dispensary physicians published advertisements arguing the advantages of vaccination over inoculation in safety and effectiveness. In one of these, they pledged to continue to inoculate those who demanded it, but with a caveat. People who insisted on inoculation should "acquit us from all responsibility for the distresses, anxieties, dangers, and deaths that may result

---

[66] *Charleston Medical Register*, 1802, 1–2.
[67] Hopkins, *Princes and Peasants*, 8–9, 77–78; Miller, *Letters of Edward Jenner*, 119, n.2; Glynn, *Smallpox*, 95–142.
[68] *The Medical Repository*, 255–258; John Vaughan to Philip Tidyman, Dec. 11, 1801, April 7, 1802, Letters of John Vaughan to Philip Tidyman, 1801–1802, COCSC, Mss. 34–135; Ramsay to John Vaughan, April 14, 1803, in Brunhouse, *Ramsay*, 155.
[69] Miller, *Letters of Edward Jenner*, 118, 119, n. 3; Ramsay, *History of South Carolina* 2: 44–45; Waring, *Medicine in South Carolina, 1670–1825*, 218.
[70] *Charleston Medical Register*, 1802, 7; Miller, *Letters of Edward Jenner*, 128; Ramsay to John Coakley Lettsom, Oct. 29, 1808, in Brunhouse, *Ramsay*, 163.
[71] Glynn, *Smallpox*, 200–227; Fenner, Henderson, et al., *Smallpox*; Leon Banov, *As I Recall: The Story of the Charleston County Health Department* (Columbia, SC: R. L. Bryan, 1970).

from yielding to your prejudices." When the disease became epidemic again in 1805, the doctors openly declared the superiority of vaccination.[72]

Ramsay used several arguments against inoculation in writings during and after the epidemic. Ironically, one had been used by opponents of inoculation since its introduction, namely that it caused the disease to spread: "Charleston has abounded with cases of the natural small pox following the inoculated small pox."[73] Vaccination was not only safer than inoculation – it produced less discomfort and disruption of everyday life: "The subjects of it were seldom laid up, or ceased a single day to perform their usual business. Pustular eruptions, to any considerable degree, were very uncommon, and never dangerous." None of the hundreds of people vaccinated contracted smallpox, but four inoculated children died.[74]

In addition to overcoming inoculation, vaccination faced many of the same obstacles as had inoculation. Many people were reluctant to undergo the procedure for religious reasons or unless they felt an immediate threat from smallpox. In the aftermath of the 1802 epidemic, Ramsay wrote: "We have few cases of vaccination among us at present. The smallpox [has] disappeared and the dread of that disorder drives many to inoculation either old or new." Most of the susceptible people receptive to vaccination had already received it. Others opposed the procedure in principle or now thought it unnecessary. Ramsay fumed that if smallpox was not eliminated it would be due to the "carelessness, ignorance, and prejudices of the people." John Shecut also blamed the populace. Many people failed to get vaccinated when the disease was not present because they felt no immediate danger. They waited until the disease was epidemic, and then it was often too late. Popular concerns about vaccination, however, were sometimes legitimate. As in other places, acceptance of vaccination was hindered by some practitioners using spurious vaccine, vaccine that was no longer effective, or actual smallpox matter. Cowpox was a relatively rare disease that had to be imported over long distances, and keeping the virus effective for long periods was a problem, especially in hot climates. Claims of smallpox cases occurring among the vaccinated added to the skepticism. Charleston's vaccinating doctors tended to lay the blame on unqualified practitioners: quacks, charlatans, and the ignorant. Nevertheless, in 1812, the Medical Society announced that vaccination was "progressing" in the city.[75]

---

[72] *Palladium of Knowledge: or, the Carolina and Georgia Almanac* (Charleston, 1803), n. p.; *The Courier*, April 9, 1805. See also, *The Courier*, March 7, 1803; Glynn, *Smallpox*, 135–136.

[73] Miller, *Letters of Edward Jenner*, 117–119, 119, n. 3.

[74] *Charleston Medical Register*, 1802, 6; Miller, *Letters of Edward Jenner* 118–119, 119, n. 3; *Charleston Times*, July 19, 1802.

[75] David Ramsay, *History of South Carolina* 2 vols. (Charleston, 1858, first edition, 1809) 2: 45; *Charleston Medical Register*, 1802, 6; John L. E. W. Shecut, *Shecut's Medical and Philosophical Essays* (Charleston, 1819), 179; Miller, *Letters of Edward Jenner* 118–119, 119 n. 3; MSM, Nov. 11, 1812, 20. On the spread of vaccination and the obstacles it faced

Apparently not fast enough. In 1817, as smallpox once again spread its tentacles through the neighborhoods of Charleston, the Medical Society published a full endorsement of vaccination. They claimed that the epidemic was due to neglect of true vaccination and "false confidence" in improperly performed vaccination. They denied that vaccination properly performed had failed to prevent the smallpox. Rumors to that effect were the result of incorrect methods of vaccination and confusion with the much milder chicken pox, which was circulating at the same time. The society pointed out that these problems were not unique to Charleston and constituted a strong argument for confining the operation to medically trained professionals. The society's members were uniformly convinced that the vaccine was effective. On this occasion, they refused to perform inoculation except to gratify friends after vaccination, the result of which only strengthened their faith in the vaccine.[76]

Vaccination gradually increased, and deaths from smallpox declined substantially in the nineteenth century. But vaccination was not made compulsory until 1905, and some people continued to oppose or neglect it. The need to periodically revaccinate was not widely accepted for many years. Southerners were slower to adopt the procedure than northerners, and blacks – dependent on their masters for the procedure – were less likely to get vaccinated than whites. The Civil War brought an upsurge in smallpox. In 1865 and 1866, it killed hundreds of people in Charleston and almost 2,000 blacks on nearby James Island, where many refugees had congregated.[77] Nevertheless, the worst ravages of the disease had been overcome. During the nineteenth century, yellow fever and malaria were the great scourges of the lowcountry and they continued to shape perceptions and realities within the region.

globally, see the articles in "Special Issue: Reassessing Smallpox Vaccination, 1789–1900," *Bulletin of the History of Medicine*, 83 (2009), 1–190.

[76] *Report on the Failures Attributed to the Vaccine in Charleston* (Charleston, 1817), 2–8; MSM, Jan. 1, 1817, 86–91.

[77] Glynn, *Smallpox*, 126–134, 139; Waring, *Medicine in South Carolina, 1825–1900*, 40.

Commerce, Contagion, and Cleanliness

I trust that the learned practitioners of Europe and America ... will easily detect the fallacy of the doctrine of the contagious nature of the yellow fever; and that disease being proved ... not contagious, will no longer subject our city to the fear, or the terrors of foreigners, and to the injurious effects that such a belief has upon our commerce, our wealth, and our population.

John L. E. W. Shecut, 1819

It is the object and interest of all commercial societies to establish, if possible, the non-contagious character of all diseases; and for the very plain reason, that the restrictions necessary to prevent the extension of such diseases, are calculated to interrupt free intercourse between commercial cities.

Benjamin B. Strobel, 1840

A COMMERCIAL PROBLEM

In the nineteenth-century South, as Margaret Humphreys has noted, "yellow fever was above all a commercial problem."[1] That was also true before the nineteenth century for ports all along the Atlantic coast, but during the early nineteenth century it became an acute commercial problem for Charleston, as the local economy began to stagnate and then decline. Although the disease killed many more people in other places, especially New Orleans, the economic malaise of Charleston and its hinterland magnified the perception of yellow fever as a commercial catastrophe. During the eighteenth century, smallpox could also shut down the port and cut off trade by land and sea. But there was a major difference. Smallpox struck Charleston less often than yellow fever and it was easily recognizable. Although it was sometimes confused with other eruptive diseases such as chicken pox and measles, the error was usually quickly rectified. Yellow fever, however, was often mistaken for other

---

[1] Margaret Humphreys, *Yellow Fever and the South* (Baltimore and London: Johns Hopkins University Press, 1992), 2.

diseases. It was much easier to debate the presence or absence of yellow fever than that of smallpox, and to argue about when and if quarantine measures were needed. Even when the presence of yellow fever was confirmed, uncertainty about its origins and means of spread led some observers to argue that it was not contagious or imported and that quarantine could do nothing to prevent it. Such a view was naturally attractive to many people whose livelihoods depended on maritime commerce. In most places where the disease was a matter of concern, these issues split the early nineteenth-century medical profession, but in Charleston there was no real split at all. Between about 1800 and the 1850s, anticontagionist and antiquarantine positions monopolized medical thinking. Almost to a man, Charleston doctors argued that quarantine was useless, unnecessary, and economically disastrous, and that sanitary improvement was the key to preventing yellow fever. The shift toward sanitation, however, had little, if any, effect. Epidemics struck the city repeatedly. By the 1850s, some doctors in Charleston and other places in the South began to change their minds and urge the reinstatement of stringent quarantine, citing its apparent success in banishing yellow fever from northern cities.

Quarantine had strong medical approval until after the Revolutionary War. Although the state relaxed quarantine against smallpox after independence, Charleston doctors continued to urge its use against other contagious diseases.[2] After 1800, however, they decided that a rigid quarantine was unnecessary for yellow fever. Paradoxically, the doctors' call for relaxing quarantine in the case of yellow fever coincided with rising concern about the disease. The concern arose less from the suffering and death the disease brought – although that was not completely ignored – than from yellow fever's effect on the city's and region's commerce. The greatest problem caused by yellow fever, the Board of Health declared in 1829, was that it was "the disease from which Charleston has suffered most in reputation, and consequently in prosperity."[3] This was never truer than in the first half of the nineteenth century. In the previous century, northern cities often suffered from yellow fever. In the early nineteenth century, the disease gradually retreated from the North, but remained a frequent visitor to parts of the South. It produced months of economic stagnation and discouraged people and businesses from coming to the region during the fever season or at all. As a rice merchant put it in 1838, yellow fever "has acted like a cramp on all business. Without it, and we would have worked off the old crop [of rice] at famous prices, but as it is now, we can scarcely sell, and everything seems out of joint."[4] The disruption to trade caused by epidemics was intolerable, and to some leaders the main problem was not so much the disease as the rigid quarantine regulations that followed announcement

[2] *The Courier*, Aug. 27, Sept. 24, 1806; MSM, June 1, 1804, Sept. 16, Dec. 2–3, 1805; Thomas Y. Simons, *A Report on the History and Causes of the Strangers or Yellow Fever of Charleston* (Charleston, 1839), 8–11, 15–17.

[3] *Communication from the Chairman of the Board of Health* (Charleston, 1829), 12;

[4] J. H. Easterby, ed., *The South Carolina Rice Plantation* (Columbia: University of South Carolina Press, 2004; 1945), 408.

of an outbreak It is not surprising that many officials, merchants, shippers, exporters, and planters were attracted to medical theories that denied that yellow fever was contagious. If it was not contagious, it was unlikely to be imported, and quarantine was a useless restriction.[5]

With the medical corps and powerful commercial interests united behind opposition to quarantine, it is not surprising that doctors were reluctant to air contrary opinions. A "premature" declaration of yellow fever or a suggestion that it might be imported could bring down the wrath of the medical and commercial communities on the offending physician. Benjamin Strobel discovered this when he diagnosed yellow fever cases among sailors in the Marine Hospital in early June 1839 and argued that they had brought the disease into the city from their ships: "[W]hat was our reward for faithfully performing that duty? For more than a month, we absolutely lived in an atmosphere of 'curses *deep*, tho' not *loud*.'" Strobel charged that the concealment of yellow fever for commercial reasons had been common in Charleston: "[T]ruth and justice have been too often sacrificed to expediency and policy, and never more so than in reference to the yellow fever. Has it not occurred, when the disease actually invaded us, that there were men who regardless of the lives of others, and listening only to the sordid suggestions of avarice, have endeavored to conceal the fact?"[6]

The eighteenth-century approach to yellow fever had been different. The colonial government and most doctors agreed that quarantine was necessary to prevent the importation of "contagious and malignant distempers." In 1698, after a major smallpox epidemic, the assembly passed a law requiring arriving ships to anchor a mile from the entrance to the harbor. The captains were to inform the harbor pilot of their port of origin and if any contagious disease was on board. If such disease existed, the ship had to remain at anchor near the harbor entrance, presumably until the sickness abated.[7] In 1707, the colonial assembly approved the construction of a pest house on the northern end of Sullivan's Island. The rationale was that confining passengers and crew on ships for long periods of time would be financially hurtful to the ships' owners and masters, and hinder the trade of the province. Several other pest houses were built on Sullivan's and other nearby islands during the eighteenth and early nineteenth centuries. These institutions were often poorly funded and maintained, and at times no pest house was in use because of poor

---

[5] Humphreys, *Yellow Fever and the South*, 2–5; Peter Coclanis, *The Shadow of a Dream: Economic Life and Death in the South Carolina Low Country, 1670–1920* (New York and Oxford: Oxford University Press, 1989); Peter Baldwin, *Contagion and the State in Europe, 1830–1930* (New York: Cambridge University Press, 1999); Erwin Ackerknecht, "Anticontagionism between 1821 and 1867," *Bulletin of the History of Medicine* 22 (1948), 117–153.

[6] Benjamin B. Strobel, *An Essay on the Subject of Yellow Fever Intended to Prove its Transmissibility* (Charleston, 1840), 9.

[7] *Stats.*, 2: 152.

conditions or destruction by storms and war.[8] In September 1752, a massive hurricane blew one of them away, killing most of its inmates. In 1754, the assembly ordered a new pest house built on Sullivan's Island, which opened a year or two later. Soon after its opening, Henry Laurens reported that it was "in good order," but its condition quickly deteriorated. When hundreds of French Acadians were landed on the island in February 1756, many quickly became seriously ill and some died, probably from dysentery and inadequate care.[9] A patriot force demolished the pest house in 1775 on the grounds that the royal governor, Lord William Campbell, was using it as a refuge for slaves who "had deserted to the [British] enemy" and were committing robberies in nearby Christ Church Parish. After the Revolutionary War ended in 1783, a new pest house was built at Sullivan's Island, but it was not in use very long. In the 1790s, the island became a summer refuge for people trying to avoid yellow fever in Charleston, and residents successfully petitioned to have the pest house closed. City council ordered another one to be built on James Island, near Fort Johnson, in the late 1790s. It was replaced by another, built on Morris Island in the 1830s.[10]

During the eighteenth century, doctors generally viewed yellow fever as an imported and contagious disease. James Kilpatrick claimed that the epidemic of 1739 was "probably imported from Africa or the Caribbean."[11] John Lining argued that it had always been imported from the West Indies: "[W]henever the disease appeared here, it was easily traced to some person who had lately arrived from the West-Indian Islands, where it was epidemical."[12] At least one doctor, John Moultrie, Jr., dissented from this view. In his medical dissertation of 1749, Moultrie argued that people favored the importation theory because it placed blame for the disease elsewhere. Everyone wanted "to escape the disgrace attaching to a most fearful disease." But the conditions that produced yellow fever in the West Indies also existed in the southern parts of North America. If it was more common in the islands, it was because the heat in them was more intense and longer-lasting. Moultrie doubted – correctly – that the disease could spread unless the air was suitable for producing it. He attributed the fever to the corruption of the air combined with excessive exertion.

[8] Nicholas Trott, "The Temporary Laws of South Carolina, An Act for the Raising a Publick Store of Powder for the Defense of this Province," 1707, Ms., 18–25, SCDAH; *Yearbook, City of Charleston* (Charleston, 1880), 75–76; *JCHA*, 7: 161, 11: 122, 124, 139–140.

[9] *JCHA*, 14: 123, 139, 151, 158, 200; BPRO/SC, 27: April 14, June 16, 19, 1756.

[10] *Stats.* 4: 572, 615–618, 668; *Journals of the Privy Council 1783–1789*, ed. by Adele S. Edwards (Columbia: University of South Carolina Press, 1971), 84, 91, 334, 365; *HLP*, 10: 546, 576; *Ordinances of the City Council of Charleston* (Charleston, 1807), No. 173, May 12, 1800, 191–193; Waring, *History of Medicine in South Carolina, 1825–1900*, 67.

[11] James Kilpatrick, *Essay on Inoculation* (London, 1743), 56–57.

[12] John Lining, "A Description of the American Yellow Fever," *Essays and Observations, Physical and Literary* (Edinburgh, 1756) 2: 373–374; Benjamin Rush, *Observations upon the Origin of the Malignant Bilious, or Yellow Fever* (Philadelphia, 1799), 17.

The local topography was to blame for the corruption. The huge forests were full of "poisonous" trees and numerous "swamps, pools, and subterranean places," and summer heat lifted their "copious exhalations and putrid miasmas" into the air, creating conditions that propagated yellow fever.[13]

Moultrie was also skeptical about the contagiousness of yellow fever. "Almost all authorities" believed in contagion, he declared, and he appeared to agree in part. The corrupted air endangered everyone, but those nursing the sick were especially vulnerable. At first glance, this might be seen as support of contagion, but Moultrie meant that those who tended the sick received an extra dense concentration of the corrupt air – "the sharp, semi-putrid exhalations" – that issued from the bodies of the sick. At the same time, he admitted that many people "in close contact with the ill escaped unaffected." There had to be something that protected them against the effects of the concentrated miasma. Unlike Lining, Moultrie did not believe that one attack conferred immunity, so he could not explain their escape that way. Advocates of human contagion faced the same problem. It was not only that some people close to the ill never got the disease. It was also that people who never came in direct contact with an infected person contracted it.[14]

Nevertheless, before 1800, the dominant view was that yellow fever was imported and contagious, and that quarantine was justified. In Europe, quarantine was a well established method of preventing the importation of contagious diseases, having been pioneered by Italian city-states in the fifteenth and sixteenth centuries to prevent or contain plague.[15] South Carolina Governor James Glen summed up a common view after a yellow fever epidemic in 1745: "[I]t is apprehended the late grievous distemper ... was brought from abroad."[16] The colonial quarantine acts explicitly stated that imported, contagious diseases were the main health threat to the colony. One of 1712 declared that "great numbers of the inhabitants of this Province have been destroyed by malignant, contagious diseases, brought here from Africa and other parts of America." The framers unaccountably absolved Europe from blame. The act appointed a health officer whose task was to inspect ships and question masters to determine whether anyone on board had died or become ill from "plague, smallpox, spotted fever, Siam distemper, Guinea fever, or any other malignant contagious disease." If the health officer discovered any

[13] Joseph I. Waring, "John Moultrie, Jr., M.D., Lieutenant Governor of East Florida, His Thesis on Yellow Fever," *The Journal of the Florida Medical Association* 54 (1967), 774–775.

[14] Waring, "Moultrie's Thesis on Yellow Fever," 775. William Hillary, a Barbados doctor, also questioned the contagiousness of yellow fever, in *Observations on the Changes of the Air and the Consequent Epidemical Diseases, on the Island of Barbados* (London, 1759), 145–146.

[15] Sheldon Watts, *Epidemics and History: Disease, Power and Imperialism* (New Haven, CT and London: Yale University Press, 1997), 15–23; Ann G. Carmichael, *Plague and the Poor in Renaissance Florence* (Cambridge: Cambridge University Press, 1986); Carlo Cipolla, *Cristofano and the Plague* (Berkeley: University of California Press, 1973).

[16] *JCHA*, 6: 12, Dec. 6, 1745; Journal of His Majesty's Council of South Carolina, Minutes, Dec. 6, 1745, SCDAH; *SCG*, Dec. 9, 1745.

such diseases, he could order the ship into quarantine for twenty days, require the master to cleanse the ship and cargo, and send diseased persons to the pest house. The act punished violations of quarantine with fines, whipping, or forfeiture of slaves.[17] Subsequent quarantine acts followed a similar pattern, adding additional precautions and punishments. The later acts also applied to the ports of Georgetown and Beaufort. Georgia established a quarantine system in the 1750s.[18]

Repeated epidemics of yellow fever and smallpox led to concern about the effectiveness of quarantine. In 1744, Governor James Glen told the assembly that ships from "suspected places" performing quarantine at Sullivan's Island were not being guarded carefully enough.[19] The assembly passed a new quarantine act that focused primarily on tightening up control over slave ships. The act's preamble declared that the health of the province had improved since 1740, when the assembly had placed a prohibitive duty on the importation of Africans in response to the Stono Rebellion. The improvement did not convince the assembly to maintain the duty, however. Instead, they decided that contagious diseases could be kept out by stricter quarantine of imported slaves. The act of 1744 required all ships bringing slaves for sale to anchor offshore near Sullivan's Island for ten days. During that time, the slaves were to be kept on shore, or be put on shore for at least six hours a day for five days, to allow the ships and slaves to be purified and cleansed of "any infectious distemper." Selling slaves without having obeyed this regulation was punishable by forfeiture of the slaves.[20] This and most future colonial quarantine acts were based on the assumption that slave ships were the main source of malignant diseases. Not everyone agreed. In 1756, a committee that reviewed the quarantine acts called for stricter regulations on ships carrying white passengers. The danger from whites, they argued, was the same as that from blacks, because their bodies and clothing could also harbor "contagious and malignant distempers."[21]

Tinkering with the quarantine acts continued throughout the colonial period. In 1747, the assembly increased fines for neglect or violation of the law and appointed six (later increased to nine) port physicians to inspect ships from places where contagious diseases were known to exist. By dividing the job among several doctors, the assembly obviously hoped to achieve more careful inspections.[22] This measure also failed to stop yellow fever, and in 1749, the assembly tried another approach. A petition from a group of citizens argued that the disease might originate locally from the large numbers of sick sailors crowded into the town from merchant ships and British warships. The petition

[17] *Stats.*, 2: 382–385.
[18] *Stats.*, 3: 127–130.
[19] *JCHA*, 4: 527, 531–535, 5: 159, 164–170, 184, 196, 480, 483–484; Council Journal, Minutes, Feb. 19, 1744, SCDAH.
[20] *Stats.*, 3: 773–774.
[21] *JCHA*, 14: 106, 11: 188–189, 217.
[22] *JCHA*, 6: 12, 7: 259, 325, 379; *Stats.*, 3: 694–696, 4: 28.

did not claim that the sailors themselves had brought yellow fever, but that a dense body of sick people could corrupt the atmosphere sufficiently to produce the fever. The petitioners questioned the common view that yellow fever was an exclusively imported disease. As we have seen, John Moultrie, Jr. argued the same view in that year. It is probable that the idea had been circulating in the town before Moultrie went to Edinburgh to study medicine. Many people believed that the fever came from West Indies, the petitioners noted, but it could also have been generated locally by sick sailors "crowded into some old rotten punch houses without either tolerable accommodations or attendance." The noxious effluvia arising from their bodies might corrupt the air of the town and "produce a malignant fever, though none were imported; or at least to spread and propagate it; if any such were." The last phrase indicates that the petitioners were not rejecting importation altogether.

The solution, they believed, was to establish a hospital for sick sailors outside the town. The assembly responded with an act that empowered St. Philip's Parish to buy or rent a house, "at a proper distance" from Charleston, to serve as a hospital for sick sailors and other transients. Without knowing why, the petitioners were right to suggest moving the sick away from the crowded town. If the newcomers were infected with yellow fever, mosquito vectors could easily transfer it from them to nearby inhabitants. In claiming that yellow fever could arise locally, the petition and act of 1749 in some ways presaged the turn away from quarantine in the early nineteenth century. The act also stressed the commercial losses epidemics caused: Malignant diseases had been "greatly detrimental to the trade and commerce of this Province."[23] It is perhaps not coincidental that the term "yellow fever" itself virtually disappeared from public discourse for half a century after this act was passed.

Nevertheless, the South Carolina colonial assembly continued to focus on tightening up the quarantine acts. To judge by complaints and changes in the law, they were often evaded. In 1756, a committee of the assembly reported that enforcement of quarantine had improved but that evasion of it was still too common.[24] In May 1774, a letter to the *South Carolina Gazette* complained that slave ships were being permitted to come into the harbor before they had performed the required quarantine. The evasion, he feared, would expose the town's inhabitants "to some terrible calamity worse than the rage to buy negroes."[25] This source of imported disease was partly closed in 1787 when the state legislature prohibited importation of slaves into South Carolina. Slaves continued to come in through Georgia, however. The prohibition was renewed several times before the slave trade was reopened in 1803 for four more years.[26]

[23] *JCHA*, 9: 200; *Stats.*, 3: 720–723; Waring, *History of Medicine in South Carolina, 1825–1900*, 109–110.
[24] *JCHA* 14; 105–107; Council Journals, July 1, 31, Sept. 16, 1745, SCDAH.
[25] Donnan, *Slave Trade*, 4: 467, n2.; *SCG*, Feb. 2, 1769, July 30, Sept. 10, 1772, May 1774.
[26] *Stats.*, 7: 433–434, 436, 444, 447, 449; Donnan, *Slave Trade*, 4 : 494, note 3.

By the mid-1750s, the quarantine acts were enforced more strictly than ever before, if we can believe Henry Laurens. In 1755 and 1756, he had more than 1,300 slaves under quarantine. He warned Gedney Clarke of Barbados that if he had a ship with any contagious disease aboard that he should not even consider sending it to Charleston. Laurens's correspondence from the mid-1750s and 1760s is filled with references to slave ships performing long quarantines, and the problems it caused for the sellers. Laurens was not opposed to quarantine itself. In 1774, he accused the British government of using "arbitrary power" to annul a strict quarantine act the Virginia assembly had passed. The act was designed to protect against the alleged threat of contagious disorders arriving on ships transporting convicts from Britain. Laurens complained that the action of the British government threatened "the health and natural liberty of a whole colony of Americans." It is clear from his letters that he knew that the slave trade also threatened the health of his own region. As to liberty, he did not say.[27]

The assembly passed the last quarantine act of the colonial period, a consolidating statute, in 1759. It, too, blamed contagious diseases primarily on the importation of African slaves, although it did not totally neglect European sources. The provisions of the 1759 act, with minor changes, were later incorporated into the quarantine acts passed by the state assembly after the Revolutionary War. With the move of the capital to Columbia soon after that, the power to order quarantine devolved to the city councils of Charleston and the other ports.[28]

QUARANTINE REJECTED

Around 1800 most Charleston doctors rejected the view that yellow fever was imported and contagious. They were undoubtedly influenced by Benjamin Rush's conclusion that the yellow fever that struck Philadelphia in 1793 had domestic origins and did not spread from person to person. Rush declared that yellow fever was related to and arose from the same causes as intermittent and remittent bilious fevers: miasmas arising from decomposing organic matter in hot weather. Yellow fever could develop anywhere that the right conditions of heat, moisture, and organic decomposition existed: the filth of the docks, the foul air of ships, sewers, privies, gutters, dirty cellars and yards, impure pump water, putrefying organic matter. Some northern doctors never accepted Rush's anticontagionist position. Even those who did often continued to advocate quarantine as a precaution or because they believed yellow fever could sometimes be imported. Charleston's doctors, however, accepted

[27] Donnan, *Slave Trade*, 4: 316, 320–321, 325, 336–337, 348–349, 359–361; *HLP*, 1: 294–295, 2: 41, 78, 223–224; 233; 275–277, 299–301, 472–473; 4: 507, 9: 348.

[28] *JCHA*, 11: 252, 363–366; *Stats.*, 3: 771–773; 4: 78–86; 572–574, 615–618; 668; 5: 284–285, 315; 6: 472–474; *Digest of the Ordinances of the City Council of Charleston* (Charleston, 1818), appendix, 26–27, 205.

Rush's views almost universally. In 1802, Ramsay noted that the "disputes about the origin of yellow fever, which have agitated the northern states, have never existed in Charleston." The doctors and inhabitants were agreed it "was neither imported nor contagious."[29] Ramsay was not exaggerating the unanimity of the doctors at least. In the midst of the yellow fever epidemic of 1799, the Medical Society agreed, by a vote of ten-to-one, that the disease was not contagious. Later that year, they voted unanimously that it was neither imported nor contagious.[30] The doctors' position soon became widely known and accepted. When Francois Michaux arrived in Charleston in 1802, he learned that locals believed that yellow fever was not contagious, in contrast with people in New York and Philadelphia. He also reported – perhaps unwittingly – the major reason for the difference: Inhabitants of the northern cities were "as apt to contract it as foreigners."[31] In other words, the widespread immunity of Charlestonians to yellow fever made it easier for them to accept that it was not contagious, whereas the widespread susceptibility of most people in northern cities inclined them toward the view that it was. The vulnerability of the inhabitants of northern cities also made them more likely to err on the side of caution in regards to quarantine. Yellow fever epidemics in northern cities may have been rarer than in Charleston and other southern cities, but they often infected and killed a much larger number of people, as in Philadelphia in 1793.

Most Charleston doctors remained anticontagionist between 1800 and the 1850s. In 1819, John Shecut declared that all doctors but one agreed that yellow fever was never contagious in Charleston at least.[32] About the same time, Joseph Johnson told the Medical Society "we all believe that yellow fever is not contagious *here*" (emphasis added). Shecut and Johnson may have been trying to bridge the gap between northern contagionism and southern anticontagionism. Another local doctor, Matthew Irvine, was less compromising. He viewed contagionism as an error propagated by the boards of health of northern cities. Many doctors in other American and European cities agreed with the Charleston doctors. Yet, contagionist ideas continued to be supported by influential physicians elsewhere, especially in New York and Philadelphia.[33]

[29] David Ramsay, "Facts concerning the yellow fever, as it appears at Charleston (South Carolina)" *Medical Repository* 4 (1801): 217–220; David Ramsay, *An Eulogium upon Benjamin Rush, M. D.* (Philadelphia, 1813), 28–31. Benjamin Rush, *Observations upon the Origin of the Malignant Bilious, or Yellow Fever* (Philadelphia, 1799), 3–5; William Currie, *An Impartial Review of Dr. Rush's Late Publication Entitled "An Account of the Bilious Remitting Fever"* (Philadelphia, 1794); Lloyd G. Stevenson, "Putting Disease on the Map: The Early Use of Spot Maps in the Study of Yellow Fever," *Journal of the History of Medicine and Allied Sciences* 20 (1965), 229–233.

[30] MSM, May 23, Aug. 24, 29, 1799, July 1, 1800.

[31] Francois Andre Michaux, *Travels to the West of the Allegheny Mountains* (London, 1805), in Reuben Gold Thwaites, ed., *Travels West of the Alleghanies* (Cleveland, 1904), 120.

[32] MSM, Sept. 15, 1817; Shecut, *Medical and Philosophical Essays*, 115.

[33] MSM, Sept. 1, 1820, 165, Sept. 6, 1824, 247; Thomas Y. Simons "Observations on the Yellow Fever, as it occurs in Charleston, South Carolina," *Carolina Journal of Medicine, Science,*

Once Charleston's doctors adopted the anticontagionist position, they logically advocated a relaxation of quarantine. Until 1799, the Medical Society had supported the quarantine laws and called existing laws inadequate. In 1794, they even recommended more stringent regulations against vessels coming from the West Indies.[34] By 1799, they were backing off that position. They supported continued quarantine that year but indicated the direction their ideas were heading: "We consider our greatest danger to be from domestic sources."[35] The following year, they explicitly rejected the need for quarantine. They advised the authorities that because yellow fever had domestic origins and was not contagious, relaxing the quarantine laws was safe.[36] A few years later, Ramsay called quarantine an absurd and useless restriction on commerce "founded in the ignorance and error of a comparatively unenlightened period." By 1809, he noted approvingly that the execution of the laws was sufficiently eased to avoid major inconvenience to shipping.[37]

Most of Ramsay's colleagues agreed. In 1805, Tucker Harris declared that "scarcely one" physician in the city doubted the domestic origin of yellow fever, and added that if their view was correct, "all quarantine laws respecting it must be nugatory." Why did the city have no yellow fever in 1793, 1798, and 1803, he asked, when commerce with the West Indies went on as usual? Why did New York and Philadelphia have epidemics in years Charleston did not, and vice versa, when both traded with the latter?[38] The Charleston *Courier* joined the parade. Yellow fever, it noted, had appeared in ports before any ships had arrived with the disease on board, "before there was the smallest probability of its having been introduced from abroad." The refrain was repeated endlessly: Quarantine hurt the local economy without solving the problem. If yellow fever was not imported, quarantine was superfluous. If it was imported, quarantine had proved ineffective because the disease kept coming back. Quarantine was also inhumane. People were isolated miles away from regular medical attendance. Humanity dictated that they be allowed to come into the city and receive proper treatment at the Marine Hospital or be provided with a comfortable and well-equipped lazaretto. Contagionism was also chauvinistic. As John Moultrie, Jr. had argued, people rejected the

and Agriculture 1 (1825), 4; F. M. Robertson, *A Report of the Origin and Cause of the Late Epidemic in Augusta, Georgia* (1839), 29–30; Matthew Irvine, *Irvine's Treatise on the Yellow Fever* (Charleston, 1820), 3–6; Samuel Henry Dickson, *Essays on Pathology and Therapeutics* 2 vols. (Charleston, 1845), 1: 339; William Currie, *Philadelphia Medical and Physical Journal*, 2 (1805), 35–39; Baldwin, *Contagion and the State*; Stevenson, "Putting Disease on the Map," 229–233.

34 MSM, July 26, 1794, May 1, 1795.

35 MSM, May 15, 1799, 94–95, Aug. 29, 1799, 97.

36 MSM, June 23, 1800, 101; David Ramsay, "Facts concerning the yellow fever, as it appears at Charleston (South Carolina)," *Medical Repository* 4 (1801): 217–220.

37 David Ramsay, "Remarks on the yellow fever and epidemic catarrh, as they appeared in South Carolina during the summer and autumn of 1807," *Medical Repository* 2d ser. 5 (1808): 234; Ramsay, *History of South Carolina*, 2: 48.

38 Harris, "Yellow Fever of Charleston," 29–33.

domestic theory of yellow fever because it seemed an insult to their homeland. It was more comforting to lay the blame elsewhere.[39]

As in the North, a few lowcountry doctors rejected contagionism without rejecting quarantine. They argued that the noxious atmosphere of yellow fever could in some way reproduce itself. As Joseph Johnson put it in 1820, "this comes so near to the generation of contagion, that the quarantine regulations are very prudently enforced."[40] Doctors who advocated relaxation of quarantine, however, dominated thinking on the subject until the 1850s. In 1817, the president of the Medical Society, James B. Finley, reiterated the society's opinion that yellow fever was not contagious and added that he hoped this opinion would remove "all unnecessary embarrassments from the commerce of our city." He might have been embarrassed to know that one of his acquaintances, Hetty Heyward, wrote that Finley had contracted the disease after treating many patients with it and that his own family believed "he could not escape."[41]

A SANITARY SOLUTION

In 1820, Dr. Matthew Irvine of Charleston decided that he must write an essay on yellow fever. Contagionist doctrine, he argued, was gaining wide acceptance among physicians in New York, Philadelphia, and Baltimore, a trend he viewed as dangerous for the country. It would produce quarantine restrictions harmful to the nation's commerce and interrupt communication between the different states of the Union. It would also tend to produce a relaxation of sanitary regulations, the surest defense against the disease.[42] Irvine's view was common in his city. During the first half of the nineteenth century, most Charleston doctors held that the best way to prevent epidemic disease, and especially yellow fever, was to improve sanitation. In this they were following in the wake of many doctors elsewhere in the western world. Inspired by scientific advances and Enlightenment notions of progress, some doctors fostered an international campaign to prevent disease by combating its local environmental origins. Advocates saw themselves – somewhat incorrectly – as followers of the "divine" Hippocrates and Thomas Sydenham, the "English Hippocrates." They cited Hippocrates' admonition that one must study the climate, waters, diet, and topography of a place in order to understand and properly treat its diseases. Hippocratic revivals were nothing new,

---

[39] *The Courier*, Aug. 27, Sept. 24, 1806; MSM, June 1, 1804, Sept. 16, Dec. 2–3 1805; Dr. Thomas Y. Simons, *A Report on the History and Causes of the Strangers or Yellow Fever of Charleston* (Charleston, 1839), 8–11, 15–17.

[40] MSM, Sept. 1, 1820.

[41] *The Courier*, Sept. 9, 1817; Hetty Heyward to Mother, Sept. 13, 1817, Heyward and Ferguson Family Papers, COCSC. Whether Finley contracted yellow fever or not is unclear, but he was forced to retire from the chair of a meeting of the Medical Society of on Sept. 15, 1817 in the midst of an epidemic because of "indisposition."

[42] Matthew Irvine, *Irvine's Treatise on the Yellow Fever* (Charleston, 1820), 3–4.

but eighteenth-century physicians added a new twist of optimism. They contended that it was possible for humans to alter the disease environment for the better and thus eliminate the sources of many illnesses. Advocates of this environmental approach generally held that disease originated in miasmas or "bad air" (*mal'aria*) produced by the decomposition of organic matter, vegetable, animal, and human. Marshes, swamps, filthy streets, clogged drains and sewers, animal pens, and urban cemeteries were all sources of miasmatic poisons. To combat these sources of disease, it was necessary to remove decomposing matter from the vicinity of human habitations, and to provide good ventilation, proper drainage, and an adequate supply of clean water. The result would be a healthier, larger, and more productive population.[43]

Attempts to ensure public health through sanitary regulations dated from the origins of the Carolina colony. The Lords Proprietors were concerned about the colonists' health, because the economic success of their project required a substantial settled population. The colonists themselves soon became concerned about the dangers of miasmas produced by their own concentration in Charleston. At the time of the colony's first epidemiological crisis in 1685, the assembly passed a statute that required owners and possessors of lots in Charleston to clear them of bushes, young pines, and weeds, for "the preservation of the good air thereof." The colonial government subsequently passed many acts designed to remove or restrict noxious nuisances such as weeds, foul privies, cattle, sheep and hog pens, and slaughterhouses. After the yellow fever epidemic of 1706, Governor Nathaniel Johnson attributed the sickness in part to "the nasty keeping of the streets."[44] In 1710, the assembly created the offices of town scavenger and clerk of the market with authority to enforce all sanitary acts. Various acts thereafter empowered commissioners to order the building of drains and cleansing of streets in Charleston.[45]

Sanitary progress was glacial. Visitors and locals often remarked on the poor condition of the streets and the lack of proper drainage. In 1741, the wardens and vestry of St. Philip's Parish complained that a dammed creek on Church Street had become "a nasty, stinking pond, a nuisance not only to that neighborhood, but to the community in general ... tending to corrupt the air and occasion sickness among them."[46] Such complaints remained common throughout the colonial period and beyond. In 1757, a letter to the *South Carolina Gazette* noted that the "mischievous consequences" of climate, topography, and inundations for rice and indigo cultivation were aggravated

[43] James C. Riley, *The Eighteenth Century Campaign to Avoid Disease* (New York: St. Martin's Press, 1987); Richard Towne, *A Treatise on the Diseases Most Frequent in the West Indies* (London, 1726), 1, 17.

[44] *Stats.*, 7: 1–2, 5–6, 9–12, 38; *JCHA*, March 6, 1706/07, 5.

[45] St. Julien Ravenel Childs, "Notes on the History of Public Health in South Carolina, 1670–1800," *Proceedings of the South Carolina Historical Association*, 18, note 22; Nicholas Trott, *The Laws of South Carolina* (Charleston, 1736), 436; *Stats.*, 3: 405.

[46] *JCHA*, 2: 510–511; *SCG*, July 9, 1750, "An Abstract of an Act ... for keeping the streets in Charles-Town clean."

by crowding, filth, and poor drainage. He urged improved drainage of the streets and low places where standing water collected, and removal of rotting carcasses and other animal filth.[47] The next year, the *Gazette* printed "A Remonstrance of the Streets of Charles-Town against the Inhabitants." In a work that might have been inspired by a dose of opium, the anonymous writer brings the streets to life to charge the citizens with a dangerous neglect of their main thoroughfares. The streets are not only outraged by their filthy condition, they also pose as defenders of the health and reputation of the city. They denounce the "little, narrow, dirty and irregular alleys and lanes opened every where through and through us ... [as] a disgrace to the town." Because of the negligence of the citizens, "we are daily abused and reviled by strangers, for being the most stinking and nasty streets in the world." The streets absolve themselves of all blame "for the diseases that may happen, or the lives, which may be lost, by such a pollution of the air, as may arise from so infamous a neglect."[48] Despite such protests, little improvement occurred. Even today, some Charleston streets are poorly drained.

After independence in 1783, Charleston was incorporated. Responsibility for its sanitary condition was henceforth in the hands of the city government and the officers and commissions it established, although the state government occasionally passed acts relating to public health that affected Charleston. The Revolutionary War had severely hurt the city economically and left it in a filthy and overcrowded condition. Like the South Carolina colonial assembly before it, city council passed numerous ordinances in the following decades designed to remove "nuisances" and establish cleanliness.[49] Something had changed, however. City officials actively sought the advice and expertise of the local doctors, and the doctors were happy to comply. The Medical Society of South Carolina made the prevention of disease through improved urban sanitation one of its main goals. Its members repeatedly urged a series of sanitary measures, including daily street cleaning, improved drainage and sewage removal, filling holes in streets and marshes, planting trees, putting greater space between houses, and providing pure water. In the late 1790s, the city council requested that the society act as a de facto board of health, giving advice on public health matters.[50]

The Medical Society's views may have been especially attractive to city officials because of their rejection of quarantine. In 1806, a series of articles in The Charleston *Courier* presented the Medical Society's views in detail. The author argued that yellow fever could be prevented through sanitary measures. If the city government implemented the Medical Society's recommendations,

---

[47] SCG, June 9, 1757; M. Foster Farley, *An Account of the History of Stranger's Fever in Charleston, 1699–1876* (Washington, DC: University Press of America), 26–28.
[48] SCG, Dec. 1, 1758.
[49] *Ordinances of the City Council of Charleston* (Charleston, 1802, 1807), 132–133, 164–165, 407–422; *Digest of the Ordinances of Charleston*, 193–194.
[50] MSM, May 1, 1795, May 23, 1799; David Ramsay, *A Dissertation on Preserving Health in Charleston and the Adjacent Lowcountry* (Charleston, 1790), 15–16.

Charleston would be the cleanest and healthiest city in the country.[51] During the next few decades, the city focused on a sanitary solution to yellow fever. In 1808, it created a commission of streets and lamps with power to implement various sanitary measures.[52] In 1815, it established a Board of Health that was required to meet at least once a week between June and November – the yellow fever season. It was instructed to publish weekly returns of interments in the city during these months. In 1818, the board gained the power to order owners of low lots to drain them or fill them up to the level of the streets. Enforcement of sanitary regulations proved difficult, however. Owners often failed to obey orders to fill lots or filled them with noxious organic matter. The Medical Society often deprecated the practice of filling up low grounds and making and repairing streets with filth and offal.[53]

Sanitary improvements had unanimous support among Charleston's doctors. But some did not think that these measures would prevent yellow fever. In 1805, Tucker Harris put it bluntly: "[W]ere our city to be kept as clean as the drawing room of a fashionable lady, and were the waters we use as pure as Helicon," it would not prevent the disease.[54] In 1840, Benjamin Strobel also questioned the effectiveness of sanitary measures in preventing the fever. Unsanitary conditions were deplorable, but they could not – by themselves at least – cause yellow fever. Epidemics invariably began on or near the docks on the Cooper River, in the southeastern part of the city. To be sure, the waterfront was a dirty area, but sections of the city where yellow fever never penetrated were just as dirty. Something besides filth was necessary to produce it.[55]

For most doctors, that something was meteorological: a peculiar state of the atmosphere. But exactly what was that peculiarity? Everyone agreed that yellow fever could not exist without a certain degree of heat and moisture, but that, too, was not sufficient. Some doctors believed that the quantity of "electric fluid" or some other substance in the air was the key factor. Since the late eighteenth-century electrical experiments of Luigi Galvani and others, many doctors had become convinced that electricity was a vital principle, perhaps the principle of life itself. This was the time when a young Englishwoman conceived a tale of the creation of a man – or monster – from dead body parts, brought to life by some means involving electricity. In real life, doctors were trying to jolt executed convicts into life with electric shocks. In the same year as Mary Shelley's *Frankenstein* appeared, 1819, John Shecut ascribed the peculiar atmospheric state that produced yellow fever to an "absence of a due proportion of the electric fluid" in the atmosphere, brought on by a below-average number of summer thunderstorms. He theorized that lightning helped neutralize or disperse disease-causing miasmas that otherwise reached fatal

[51] *The Courier*, June 14–Oct. 1, 1806.
[52] *Digest of the Ordinances of Charleston*, 407–422; Ramsay, *History of South Carolina*, 2: 48–49; MSM, May 17, 1808, June 1, 5, 1810.
[53] *Digest of the Ordinances of Charleston*, 21–27; MSM, June 2, 1817, 97, Nov. 1, 1824, 253.
[54] Harris, "Yellow Fever of Charleston," 27, 32–33.
[55] Strobel, *Yellow Fever*, 208–210.

concentrations during the heat of summer. Other doctors posited a relationship between epidemics and thunderstorms, amount of rain, or other meteorological phenomena. Of course, nothing could be done to change the weather. But Shecut argued that if electrical storms neutralized the miasmatic poisons, then reducing the sources of miasmas – draining and filling creeks and marshes, and making Charleston higher and drier – could prevent yellow fever. Shecut hoped the work of drying and elevating could be completed within a century. His timeline was about right.[56] Other doctors agreed with Shecut's goal if not his theory. Matthew Irvine urged authorities to enforce the city's sanitary ordinances if they wanted to prevent or at least reduce the effects of yellow fever. Even doctors who thought it was imported believed it could not become epidemic in the absence of the right environmental conditions.[57]

Making Charleston as clean and dry as the doctors prescribed was an elusive goal. It required not only increased taxation but also interference – not always justified – with people's lives and properties. One of the favorite measures of nineteenth-century sanitarians in Charleston, as elsewhere, was prohibiting burials within the city, on the grounds that decaying corpses were a source of miasmatic poisons. The idea outraged the clergy and their congregations. After the yellow fever epidemic of 1858, a city council committee proposed an ordinance designed to end interments in the churchyards. The proposal provoked a memorial and report, signed by many of Charleston's leading citizens, sternly rebuking the idea. They claimed – correctly – that urban burials had no connection with yellow fever or other diseases. They also noted – again correctly – that the doctors themselves disagreed about the cause of yellow fever.[58]

City officials may have been well intentioned, but the sanitary improvements they secured were marginal. In 1829, the Board of Health described a city abounding in nuisances that more than a century of sanitary legislation had not removed: narrow unpaved streets; inadequate drains; filthy cellars and cesspools; abundant cow yards and hog pens; poor-quality water. The board blamed complacency produced by the occasional years in which yellow fever was absent or mild, combined with a fatalistic resignation during epidemics and the belief that adult natives and long-time residents were immune. The citizens, the board insisted, had a duty to "render this city, to children and strangers, what it is now to its resident inhabitants, one of the most healthy abodes" in the world. The board called for a comprehensive plan to secure

[56] Shecut, *Medical and Philosophical Essays*, 26–27; Ramsay, *History of South Carolina*, 2: 39–42; James Tinsley, *A New Theory of the Yellow Fever* (Charleston, 1819); MSM, Sept. 1, 1820, 165; Joseph Johnson, "Some Account of the Origin and Prevention of Yellow Fever in Charleston, South Carolina," *Charleston Medical Journal and Review*, 4 (1849), 154–155.

[57] Irvine, *Yellow Fever*, 55–56; Samuel Henry Dickson, "Account of the Epidemic which prevailed in Charleston, S. C. during the summer of 1827," *The American Journal of the Medical Sciences* (1828), 2: 6–8; Strobel, *Yellow Fever*, 11; *Report of the Committee of the City Council of Charleston, upon the Epidemic Yellow Fever of 1858* (Charleston, 1859), 25–27.

[58] *Report of the Committee of the City Council of Charleston upon Interments within the City, and the Memorial of the Churches and Citizens* (Charleston, 1859), 3–8.

the removal of nuisances through improved drainage and filth removal, and cleaning up of unsanitary cattle pens. They called for more open spaces and improvement of water supplies. These improvements, they conceded, would require large increases in funding and personnel.[59]

That kind of financial commitment was not forthcoming. Instead, city authorities tried to prevent pestilence by seasonal calls for cleanliness and disinfection of the air. During warm weather, the Board of Health placed notices in the newspapers calling for the prompt removal or disinfection of putrefying substances. In addition to the usual recommendations of cleansing drains and filling holes, they urged the throwing of disinfectants such as quick lime into privies and graves. During the epidemic of 1817, the Medical Society recommended alkaline disinfectants such as lime, potash, and wood-ashes. When these methods of prevention failed, the society urged people to use acid fumigations made up of water, table salt or niter, and sulfuric acid to disinfect houses, buildings, and the holds of ships. City council asked the society whether its members believed burning tar or charcoal would help. They thought it doubtful, but the city did it anyway, surely because it had been a standard response to urban epidemics for centuries. Benjamin Strobel recalled such attempts to destroy or neutralize the miasma during his youth: "We well remember the burning of tar, the sprinkling of lime, and various other means adopted in the vain hope of arresting the scourge."[60]

The sanitary condition of Charleston may have improved marginally during the antebellum period, but it is difficult to detect any significant lasting change. In the aftermath of the yellow fever epidemic of 1838, a city report blamed overcrowding near the wharves and bad well water. Mayor Henry Laurens Pinckney charged that the city's water was a pestilent brew containing "not only the soluble filth, and excretion of men and animals, but the very mortal remains of our citizens."[61] A flurry of cleaning activity followed: Low lots were filled, new drains built, potholes fixed, streets swept more regularly, and the number of scavengers' carts increased. In 1839, The Charleston *Courier* attributed another epidemic to some putrid bacon and rotten cotton seed found in a vacant lot. It was cleaned up, but the disease continued its sway for weeks.[62]

In 1849, after a decade relatively free of yellow fever, Joseph Johnson remarked that the "cleanliness of the city was remarkable." He lauded new building codes that prohibited cellars, the planting of trees in the streets, and the widening and ventilating of narrow lanes and alleys. Yet epidemics struck the city that year and repeatedly during the 1850s. Poor sanitation was still being blamed. In 1858, after the highest yellow fever death toll of the century,

[59] *The Courier*, May 20, 1818; *Stats.*, 7: 144; *Communication from the Chairman of the Board of Health* (Charleston, 1829), 3–16.
[60] *The Courier*, Aug. 9, Sept. 18, 1817, Aug. 30, 1824, Aug. 27, 1838; MSM, Sept. 4, 1817, 101; Strobel, *Yellow Fever*, 201.
[61] Fraser, *Charleston!*, 217.
[62] *The Courier*, Aug. 22, 1839.

the Medical Society and a city committee agreed that neglect of sanitation had caused the epidemic. Sanitary conditions deteriorated further during the Civil War and after. At the time of Charleston's last major epidemic of yellow fever in 1871 and into the early twentieth century, citizens and visitors were deploring the filthiness of many parts of the city.[63] But before then, ideas about preventing the scourge had begun to shift again.

"THIS DREADFUL FOREIGN SCOURGE"

During the yellow fever epidemic of 1838, *The Courier* expressed astonishment at the conduct of the authorities of Wilmington, North Carolina. They had declared quarantine against Charleston: "Can it be possible that the citizens of a southern town, within 14 hours sail of Charleston, are so little acquainted with the disease that afflicts us, as to suppose that they would be affected by it, by allowing passengers to land? That their hotels were closed against travelers, from the fear of infection?" *The Courier* added incredulously, "even the negroes were cautioned not to go near the boat from Charleston, for fear they should catch the fever." Were the citizens of Wilmington not aware that blacks were immune to the disease?[64]

The following year, a Charleston doctor argued that Wilmington's action was not at all bizarre. In 1839, another epidemic convinced Benjamin Strobel, physician at the Marine Hospital, that yellow fever could be imported. He sidestepped the thorny issue of personal contagion, conceding that the evidence on that was ambiguous. Instead, he insisted that yellow fever was in some unknown way "transmissible" from place to place. It could be shown to move along shipping and trade routes. Strobel did not deny that it could originate locally or that local atmospheric conditions always played a role in its propagation. Yet his investigation of the epidemic of 1839 convinced him that the disease had often been imported in ships arriving from the West Indies. His effort to trace the spread of the disease from the ships through the city's neighborhoods was an impressive piece of epidemiological detective work, using spot maps for tracing cases (see Figure 12.1). It did not establish the case for importation "beyond a shadow of a doubt" as he claimed, but it certainly angered many of his medical colleagues. His main conclusion – that the evidence warranted "a rigid and effective quarantine" – was shared by many physicians and health boards in the North but was anathema in his native city and other southern ports. He conceded that it might take a long time for his view to prevail in Charleston because so many commercial interests and

---

[63] *Yearbook, City of Charleston*, 1880, 30–33, 39, 75–77; Leon Banov, *As I Recall: the Story of the Charleston County Health Department* (Columbia, SC: R. L. Bryan Co., 1970), 7–11; Waring, *Medicine in South Carolina, 1825–1900*, 67; E. Chernin, "The Disappearance of Bancroftian filariasis from Charleston, South Carolina," *American Journal of Tropical Medicine and Hygiene* 37 (1987), 111–114.

[64] *The Courier*, Sept. 13, 1838.

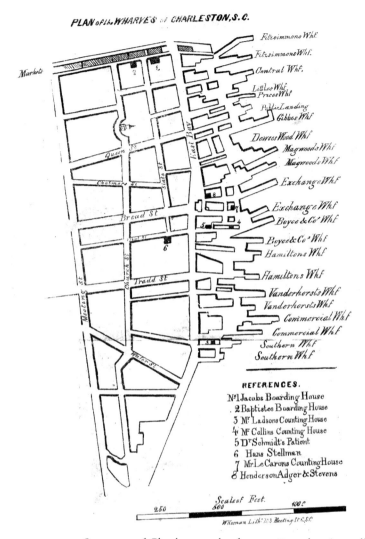

FIGURE 12.1. Spot map of Charleston wharf area, 1839, showing yellow fever cases, from Benjamin Strobel, *An Essay on the Subject of Yellow Fever Intended to Prove its Transmissibility* (Charleston, 1840) (Courtesy of the Waring Historical Library, MUSC).

prejudices were arrayed against it: "Boards of health, the mercantile interests, and the captains of vessels in their employ, all seem linked together for the purpose of concealing the existence of the disease, until it has made such progress and become so manifest, as to announce itself." Opponents of quarantine were not only placing economic interests above the public health; they were exploiting public ignorance to maintain the status quo: "[W]hilst error and delusions are propagated gratuitously at the public expense – truth creeps into notice, often amidst the revilings and denunciations of the rabble for whose benefit it is designed." Strobel's apostasy, accusations of collusion, and language – "delusions," "rabble" – aroused anger in some quarters. These factors surely contributed to a rupture with his medical colleagues. In 1841, he was dropped from the rolls of the Medical Society for nonpayment of dues. He died in 1849, just as medical opinion in Charleston and in other southern cities was shifting toward his views.[65]

One prominent Charleston doctor supported Strobel in 1839: Samuel Henry Dickson, professor of medicine at the Medical College of South Carolina. A few years later, Dickson noted that the unanimity of views about yellow fever's origins among Charleston's doctors was breaking down. The change did not mean complete rejection of the theory of local origins, but rather acceptance that the disease was sometimes imported from the West Indies. In Dickson's view, one of the things that undermined the theory of local origins was the irregular periodicity of epidemics in Charleston. If it was truly endemic, as advocates of local origin claimed, why did it not appear more regularly? Dickson argued that Charleston was probably located at the "extreme northern limit of spontaneous production" of yellow fever; that is, under favorable conditions it might arise locally, but was often killed off by Charleston winters. Strobel's evidence was not conclusive, but it was "highly probable ... that yellow fever is contagious and communicable" where populations were dense and temperatures sufficiently warm. Given these realities, it was foolish to relax quarantine restrictions, "absurd and inconvenient" as they might be. In 1849, Joseph Johnson, president of the Medical Society, argued that yellow fever could be introduced by ships from infected ports. It had sometimes been carried inland by people who had become infected in Charleston. During the 1850s – a decade of severe epidemics – more and more doctors began to call for an effective quarantine against yellow fever. In the mid-1850s, the Medical Society announced that it would no longer oppose strict enforcement of the quarantine laws. In 1858, Charleston attorney Edward McCrady noted that the return of epidemic yellow fever in 1849 had coincided with the start of direct steamship communication between Havana and Charleston.[66]

In the same year McCrady's piece appeared, Dr. Bennet Dowler of New Orleans complained that "a small minority of the medical faculty" in southern states were influencing cities and states to "enforce oppressive quarantine laws."[67] Pressure to enforce the laws was indeed increasing in Charleston. After

[65] Strobel, *Yellow Fever*, 8–9, 126–128, 216; Waring, *Medicine in South Carolina, 1825–1900*, 222–226, 304–305; Stevenson, "Putting Disease on the Map," 253–256; Humphreys, *Yellow Fever*, 21–24.

[66] Samuel Henry Dickson, *Essays on Pathology and Therapeutics* 2 vols. (Charleston, 1845), 1: 338–343; Johnson, "Origin and Prevention of Yellow Fever in Charleston," 156–159; Humphreys, *Yellow Fever*, 20–25.

[67] Bennet Dowler, "The Yellow Fever in Charleston in 1858," *New Orleans Medical and Surgical Journal*, 16 (1858), 600.

the epidemic of 1858, the city council appointed a committee to investigate the origins and spread of yellow fever. In its report, the committee noted that a "respectable part of the citizens" believed that the disease could be prevented by quarantine; and that on the other hand, "a large and intelligent portion" of them were convinced that only the most rigid sanitary regulations could prevent it. The committee polled some of the oldest doctors in town on the controversy, those who had been in practice at least twenty-five years. Of the ten doctors who replied to the committee, five believed that yellow fever was never imported, four argued that it sometimes was, and one had no opinion. Most believed that the disease could or did originate locally, but a few thought imported cases could make it more virulent, more infectious, and possibly also contagious. The committee took no stand on the issue of importation, although they did agree that yellow fever had existed in Ancient Greece – an announcement that must have comforted many people.[68]

One of the most important converts to importation in the 1850s was Dr. William Hume, long a staunch believer in the domestic origins of yellow fever. A science professor at The Citadel, the state military academy, Hume had labored for years to prove that the disease was native to Charleston and produced by specific meteorological conditions. But in 1854, he confessed that his study of the meteorological conditions of epidemic and healthy years had convinced him that no clear correlation existed between weather patterns and yellow fever epidemics. Weather conditions in epidemic and healthy years had often been virtually identical, as had the sanitary conditions in the city. After failing to predict an epidemic in 1852, and incorrectly predicting one in 1853, Hume sought another explanation. Although local weather and sanitary conditions might be necessary to the production of the disease, he concluded, they were not sufficient to explain its origins or the variability in its visitations. The exciting principle of the disease must come from elsewhere, and the evidence overwhelmingly pointed to ships from infected ports. John Lining had been right and Benjamin Rush wrong.

Hume wrote many articles and reports urging the city to enforce strict quarantine. He even suggested excluding ships from the West Indies for several months a year. Failure to do this, pleading commercial needs, was equivalent to poisoning local wells for profit. In any case, the claim that quarantine would destroy Charleston's West Indian trade was false. Strict quarantine in New York had kept the fever at bay for nearly twenty-five years without a significant increase in the price of sugar there. Moreover, any price increase would be borne by consumers, not merchants. Hume concluded that Charleston was too far north to generate yellow fever locally because it did not occur every summer, in contrast to Havana, which he saw as the main source of Charleston's epidemics. Sporadic cases might arise locally, but could not produce epidemics by themselves. Hume recommended that quarantined

<hr />

[68] *City Council of Charleston, on the Origin and Diffusion of the Yellow Fever in Charleston in the Summer of 1858* (Charleston, 1858), 4, 23–46.

ships and their cargoes be fumigated before being allowed to dock at the city
wharves. Charlestonians, especially blacks, being largely immune to the fever,
would be excellent for the work of transferring and disinfecting cargoes.
Strangers should be prohibited from it.[69]

By the 1850s, the Charleston mercantile community was openly divided
on quarantine. In May 1854, a petition from "dry goods merchants" led the
city council to propose a new ordinance tightening up quarantine. It aroused
strong opposition from merchants engaged in maritime commerce, especially
with the West Indies. A letter to *The Courier* claimed that the proposed regulations, which included a thirty-day quarantine of all ships arriving from
infected ports, would be an unwarranted hindrance to the city's seaborne
commerce. It could be justified only if it was proven that the disease was
imported. That could be done only by implementing quarantine by land as
well as by sea. The author proposed the establishment of a strict 'cordon
sanitaire' around the city, blocking the arrival of goods and persons by rail-
road. If that policy succeeded in preventing the disease, he would "rejoice"
even though it would mean the death of maritime commerce in Charleston
and the South. The stakes were high. Seaborne commerce was the only thing
that would "secure the commercial independence of the South" – a matter of
great concern to many southerners in the 1850s.[70]

A few days later, an advocate of quarantine replied that yellow fever was
undoubtedly transportable by ship in some fashion, through fomites such as
fur, hair, or cloth, or by persons. He added that it was possible to establish an
effective quarantine; that such regulations were for the benefit of all; and that
however burdensome, they would be less injurious to the community than the
"invasion of a pestilential epidemic." The writer, a doctor, claimed that few
people in the medical profession would now dispute these propositions – a
remarkable change from the situation only twenty years before. He noted that
many cities to the north that had once suffered severely from yellow fever epidemics were now exempt from them because they enforced a strict quarantine.
When yellow fever broke out in Charleston in the summer of 1854, another
citizens' petition demanded effective quarantine regulations. It was the only
way, they claimed, to prevent "this dreadful foreign scourge." Moreover,
they claimed, "an efficient quarantine would only impede a small portion
of Charleston's trade, while the epidemic has paralyzed the entire business

---

[69] William Hume's articles include the following: "Report to the City Council of Charleston,
on a Resolution of Inquiry, relative to the Source and Origin of Yellow Fever," *Charleston
Medical Journal and Review*, 9 (1854), 145–164; "An Inquiry into some of the general and
local causes to which the endemic origins of Yellow Fever has been attributed by myself and
others," *Charleston Medical Journal and Review*, 9 (1854), 721–727; "On the Germination
of Yellow Fever in Cities," *Charleston Medical Journal and Review*, 13 (1858), 154–157,
177; "The Yellow Fever of Charleston, considered in its relation to West India commerce,"
Charleston Medical Journal and Review, 15 (1860), 1–32. See also, Waring, *Medicine in
South Carolina, 1825–1900*, 248–249.

[70] *The Courier*, May 29, 1854.

of the city."[71] Following the epidemic, city council passed an ordinance to make quarantine more effective. The ordinance applied the strictest regulations during the warm months to ships coming from infected ports or tropical and subtropical regions. It gave the port physician wide powers to order ships, passengers, and cargo to be cleansed and ventilated and to destroy any cargo he considered incapable of purification.[72]

By the 1850s, quarantine had an attraction beyond its possible health benefits. Hume argued that a moratorium on trade with the Caribbean during the yellow fever months would attract white immigrants and capital. Opponents of quarantine apparently believed that "the importation of one thousand hogsheads of sugar and molasses advances the prosperity more than the immigration of one thousand Irish and German candidates for permanent citizenship." He charged that the immunity of many natives from the disease had made some of them a bit callous toward the suffering of strangers, especially when the latter's health competed against the needs of commerce.[73] Experience had shown that "an increase of population is incompatible with the prevalence of a mortal pestilence.... It destroys those who settle and deters others from settling." Hume's argument had an elitist side. Under existing conditions, only "the ignorant, the destitute, or the desperate" would risk Charleston's climate, whereas "the more desirable and useful will settle other and safer regions ... Capitalists and foreign merchants avoid us, while petty German traders and Irish laborers supply their places." At the same time, he accused locals of chauvinism, or worse: They resented immigrants and even welcomed yellow fever as a means of reducing the number of "undesirables" in the population.[74]

Hume was responding to a common concern: the slow rate of population growth in Charleston and South Carolina compared to other cities and states, and the fact that whites were a minority in the state. The lagging population was partly the result of out-migration – mainly to the richer cotton lands to the west – which had accelerated after 1820. The censuses of 1850 and 1860 showed that about 40 percent of people born in South Carolina were living in other states. Most of them had gone to the Lower South states to the west: Georgia, Alabama, and Mississippi. South Carolina had a higher rate of out-migration than the nation. The out-migrants greatly outnumbered in-migrants from other states, fourteen to one. Immigration from Europe also dropped to a trickle during the antebellum period, in contrast to many other states, especially in the North and Midwest. In 1850 and 1860, more than 90 percent of South Carolina's people had been born there, making it one of the most insular states in the country. Diseases, especially yellow fever and

[71] *The Courier*, June 6, Sept. 30, 1854.
[72] *Ordinances of the City of Charleston, in Relation to Pilots and Pilotage, and Quarantine* (Charleston, 1859), 14–16; Humphreys, *Yellow Fever and the South*, 21.
[73] Hume, "Source and Origin of Yellow Fever," 160.
[74] Hume, "Yellow Fever of Charleston, considered in its relation to West India commerce," 1–2; Waring, *Medicine in South Carolina, 1825–1900*, 34.

malaria, discouraged immigration. It also killed many newcomers and caused others to leave. Had Charleston attracted and kept more immigrants, however, it would also have had a higher mortality rate.[75]

Ironically, the view that yellow fever was imported became widely accepted after the Civil War. In 1883, a work designed to promote opportunities for work and business in South Carolina declared flatly that yellow fever was not endemic there. It required a "fresh importation every year."[76] Importation theory was now the friend of economic progress. Ironically, by the time the authors wrote this – although no one could know it – the reign of yellow fever was over in South Carolina. The last recorded epidemic was in 1877. How much that development owed to improved quarantine is unclear. The decline of Charleston's seaborne trade in the late nineteenth century may have done more than anything to lift the curse of yellow fever. Southern ports that attracted large numbers of vessels from the Caribbean region – and places that traded with them – continued to suffer yellow fever epidemics for decades longer. The bustling port of New Orleans experienced the last epidemic in the United States in 1905 – five years after the Reed Commission demonstrated the mosquito vector theory of transmission. Economic misfortunes sometimes produce unexpected benefits.

[75] Alfred G. Smith, *Economic Readjustment of an Old Cotton State: South Carolina, 1820–1860* (Columbia: University of South Carolina Press, 1958), 25–26; Tommy Rogers, "The Great Population Exodus from South Carolina," *SCHM* 68 (1967), 14–21; James David Miller, *South by Southwest: Planter Emigration and Identity in the Slave South* (Charlottesville and London: University Press of Virginia, 2002).

[76] Harry Hammond, ed., *South Carolina, Resources and Population, Institutions and Industries* (Charleston, 1883), 22; Humphreys, *Yellow Fever and the South*, 12; James Haw, "'The Problem of South Carolina' Reexamined," *SCHM* 107 (2006), 9–10.

13

A Migratory Species

I perceive by the loss of my strength that I have but a short time to live. If my superiors think I may be of any use here ... I am content to live and die in this place under their favourable protection. But if they would think convenient to employ me in any thing I can do in Barbados ... I will submit so much the more cheerfully because in those hot climates I have formerly enjoyed more health, than I did here where in ten years time I have had I really believe by computation six years or more sickness.

Francis Le Jau, 1716

The 'yawning grave' has received whole families within a few hours of one another – but this usually happens to strangers. In June, most people who can afford it leave for the eastern states or elsewhere, to avoid the pestilence. Some ... merely remove to Sullivan's Island.

Isaac Holmes, 1823

I am miserable; where are we to fly? Like hunted deer – this is the only thicket that promised safety. Oh! Death! That mighty hunter, should it earth us GOD grant we may be prepared.

Adele Vanderhorst?, 1838

PERIPATETIC PLANTERS

In the 1850s, a Charleston planter told Fredrick Law Olmsted, "I would as soon stand fifty feet from the best Kentucky rifleman and be shot at by the hour, as to spend a night on my plantation in summer."[1] The sentiment, if not the exact wording, had been common for many decades. The threat of fevers transformed the white elite into a migratory species. Every summer and autumn, many of them left their plantations or Charleston for healthier locales, or those they perceived to be healthier. The elite's efforts to avoid the lethal diseases their economic pursuits had produced often involved moves

---

[1] Frederick Law Olmsted, *A Journey in the Seaboard Slave States* (New York, 1856), 419.

from town to country, country to town, lowcountry to backcountry, and South Carolina to the North or Europe. Patterns of migration varied and changed over time. The distances might be short or long. Sometimes migrating involved merely relocating temporarily or permanently farther away from the fever-inducing swamps and rice fields. Planters might come to Charleston to avoid "the country fever." People in Charleston might flee to the nearby countryside to avoid yellow fever. Folk who could afford it sometimes went much farther – to the northern colonies or states, Bermuda, the Bahamas, or Europe. After the Revolution, planters often sought health in the nearby pine-barrens, at the seashore, or on the uplands to the northwest.[2]

By the early nineteenth century, the gentry's seasonal abandonment of their plantations had become so prevalent that the Episcopal Church ceased to provide Sunday services in some parishes for at least five months. "From the unhealthiness of the lower country," Frederick Dalcho wrote in 1820, "our planters leave the parish in the summer, and divine service is only expected from November to June." The elite debated when it was prudent to leave the plantations. In 1823, the Medical Society of South Carolina appointed a committee to consider the question of whether May or June was the safer time to migrate from the country to the city. The committee answered "the earlier the better," but added that "some seasons might justify delay." In the end, the doctors decided that the best guide was "the intelligence of the individual and the advice of his friends, under the particular circumstances of the season." A few years later, Samuel Henry Dickson claimed that people were now leaving their plantations earlier than before, around the middle of May.[3]

When it was safe to return to the plantations was a question of equal importance. Answers varied from early October to late November, but again much depended on the weather. Many people argued that the key was to wait until the first black or killing frost. At the end of October 1799, John Ball wrote his son John, "We now think of retiring into the country for the winter – about the middle of November will be the time for us to go."[4] In September 1860, Robert F. W. Allston wrote from White Sulphur Springs that he had intended to take his children to school in Charleston by October 15, but rumors of yellow fever in the city made that impossible. Instead, the family would wait until

---

[2] Jill Dubisch, "Low Country Fevers: Cultural Adaptations to Malaria in Antebellum South Carolina," *Social Science Medicine* 21 (1985), 641, 645; Lawrence F. Brewster, *Summer Migrations and Resorts of South Carolina Low-Country Planters* (Durham, NC: Duke University Press, 1947); George T. Terry, "'Champaign Country': A Social History of an Eighteenth-Century Low Country Parish in South Carolina, St. Johns Berkeley County," Ph.D. Diss., University of South Carolina, 1981.

[3] Frederick Dalcho, *An Historical Account of the Protestant Episcopal Church in South Carolina* (Charleston, 1820), 263; MSM, June 16, 1823, 216–217; Samuel Henry Dickson, "Account of the epidemic which prevailed in Charleston, S. C. during the summer of 1827," *The American Journal of the Medical Sciences* 2 (1828), 3.

[4] John Ball, Sr. to John Ball, Jr., Oct. 29, 1799, Ball FP, 11/516/10, SCHS.

it was safe, presumably after a hard frost.[5] Such frosts sometimes came very late in the year, if at all close to the coast.

Because of their annual peregrinations, many planters became absentee landlords for a large part of the year. The wealthiest often spent part of the winter in Charleston to partake of the "season" of balls and plays.[6] Their warm-weather absences, however, followed from their perceptions of the environment. They came to view certain locations as inimical to health at certain times, and acted accordingly. H. Roy Merrens and George Terry argue that changing perceptions of the lowcountry disease environment and the lifestyle changes they produced were a major reason for a drop in white mortality rates after 1760. It is difficult to prove, however, that these moves were responsible for the decline. An increase in the number of people with acquired immunities to local fevers was another and more likely source of improvement. The migrants themselves disagreed about which areas were dangerous and when they became so. Some migratory strategies were not successful, and some that succeeded in the short term concealed long-term dangers.[7]

It is also important to recall that migrations to avoid fevers were largely limited to the planting and mercantile white elite. Blacks and many whites – including those left to manage plantations and businesses for the elite – did not have the option of moving away during the fever season. An example is William Cochran, who came from New York to work in a merchant house in Charleston. He died of yellow fever in September 1824, aged nineteen. His obituary states that "this amiable youth had been left to conduct the affairs, during the summer, of the respectable House of Messrs. S. and M. Allen and Co., Brokers, of this city." Presumably the Allens had left for a more salubrious place. Like many strangers, Cochran fled to supposedly safe Sullivan's Island when yellow fever became epidemic, but to no avail. The fever followed him there, or perhaps he had contracted it before he went. Most of the city's inhabitants were unable to flee even that short distance in quest of health. But as Cochran's experience showed, flight to the island was not a certain route to security.[8]

Migrating away from fever areas may have lowered mortality for some, but migration harbored its own dangers. Obviously, they could spread diseases

[5] J. H. Easterby, ed., *The South Carolina Rice Plantation* (Columbia: University of South Carolina Press, 2004; 1945), 166.

[6] Samuel Gaillard Stoney, *Plantations of the Carolina Low Country* (Charleston, SC: The Carolina Art Association, 1939), 36.

[7] H. Roy Merrens and George D. Terry, "Dying in Paradise: Malaria, Mortality, and the Perceptual Environment in Colonial South Carolina," *Journal of Southern History* 50 (1984), 546.

[8] *Marriage and Death Notices from the (Charleston, South Carolina) Mercury, 1822–1832*, comp. by Brent Holcomb (Columbia, SC: SCMAR, 2001), 70; Joyce Chaplin, *Anxious Pursuit: Agricultural Innovation and Modernity in the Lower South, 1730–1815* (Chapel Hill: University of North Carolina Press, 1993), 97; James M. Clifton, ed., *Life and Labor on Argyle Island: Letters and Documents of a Savannah River Plantation, 1833–1867* (Savannah, GA: The Beehive Press, 1978), 198.

to other areas. Moreover, people who left the region for long periods could lose – or never acquire – resistance to malarial parasites. This made future warm-weather residence in the lowcountry even more dangerous, which in turn made seasonal emigration seem even more imperative. Families who removed young children from Charleston during the yellow fever season prevented them from gaining lifelong immunity to the disease at an age when they were least likely to die from it. There is also little reason to believe that the danger of fevers to newcomers lessened in the late eighteenth century, to judge by the British experience in the Revolutionary War and evidence from the following decades. Indeed, some antebellum observers claimed that the region became unhealthier in the late eighteenth century than before.[9]

The elite's perceptions of the lowcountry disease environment were never consistent and often changed radically over time. In the early eighteenth century, the predominant view was that Charleston was unhealthier than the surrounding plantation country. In the 1750s, the conventional wisdom was reversed: People began to see the country as unhealthier than the city. After this time, increasing numbers of planting families spent all or part of the sickly season in the city.[10] Around 1800, the resurgence of yellow fever caused perceptions to shift again. For strangers and country people, Charleston regained its reputation as a dangerously unhealthy place in the late summer and fall.[11]

CHANGING AIRS AND PLACES

In 1806, Philadelphian Esther Bowes Cox was anxious about the recent illnesses suffered by her daughter, Mary Cox Chesnut. Mary was married to a South Carolina planter. Mrs. Cox was confident that Mary's health required removing from the plantation during the fever season: "[I]f your good husband takes you to Charleston, the enlivening scenes there, as well as the mildness of the climate, will have a good effect – change of place is sometimes absolutely necessary."[12] Cox was repeating one of the main justifications for travel in the eighteenth century. Doctors often advised a "change of air" as a therapeutic measure. In part this view was the result of the widespread acceptance of miasmatic theory. Heat and moisture acting on rotting organic material were the main sources of infection. Dangerous air did not have to be foul, however. It might be just air that differed markedly from what one's body was accustomed to. Whether the air of a place was foul or just different, a temporary or permanent change of air might be a prerequisite to good health or even survival. As James Lind declared, "a change of air is useful in fevers," especially "from the land to the sea air."[13]

[9] Dubisch, "Low Country Fevers," 645.
[10] Merrens and Terry, "Dying in Paradise," 546–549.
[11] David Ramsay, "Facts concerning the yellow fever, as it appears at Charleston (South Carolina),"*Medical Repository* 4 (1801), 218–220.
[12] Esther Bowes Cox, to Mary Cox Chesnut, Jan. 3, 1806, Cox-Chesnut FP, SCL.
[13] James Lind, *An Essay on Diseases Incident to Europeans in Hot Climates* (London, 1768), 147.

The importance of the air one breathed had a regional and an individual dimension. Many colonists believed that their bodies functioned best in their "native air" – failing that, a similar air such as that of the northern colonies. Sea air and temperate islands were healthy for British bodies, because they were a seafaring island people. Some people might be able to tolerate the heats of the climate after a period of seasoning, but others could survive only by migrating during the warm season. William Murray expressed a common view when he explained that "something in the climate of Carolina ... don't suit my constitution."[14] Eliza Pinckney, concerned about the poor health of some friends, declared that "a change of air must be necessary for them all."[15] In 1815, Alice Izard reported that she wished to take her daughters to Philadelphia to prevent them becoming "sacrifices to unhealthy air." She quoted a friend who had said that "no one could think of living in Carolina if it were possible for him to live at the northward."[16]

From the early eighteenth century, Anglican missionaries regularly requested a "change in air." By this they might mean a short move to a different local parish, a leave of absence to spend the warm months in a healthier climate, a transfer to a northern parish, a return to Britain, or even being sent to Barbados, Bermuda, or the Bahamas, all perceived as healthier. In 1716, Francis Le Jau requested a transfer to Barbados, where he had enjoyed much better health than in Carolina. Three years later, his colleague, Gilbert Jones, requested leave to return to England because doctors had advised him that "my native air and the sea are the only remedy that will relieve me."[17]

The missionaries' requests to leave the province for health reasons became so frequent that in 1740, Commissary Alexander Garden began denying them except to the seriously ill. At the annual visitation of the clergy, he agreed to the leave of one missionary who was suffering from dysentery but denied the applications of two others who "were merely leaving in anticipation of illness." If he acceded to such requests, Garden declared, the colony would be stripped of clergy during the summer. One of the men agreed to forego his trip but the other, Andrew Leslie, resigned and left for England, claiming that his health had been undermined by his "long continuance in this sickly colony."[18] Garden argued that the real reason for his departure was not ill health but "fear of attack by the Spaniards, Indians, or slaves." That may have been true.

[14] William Murray to John Murray of Murraywhat, Jan. 29, 1765, Murraywhat Muniments, SRO/GD219/288/17; Stephen Roe, July 8, 1739, SPG Journals, 8: 117; Chaplin, *Anxious Pursuit*, 98.

[15] "Letters of Eliza Pinckney," *SCHM* 76 (1975), 166; see also, Esther Bowes Cox to Mary Cox Chesnut, Jan. 3, 1806, Cox-Chesnut FP, SCL.

[16] A. Izard to Mrs. Manigault, Jan 5, 1815, Manigault FP, SCL.

[17] Frank J. Klingberg, ed., *The Carolina Chronicle of Francis Le Jau* (Berkeley: University of California Press, 1956), 138–139, 199–203; Gilbert Jones, May 18, 1719, SPG Letter Books, A13: 231, Feb 10, 1719/20 A14: 66; Stephen Roe, July 17, 1739, SPG Letter Books, B7, 1: 223.

[18] Richard St. John, August 14, 1749, SPG Letter Books, B16: 191–192; Andrew Leslie, Jan. 7, 1739/40, SPG Letter Books, B7, II: 243–244; William Guy, SPG Letter Books, B14: 222.

More than twenty of Leslie's parishioners had been killed during the Stono slave rebellion of the previous year.[19] But most requests for health leaves were probably genuine. In the late 1760s, Charles Woodmason attributed the high mortality among Anglican clergy in the lowcountry to their being required to stay there too long. He recommended that they be given regular leaves to restore their health in the backcountry.[20]

The white elite followed the same patterns as the Anglican clergy. They voyaged to the Bahamas, Bermuda, or Barbados to restore their health. In the fall of 1735, merchant Gabriel Manigault advised an ailing Nathanial Broughton that a voyage to the Bahamas "would be of great service to you."[21] British Major George Hanger was sent to Bermuda in 1780 to recover from what he called yellow fever. He was told that the island had the healthiest climate in the world and that "sick persons from the West Indies and the Carolinas" often went there to recover their health.[22] The northern British colonies were also popular elite refuges. Perhaps no place became more associated with lowcountry health seekers than Newport, Rhode Island, once known as "the Carolina hospital." A trip to Newport combined the advantages of a sea voyage, a stay in a sea town, and a bracing northern climate.[23] Northern cities were common destinations for elites who wished to escape or recover from the region's fevers. In the 1730s, Robert Pringle wrote that he hoped to send his wife to Boston to recover her health, "it being the opinion of our physicians and most here that a change of climate is likely to prove the most effectual...."[24] A few years after arriving in Charleston in the early 1750s, Dr. Alexander Garden retreated to New York "in search of cool air" after a severe bout of fever. He wanted to move to England, but feared he would not be able to establish a viable medical practice there. In the 1760s, he also considered going to Florida (recently acquired from Spain) or the Blue Ridge Mountains to improve his health.[25] In the 1790s, architect Gabriel Manigault decided to spend his summers in the North, after first contemplating leaving

[19] *The Fulham Papers in the Lambeth Palace Library; American Colonial Section Calendar and Indexes*, compiled by William W. Manross (Oxford: Clarendon Press, 1965), 149, nos. 58–61; Alexander Garden, [1761], SPG Letter Books, B5: 215; Levi Durand, Jan. 1, 1761, B5: 243.

[20] Richard J. Hooker, ed., *The Carolina Backcountry on the Eve of the Revolution: The Journal and Other Writings of Charles Woodmason, Anglican Itinerant* (Chapel Hill: University of North Carolina Press, 1953), 196.

[21] Gabriel Manigault to Nathaniel Broughton, Nov. 6, 1735, Manigault Papers, SCHS 11/275/5.

[22] George Hanger, *Life, Adventures, and Opinions of George Hanger* (London, 1801), 181.

[23] Waring, *Medicine in South Carolina, 1825–1900*, 39; HLP, 7: 333; Gabriel Manigault to Anne Manigault, June 4, 1774, July 21, Aug. 22, Sept. 20, 1774, Manigault FP, SCL; A. S. Salley, Jr., *Death Notices in the South Carolina Gazette, 1731–1775* (Charleston: Historical Commission of South Carolina, 1917), 31.

[24] Walter Edgar, ed., *The Letterbook of Robert Pringle* 2 vols. (Columbia: University of South Carolina Press, 1972), 1: 175, 205.

[25] James Edward Smith, *A Selection of the Correspondence of Linnaeus and Other Naturalists* 2 vols. (New York: Arno Press, 1978) 1: 345, 245, 526, 532.

the lowcountry permanently. His brother Joseph applauded his plan: "[Y]ou enjoy your health so much better there." Elite families sometimes settled in the North more or less permanently.[26]

Members of the elite did not always view northern locations as healthy. In 1771, Henry Laurens wrote that he had decided not to send his children to Philadelphia to be educated partly because he did not think it "a very health-ful spot." He claimed that putrid fevers were as common there as in Carolina, "and what is a little amazing, mosquitoes, which were not known there thirty years ago," had become an annoyance.[27] In the early 1800s, cases of fever among her family and friends convinced Alice Izard that Philadelphia's air was "not pure."[28] Migrants from the lowcountry and the West Indies had proba-bly helped make the place sicklier. Nevertheless, wealthy South Carolinians continued to go there.

Those who could afford the time and money often went to Britain or Europe. They traveled for educational, cultural, and health reasons, but it is difficult to disentangle the different motives. Elite males attended English public schools such as Eton and Winchester. Some went on to Oxford and Cambridge uni-versities, to Edinburgh to study medicine, or to London to study law. In the 1760s, there were twice as many South Carolinians pursuing the study of law at London's Inns of Court than from all the other American colonies combined. Parents sometimes sent children to Geneva because they believed London presented too many temptations to drunkenness and debauchery. Many elite males took the Grand Tour – a cultural tour through the Continent pioneered by English aristocrats. The pursuit of education and cultural refinement was the ostensible reason for much travel, but the pursuit of health was mixed with these. Sending children to Europe or the North was partly motivated by lack of educational opportunities at home, and partly by wealth and snobbery, but it was also a means to preserve them from the fevers that killed so many. Elite adults also availed themselves of the opportunities of European travel to pre-serve or restore their health. In 1809, Henry Izard wrote that he had decided to take his wife, Emma, to England because he believed it to be the only means to restore her health: "She was almost destroyed by fever the last summer, and would not get through another here I am sure – a change of climate for her and for a longer time than two or three months is absolutely necessary, and is more practicable for me by a visit to Europe, than any journey I could orga-nize to the Northward." In the 1830s, the vestry of St. John's Lutheran Church in Charleston insisted that their pastor, John Bachman, take a six-month trip to Europe to recover his health.[29]

[26] A. Izard to Mrs. Manigault, Oct. 26, 1815, Manigault FP, SCL; Easterby, *South Carolina Rice Plantation*, 76–82, 166; Daniel Kilbride, *An American Aristocracy: Southern Planters in Antebellum Philadelphia* (Columbia: University of South Carolina Press, 2006).
[27] *HLP*, 7: 473.
[28] A. Izard to Mrs. Manigault Sept. 16, 1823, Manigault FP, SCL.
[29] Maurie D. Mcinnis et. al., *In Pursuit of Refinement: Charlestonians Abroad, 1740–1860* (Columbia: University of South Carolina Press, 1999), 9–21; *SCG*, Jan. 1, 1775; Henry Izard

The elite's migrations provided opportunities for social and cultural activities that were unavailable at home. As one historian put it, "the planters of the low country achieved an urbanity which seems to have distinguished them as a class from their more rustic brethren in regions less accursed."[30] Or their more rustic brethren in their own region, he might have added. The urbanity of a few came at high cost to the many, not only in the plantation era, but well beyond. Because the elite could migrate to healthier climes to acquire education and culture, they felt less urgency to promote it at home. In 1809, Dr. Isaac Auld claimed that education on Edisto Island where he lived had suffered because of the chaos of the Revolutionary War. That was surely true, but education had suffered well before then from the effects of disease and the intertwined elite practice of sending children away to be educated. The elite continued to send their offspring away in the following decades. It is significant that Auld also lamented the high mortality on Edisto Island, especially among white children.[31]

Some lowcountry schools were established during the early colonial decades but they do not seem to have survived long. Francis Le Jau, who arrived in 1707, reported that many teachers had come to the colony in recent years, but few had kept to that occupation. Presumably they died, left, or turned to more lucrative employment such as planting. In 1710, the provincial assembly passed an act to provide for free schools run by the Anglican Church and two had opened, in Charleston and Goose Creek, by 1712. Despite the name, they charged most students tuition. The free students included some blacks and Indians in the early years. The curriculum seems to have been largely limited to religious instruction. Elite children got a basic education from tutors or the private schools that emerged in Charleston after the 1730s, and often went to the North or abroad for further education. In 1769, Alexander Garden, who mentored young John Laurens informally, told his father Henry that the low-country did not have a tutor from whom the boy could learn much and that he needed to go abroad for further education.[32]

One of the major difficulties lowcountry schools faced was attracting and retaining qualified teachers. The region's sickly reputation was an important reason, combined with poor remuneration. People who expected to make a fortune as planters or merchants might feel that the risk to their health was

to Mrs. Manigault, July 22, 1809, Ralph Izard Papers, SCL; Easterby, *South Carolina Rice Plantation*, 9; Peter McCandless, "The Political Evolution of John Bachman: From New York Yankee to South Carolina Secessionist," *SCHM* 108 (2007), 12.

[30] St. Julien Ravenel Childs, "The Phenomenon of Disease in the Genesis of the Carolina Low Country," typed ms. dated 1933, WHL, 33–34.

[31] Robert Weir, *Colonial South Carolina: A History* (Columbia: University of South Carolina Press, 1997; 1983), 248–251; Walter Edgar, *South Carolina: A History* (Columbia: University of South Carolina Press, 1998), 176–178; David Ramsay, *History of South Carolina* 2 vols. (Charleston, 1809; 1858), 2: 283.

[32] Klingberg, *Le Jau*; Klingberg, *Johnston*; Gregory D. Massey, *John Laurens and the American Revolution* (Columbia: University of South Carolina Press, 2000), 20. The SPG Papers contain many references to the free schools.

worth taking, but poorly paid pedagogues tended to calculate risks differently. In 1712, Benjamin Dennis, the Anglican schoolmaster in Goose Creek, requested a salary increase. If he had not been in the service of the Church, he declared, he would not have suffered so much sickness, fatigue, and hardship for twice the money. Although a parish school in Charleston opened in 1712, when the second master died in 1716, no schoolhouse had yet been built, and he was not replaced until 1722. The assembly chartered a school at Dorchester on the Ashley River in 1725, but it did not open until 1757. Parish schools rarely stayed in operation for long, and the problem of recruiting and retaining teachers was part of the reason. Disease sometimes shut down schools for long periods and reduced the number of students.[33]

In the 1850s Frederick Law Olmsted claimed to be "astonished by the profound ignorance and unmitigated stupidity" of some wealthy planters. That may have been unfair, and certainly the lowcountry elite contained some very well educated men. There is no doubt, however, that they ruled a poorly educated or uneducated populace. The practice of educating elite children through tutors and private schools at home or abroad established a tradition of neglect of local and public education that continued in many respects into the twentieth century and beyond. In 1811, the state assembly established a system of nondenominational free schools in the state, but it was chronically underfunded and the schools were stigmatized as charity schools. By 1860, only about one-half of the white children in the state were in school, and the institutions were often of very poor quality. Before the Civil War, only Charleston had established a public school system teaching white children of all classes, and that was in the late 1850s.[34]

Disease and perceptions of disease hurt the progress of higher education as well. Colonies to the north established colleges and universities, such as Harvard, William and Mary, Yale, Princeton, Brown, and the University of Pennsylvania. Despite the lowcountry's great wealth, efforts to establish a college in South Carolina got nowhere before the Revolution. It is impossible to say that disease directly hindered the establishment of a college, but the

---

[33] Benjamin Dennis, Dec. 16, 1712, SPG Letter Books, A8: 1; Walter J. Fraser, *Charleston! Charleston! The History of a Southern City* (Columbia: University of South Carolina Press, 1989), 30, 39; Peter Coclanis, *The Shadow of a Dream: Economic Life and Death in the South Carolina Low Country, 1670–1920* (New York and Oxford: Oxford University Press, 1989), 55–56, 145, 149.

[34] Frederick Law Omsted, *A Journey in the Seaboard Slave States* (New York, 1856), 501; McInnis, *In Pursuit of Refinement*, 4, 10–16, 21, 27–29, 33, 49, 66; George Rogers, *Charleston in the Age of the Pinckneys* (Columbia: University of South Carolina Press, 1980), 77, 97–98, 120–122; Weir, *Colonial South Carolina*, 248–252; Fraser, *Charleston!*, 103–104, 215; Robert Rosen, *A Short History of Charleston* (Columbia: University of South Carolina Press, 1997), 38–39; James Alan Marten, *Children in Colonial America* (New York: New York University Press, 2006), 110–112; James L. MacLeod, "A Catalogue of References to Education in the 'South Carolina Gazettes', 1731 to 1770, and Commentary," Ed. D. dissertation, Mississippi State University, 1972, 15–16, 19–20, 31, 58, 68–69, 195–197; Edgar, *South Carolina*, 174–176.

elite's practice of sending children away for education and health reasons surely slowed the process. The College of Charleston, theoretically founded in 1770, was not chartered until 1785, and did not begin classes until 1789. For decades, it was no more than a preparatory school for students intending to study at northern universities. South Carolina College in Columbia, founded in 1805, fared better, but it was located in the healthier middle part of the state.[35]

FLOCKING UP TO THE BACKCOUNTRY

In the late 1760s, James Lind argued that Europeans in tropical lands could protect themselves from unhealthy air by avoiding certain places during the fever seasons. It was not always necessary to go great distances. The most dangerous areas were often close to ones that offered "a secure retreat and protection." Newcomers in particular should leave the unhealthy places during the sickly months at least until they became seasoned to the climate. Lind professed astonishment that so few people had adopted so obvious a solution to the problem of tropical diseases, one "which their own observations must have everyday pointed out to them."[36]

The elite began to seek refuges closer to home during the later eighteenth century: in the backcountry, in pineland villages, or at the seaside. Beginning in the 1760s, some families trekked to higher inland areas during the fever season. The trend probably began about that time because the backcountry was beginning to fill up with settlers and fear of Indian attacks receded somewhat after the Cherokee War of 1760–1761. In the 1760s, British officer Lord Adam Gordon reported that the upper country was "all healthy and fertile land."[37] About the same time, Charles Woodmason recorded that the "gentry used annually to go off to some northern colonies for change of air" but were now "flocking up" to the backcountry "to build summer seats, and hunting boxes." Woodmason thought that the expense and danger of trips to the north by sea was a factor. He noted that one Anglican minister and his family had been shipwrecked the previous year going to Rhode Island. A visiting merchant noted the trend: "Many people move considerable distances up into the country to spend the summer and avoid the intense heats and confined air of [Charleston]."[38]

Exactly how far inland people were going for health in the 1760s is less clear. In July 1765, Anglican minister Isaac Amory decided to leave his parish,

[35] Fraser, *Charleston!*, 214–215, 236–237; Edgar, *South Carolina*, 300; J. H. Easterby, *A History of the College of Charleston, Founded 1770* (Charleston, 1935), 46–48, 55–63, 75, 83, 88–95, 136.
[36] Lind, *Diseases Incident to Europeans*, 164, 166.
[37] Newton D. Mereness, ed. *Travels in the American Colonies* (New York: The Macmillan Co., 1916), 399.
[38] Peletiah Webster, "A Journal of a Voiage [sic] from Philadelphia to Charleston in South Carolina, 1765, SCHS, 34–37; Hooker, *Carolina Backcountry*, 196.

St. John's Colleton, and retreat to the cooler "hills" until late August or early September. The hills may have been the High Hills of Santee in the central part of the state rather than the more distant Appalachian Mountains. The High Hills are, alas, not very high, only a few hundred feet above sea level at their highest point. But their sandy soil and elevation above the local rivers and swamps proved unfriendly to mosquitoes. The Hills had been settled by a group of Virginians around 1750 and soon began to attract more settlers from the north. By the time of the revolution, the region was one of the most thickly settled parts of the colony. During the Revolutionary War, both sides sent soldiers there to escape or recover from the ravages of fevers. In the late 1790s, wealthy Georgetown families began to build summer residences there. Only four deaths occurred in the High Hills in 1807 and 1808, according to David Ramsay's informants.[39] Other backcountry areas also had healthy reputations. When immigrant William Mylne arrived in the Augusta area in 1773, he observed that the people along the upper Savannah River were much healthier and more robust than those he had seen in Charleston. Others made similar observations. The author of *American Husbandry* urged migrants to South Carolina to go to the backcountry, where they could raise healthy children and "more valuable staples than rice."[40]

The lure of the elevated lands near and in the Blue Ridge Mountains became increasingly attractive to health pilgrims after the Revolution. In the early nineteenth century, many lowcountry families began to move to or vacation in the highlands. Nomads seeking health or avoiding fevers went to the foothills near Greenville, Spartanburg, and Pendleton, or on to mountain locations such as Table Rock and Caesar's Head.[41] Some went to spas in North Carolina and Virginia – notably White Sulphur Springs – during the antebellum period. Traveling to these places could be very difficult before the railroads came along. Alice Izard, who visited the spa at French Broad Springs, North Carolina, in the summer of 1815, described a tale of bad roads, excessive heat, and breakdowns of their carriage.[42]

The pristine healthiness of the backcountry did not last long. When David Ramsay proclaimed in 1796 that "Westward the country becomes more hilly, the inhabitants are more ruddy, and in general more healthy," some areas were already losing their healthy luster. Ramsay was aware of the fact. He

[39] St. Johns Colleton Parish, Vestry Minutes, 76, typescript, SCHS.
[40] "Charleston in 1774 as Described by an English Traveler," *SCHM* 47 (1945), 180; William Mylne, *Travels in the Colonies, 1773–1775*, ed. Ted Ruddock (Athens: University of Georgia Press, 1993), 44–45; George Lloyd Johnson, *The Frontier in the Colonial South: South Carolina Backcountry, 1736–1800* (Westport, CT: Greenwood Press, 1997); Harry J. Carman, ed., *American Husbandry* (Port Washington, NY: Kennikat Press, Inc., 1964; originally published in London, 1775), 274.
[41] Waring, *Medicine in South Carolina, 1825–1900*, 39.
[42] Lawrence F. Brewster, *Summer Migrations and Resorts of South Carolina Low-Country Planters* (Durham, NC: Duke University Press, 1947); A. Izard to Mrs. Manigault & Mrs. J. A. Smith, Aug 2, 1815, Manigault FP, SCL.

had written Benjamin Rush as early as 1780 that the backcountry settlers were "more sickly now than formerly."[43] As we have seen, the armies of both sides during the Revolutionary War lost large numbers of men to fevers in the backcountry. The soldiers surely helped bring them there, but settlers had already begun the process. In later works, Ramsay declared that the clearing of woods and increase of mill dams in the upper country had made it unhealthy. "Mild" intermittent fevers, initially restricted to the riverbanks and the more careless inhabitants, had become common. These had recently been replaced by more violent bilious fevers of various grades, even approaching to yellow fever. The problem of disease increased with the spread of plantation agriculture into the backcountry. Ramsay called it the "new order of circumstances." Cutting down trees and breaking up the soil, he concluded, released the dormant "exciting causes of disease," which then became active. Ever the optimist – in public at least – Ramsay predicted that this unhealthy stage would soon end. The "putrescent materials ... and mephitic effluvia" would dissipate with cultivation and the land would become healthy again.[44]

Many backcountry areas suffered heavily from malaria and sometimes yellow fever in the early nineteenth century. In the summer of 1817, Rebecca Ayers of Barnwell District wrote that sickness was "everywhere." Several neighbors had recently died and many more were near death. Her slaves were "very sick." The diseases probably included yellow fever, which struck many locations that year.[45] Members of the Manigault, Izard, and Deas families who settled in the Catawba region near Rock Hill in the early nineteenth century found the area much less salubrious than they had expected. In July 1815, Anne Deas rejoiced that her family had no house in the sickly lowcountry to tempt them to stay "too long in the spring." But their backcountry lands did not prove healthy, either. Every summer and fall, her family and their neighbors battled fevers and the experience, she announced, "has given us no favorable impression of Catawba." That fall, Alice Izard reported that there was "scarcely an instance of a family in this district that has not greatly suffered, and deaths have been much more frequent than usual." After a couple of seasons in the area, Anne declared, "We have been completely disappointed ... it is decidedly a sickly country." Alice knew the reason: "[N]ew settlements," she concluded wearily, "are always hazardous."[46]

---

[43] Robert L. Brunhouse ed., *David Ramsay, 1749–1815: Selections from his Writings*, Transactions of the American Philosophical Society, N.S. 55, Part 4 (Philadelphia: The American Philosophical Society, 1965), 64; David Ramsay, *A Sketch of the Soil, Climate, Weather, and Diseases of South Carolina* (Charleston, 1796) 27.

[44] Ramsay, *Soil, Climate, Weather, and Diseases of South Carolina*, 21; Ramsay, *History of South Carolina*, 2: 36, 305–306; Waring, *Medicine in South Carolina, 1825–1900*, 36–37.

[45] Rebecca Ayer to Louis Malone Ayer, Aug. 9, Sept. 7, 1817, Louis Malone Ayer Papers, SCL.

[46] A. I. Deas, to Mrs. Manigault, July 6, 1815, Oct. 6, 1814, M. I. Manigault to Mrs. Joseph Allen Smith, Oct. 24, 1813, A. Izard to Mrs. Manigault, Feb. 9, 1815, Oct. 19, 1815, A. I. Deas to Mrs. Manigault, Sept. 14, 1815, Manigault FP, SCL.

AVOIDING SWAMPS AND RICE FIELDS

Moving to avoid disease-causing miasmas often involved very short distances. Anglican clergy sometimes asked to be transferred from one lowcountry parish to another for health reasons, as Samuel Quincy did in 1744. His family's health had suffered badly since their arrival. His wife and eldest child were dead. Although he considered the whole colony to be unhealthy and preferred transfer to a northern climate, he hoped that a "change of air" in going to another parish would "agree with me."[47] During the later eighteenth century, many planters began to relocate their houses away from the swamps and rice ponds. Colonial planters often built their houses close to the rice fields so as to be able to oversee their slaves' work. George Milligen condemned the practice in the early 1760s: "[I]n the country ... the inhabitants in general (being more careful to acquire splendid fortunes, than to preserve their healths) build their houses near their rice-fields, or indigo-dams, where they must always keep stagnating water."[48] Charles Woodmason charged that the location of the houses of the Anglican clergy was one of the main reasons for their high mortality. Most of the parsonages, he wrote, were built "on the edge of swamps, in a damp, moist situation, which quickly kills all Europeans, not seasoned to the clime." He noted that planters were abandoning their houses next to the fields and swamps and building new ones on high and dry land.[49] The trend continued but was interrupted by the Revolution. In the 1790s, Ramsay complained that many planters still lived dangerously near their rice fields. He urged them to move their houses well away from the fields and swamps or at least build on the south side of them, because the predominant winds in the fever season were southerly. Ramsay argued that the wind wafted the miasmas of the ponds northward, but it was the mosquitoes it blew that way, we now know.[50]

COUNTRY VERSUS CITY

In the 1770s, Alexander Hewatt observed that many planters were making another sort of move away from the rice fields during the fever season. In this case, though, their destination was Charleston. Many planters had become convinced that the city was less prone to fevers than the rice plantations. Those who could afford it began to retreat to town during the unhealthy season. Those who could not, especially newly arrived laborers, "suffered much during these autumnal months," according to Hewatt.[51] This was a

---

[47] Samuel Quincy, Aug. 22, 1744, SPG Letter Books, B12: 113.
[48] George Milligen-Johnston, *A Short Description of the Province of South Carolina* (London, 1770), 44–45; Ramsay, *Soil, Climate, Weather, and Diseases of South Carolina*, 27.
[49] Woodmason, *Carolina Backcountry*, 195–196.
[50] David Ramsay, *A Dissertation on the Means of Preserving Health in Charleston, and the Adjacent Lowcountry* (Charleston, 1790), 29; Ramsay, *Soil, Climate, Weather, and Diseases of South Carolina*, 27.
[51] Alexander Hewatt, *An Historical Account of the Rise and Progress of the Colonies of South Carolina and Georgia* 2 vols. (London, 1779) 2: 135–136.

major change in perception. In the first half of the eighteenth century, the elite tended to view the country as healthier than Charleston, which suffered many severe epidemics of yellow fever, smallpox, influenza, and other diseases. The high mortality in Charleston led many people to avoid the town, or flee from it to the supposedly healthier countryside.[52] Soon after he arrived in 1706, Francis Le Jau reported that Charleston was the "worst place" in the region because it lacked cold air and good water. The country, in contrast, was "mighty agreeable" and the farther from Charleston the better it got. (He later changed his mind about the country). Until the 1750s, country people viewed Charleston as a place to be avoided during the warm months.[53]

Nineteenth-century writers often claimed that the plantations had been much healthier in the eighteenth century. In 1820, Frederick Dalcho declared that people "could reside in the country in the summer and autumn without danger, and when unusual sickness prevailed in the town, the country was resorted to as a place of health. Neither can now be done with impunity." Dalcho attributed the change to the clearing of trees in the swamps for rice cultivation, but this was hardly new. Dr. Joseph Johnson and architect Robert Mills agreed about the change but traced it to the faulty development, abandonment, and neglect of inland swamp rice fields. Johnson advocated the draining of swamp rice fields, ponds, and canals and planting them with hay and corn.[54]

Some nineteenth-century writers made the rice plantations of the eighteenth century sound like an Arcadian paradise. Samuel Dubose, who was born in 1782, wrote in the 1850s that the land bordering the Santee River was remarkably healthy until after the Revolutionary War. It was "the garden spot of South Carolina" and a "second Egypt." Many Charleston families would spend weeks on the Santee River in July and August "without any apprehension of danger" and "no consequences injurious to health." After 1790, "the climate became more sickly," and the people along the swamp "suffered severely from agues and fever."[55] Frederick Augustus Porcher claimed that eighteenth-century planters had no fear of the country in summer at all. The unhealthiness of the eighteenth-century rice plantation country had "been

---

[52] Samuel Gaillard Stoney, ed., "The Memoirs of Frederick Augustus Porcher," *SCHM* 44 (1943), 135.

[53] Klingberg, *Le Jau*, 23–25; Thomas Hasell, March 12, 1712, SPG Letter Books, A7: 400; Charles Boschi, Oct. 30, 1745, SPG Letter Books, B12: 112; "John Tobler's Description of South Carolina (1753)," *SCHM* 71 (1970), 146.

[54] Frederick Dalcho, *An Historical Account of the Protestant Episcopal Church in South Carolina* (Charleston, 1820), 36n; Joseph Johnson, "Letters Addressed to the Agricultural Society of South Carolina on the means of improving the health of the Lower Country," *Carolina Journal of Medicine, Science, and Agriculture* 1, 131–138; Robert Mills, *Statistics of South Carolina* (Charleston, 1826), 140.

[55] Samuel Dubose, *Reminiscences of St. Stephens Parish, Craven County* (Charleston, 1858) reprinted in *A Contribution to the History of the Huguenots in South Carolina* by Thomas Gaillard, M.D. (New York, 1887; reprinted Columbia, SC: The R. L. Bryan Company, 1972), 37–38, 80–81.

greatly exaggerated." Even the deterioration of health after the 1780s was more perceptual than real. It was the result of improvements in the health of Charleston combined with an increased fear of fevers in general, a fear that Porcher considered unjustified.[56]

These claims smack of the myth of a colonial golden age that is not yet completely discredited. They conflict with eighteenth-century evidence and the actions of the elite, who began to avoid the rice-growing areas during the fever months in favor of Charleston well before the Revolution. It is true that some people viewed the country as healthier than Charleston into the late eighteenth century. In 1774, when visiting Lutheran minister Henry Melchior Muhlenberg and his family were struck with fever and flux, their host took them into the country in the evening "to get some fresh air."[57] Doctors made subtler if not more accurate distinctions. Lionel Chalmers claimed that the country was healthier than Charleston in the summer but less healthy during the autumn. Alexander Garden thought there was little difference between town and country in terms of health: Traveling from one to another during the fever season was the great danger.[58]

Around the middle of the eighteenth century, the perception that Charleston was healthier than the country became common. Doctors began to advise Anglican missionaries that going from their country parishes to Charleston might improve their health.[59] The missionaries themselves reported that their rural congregations were diminishing because so many families were moving into town seasonally or altogether for their health.[60] In 1760, British officer James Grant argued that his men should be housed in the barracks just

---

[56] Samuel Gaillard Stoney, ed., "The Memoirs of Frederick Augustus Porcher," *SCHM* 44 (1943), 135–136; Frederick A. Porcher, *Historical and Social Sketch of Craven County, South Carolina* (first published in *Southern Quarterly Review*, April 1852, reprinted in Thomas Gaillard, *Contribution to the History of the Huguenots in South Carolina*, 159, 164–165; Jill Dubisch, "Low Country Fevers: Cultural adaptations to malaria in antebellum South Carolina," *Social Science Medicine* 21 (1985), 644; Stoney, *Plantations of the Carolina Low Country*, 34; Maurie D. Mcinnis, *The Politics of Taste in Antebellum Charleston* (Chapel Hill: University of North Carolina Press, 2005), 10; Stephanie E. Yuhl, *A Golden Haze Of Memory: The Making of Historic Charleston* (Chapel Hill: University of North Carolina Press, 2005), 10, 44, 68, 175.

[57] *The Journals of Henry Melchior Muhlenberg*, translated by Theodore G. Tappert and John W. Doberstein, 3 vols. (Philadelphia: The Muhlenberg Press, 1945), 2: 572.

[58] Lionel Chalmers, *An Account of the Weather and Diseases of South Carolina* 2 vols. (London, 1776) 1: 14 ; Alexander Garden to Richard Bohun Baker, Nov. 26, 1764, Baker-Grimke Papers, SCHS, 11/535–536; John Drayton, *A View of South Carolina* (Charleston, 1802), 24–25.

[59] Anne Simons Deas, *Recollections of the Ball Family of South Carolina and the Comingtee Plantation* (Charleston: South Carolina Historical Society, 1978, c.1909), 46–47; Mr. Orr, Sept. 1749, SPG Journals, 11: 230; Alexander Garden, Jr., Oct. 31, 1759, SPG Letterbook, B, 1746–1768.

[60] Mr. Harrison, May 12, 1759, SPG Journals, 13: 226; St. Julien Ravenel Childs, "The Phenomenon of Disease in the Genesis of the Carolina Low Country," Ms., dated 1933, WHL, 24; Alexander Garden, Jr., April 15, 1766, SPG, B: 5, 221.

outside Charleston rather than encamped at Moncks Corner, because the
town "has always been reckoned the most healthy place in the province except
the back settlements." His phrase "always been reckoned" was wrong, but it
indicates that the opinion was already common. Grant's fellow officer, Lord
Adam Gordon, noted that most elite families had established a residence in
Charleston where they spent "the three sickly months in the fall." The town
was now the healthiest place in the province: "fevers and other disorders are
both less frequent in it, and less virulent in their symptoms; this is attributed
to the air being mended by the number of fires in town, as much as to its cool
situation, on a point."[61] Dr. George Milligen, perhaps Gordon's source, said
much the same thing. So did Benjamin West, who came from Massachusetts
in the late 1770s. By then it had become routine to explain Charleston's relative healthiness as due in part to smoke from domestic fires. The idea that
smoke equals health may seem odd today, but many people believed that fire
purified the air. Fires had long been used to combat pestilence.[62] But the town
had never been as malarial as the nearby countryside because Charleston was
surrounded by salt water, and yellow fever had become less of a problem due
to widespread immunity among the population.

People who could afford to go to Charleston were beginning to view a summer
in the country as wantonly reckless. In 1771, Elizabeth Manigault wrote of
her hope that her family's new town house would be finished soon enough
for them to come to Charleston "before the sickly time." Malarial areas were
now being accurately perceived as particularly dangerous to pregnant women.
By the time of the Revolutionary War, many elite families routinely moved to
Charleston in the warm months. In 1781, Eliza Wilkinson told a British officer
that she had always spent sickly months in Charleston, but had patriotically
refused to go there since the British captured the city in May 1780.[63]

A few years later, Henry Laurens noted that the migration of the lowcountry planters was the reverse of that in other regions: "In other countries
people go into the country for the summer, in this we come to town." Charles
Cotton, an Englishman who came to the region in 1799, found this pattern
"extraordinary; the gentry instead of retiring to the country during the summer, as is practiced in all the other great towns, spend that time in Charleston

[61] James Grant to Lord Amherst[?], Dec. 20, 1760, WO34/47; Mereness, *Travels in the American
Colonies*, 397, 399.
[62] Milligen-Johnston, *A Short Description*, 44–45; Benjamin West, *Life in the South, 1778–
1779: the Letters of Benjamin West*, ed. by James S. Schoff (Ann Arbor, MI: The William L.
Clements Library, 1963), 23, 35; Ramsay, *Preserving Health*, 30; Charles Kovacik, "Health
Conditions and Town Growth in Colonial and Antebellum South Carolina," *Social Science
and Medicine* 12 (1978), 131–136.
[63] "Papers of Gabriel Manigault, 1771–1784," ed. by Maurice A. Crouse, *SCHM*, 64 (1963),
2; *HLP*, 6: 52–53; "Letters of Eliza Pinckney, 1768–1782," *SCHM* 76 (1975), 143; Richard
Hutson to Isaac Hayne, May 27, 1776, Richard Hutson Letterbook, Langdon Cheves III
Papers, SCHS, 12/99/2, copies of original letters; Chaplin, *Anxious Pursuit*, 98; *Letters of
Eliza Wilkinson*, ed. by Caroline Gilman (New York: 1839), 104.

for health's sake. They are now flocking in very fast." When in the 1790s David Ramsay recommended that planters move to Charleston in the summer, he was merely repeating advice many people had been following for decades.[64] Ironically, the advice was now less good. During the 1790s and after, people often fled the country fever only to run into resurgent yellow fever in the city, leaving them with an agonizing dilemma.

The health advantages of Charleston over the country in the late eighteenth century were relative at best and partly perceptual. People as always had different perceptions based on their experiences. Scottish immigrant William Mylne arrived in Charleston in the fall of 1773 and immediately contracted a severe fever that he claimed had nearly killed him. After recovering, he moved to a farm near Augusta. There he suffered several bouts of intermittent fever and left. Nevertheless, he refused offers to settle in Charleston where he believed he could not survive for six months.[65] David Ramsay, who arrived in the city about the same time as Mylne, had the same reaction at first. But by the 1790s, he was declaring Charleston a much healthier place thanks to improved drainage and removal of rice cultivation to areas farther from the town. These things probably helped, but as should be obvious by now, Ramsay's claims about the region's healthiness were suspect. His perceptions had probably changed more than the reality. Moreover, his announcement of the new healthy Charleston inconveniently coincided with the resurgence of yellow fever.[66]

Ironically, the perception that Charleston was healthier than its hinterland probably contributed to that resurgence. The belief attracted people susceptible to the disease and thus provided potential victims. Country folk also sometimes brought malaria with them. In the summer of 1815, Anne Deas reported that Charleston was "sickly, chiefly with fever brought from the country."[67] During the yellow fever epidemic of 1827, Dr. Samuel Henry Dickson claimed that malaria was most often a problem in the city when yellow fever was also present. Most cases of malaria originated, he argued, outside the town, often in the suburban Charleston Neck just north of the city limits, where "intermittents and remittents abound, no season being free of their presence." For sufferers it probably mattered little where a disease originated. Anne Hart summed up the dilemma of many lowcountry residents when she lamented: "I left the country on account of sickness, but go where I will afflictions abide with me." In the late summer of 1799, John Ball remained for weeks on his plantation at risk of malaria while yellow fever raged in Charleston. In such circumstances, to move or not to move must have seemed like Hobson's choice.[68]

[64] "Letters from Henry Laurens," *SCHM* 24 (1923), 9; "Letters of Charles Caleb Cotton," *SCHM* 51 (1950), 132–144, 217; Ramsay, *Diseases of South Carolina*, 21.

[65] Mylne, *Travels in the Colonies*, 20, 44–45.

[66] Ramsay, *Diseases of South Carolina*, 21, 25; Ramsay, *History of South Carolina*, 2: 38–42.

[67] A. I. Deas, to Mrs. Manigault, July 6, 1815, Manigault FP, SCL.

[68] Dickson, "Epidemic in Charleston during the summer of 1827," 2; Anne Hart to Oliver Hart, March 31, 1785, Oliver Hart Papers SCL; John Ball, Sr. to John Ball, Jr., Sept. 7, 1799, Ball FP, 11/516/10, SCHS.

PINEY TOWNS

At the end of eighteenth century, the elite discovered two nearby locations where they hoped to avoid fevers: the pinelands and the barrier or sea islands. In 1790, David Ramsay suggested that planters could improve their health by moving away from the swamps and rivers to the nearby pinelands. He argued that the resin of the pine trees increased the healthiness of the air: "It is an old and well authenticated observation that persons, whether white or black, employed in burning [pine] tar-kilns, are always healthy." The observation may have had some validity. Burning tar probably deterred mosquitoes, but the well-drained sandy pineland soils were the chief deterrent. Ramsay did not understand the role of mosquitoes but he did declare that the sandy soil was healthier than the black muck of the rice lands. The irony – that the richest soils of the lowcountry were the most "unwholesome" whereas the poorest were relatively healthy – did not escape him: "Health and wealth seem to be at variance." He could have been writing an epitaph for the lowcountry.[69]

Some planters took up Ramsay's suggestion about the pinelands almost immediately, or perhaps had already thought of it. Beginning with the estab-lishment of Pineville in St. Stephen's Parish by James Sinkler in 1794, summer villages inhabited by planters' families mushroomed in the pinelands. They included the communities of Pinopolis, Summerton, Summerville, Walterboro, and many others. Pineville, about fifty miles northwest of Charleston, was about two miles south of the Santee swamp. In 1808, the village contained 22 houses and about 150 white and 300 black residents. Robert. F. W. Allston wrote in 1854 that the pineland retreats were frequented by planters on the Peedee, Black, and Sampit Rivers for their relative freedom from oppressive nights and "the annoyance of mosquitoes." In the 1850s, Samuel Dubose claimed that no development had done more to contribute to the welfare of the lower country than the establishment of the pineland communities. They allowed the planters and their families to enjoy health and yet remain near their plantations. Dubose claimed that the resort to pineland summer resi-dences had "prevented the depopulation of the country."[70]

Dubose's contemporary, Frederick A. Porcher, had a less positive view of the pineland retreats. He recalled that highly mortal fevers had struck Pineville in 1817, 1819, and 1833–1836. The fevers probably included yellow fever. In the early nineteenth century, yellow fever spread from Charleston to other loca-tions in the lowcountry and midlands. *The Southern Patriot* reported several deaths in the pineland villages in September 1819 that could well have been yellow fever, then raging in Charleston. Porcher's description of several deaths

---

[69] Ramsay, *Preserving Health*, 29.
[70] Ramsay, *History of South Carolina*, 2: 54–55, 293–294; Stoney, *Plantations of the Carolina Low Country*, 36; Stoney, "Memoirs of Frederick Augustus Porcher," 136; Dubose, *Reminiscences of St. Stephens Parish, Craven County*, 81–82; Easterby, *South Carolina Rice Plantation*, 9, 62; Waring, *Medicine in South Carolina, 1825–1900*, 38–39.

in Pineville in 1833 also evokes yellow fever: A friend, John Ravenel, came down with what appeared to be a mild disorder. Then, the fever, "after toying with him for a few days … suddenly seized him with a rigour so intense that nothing could allay it and in an hour or two he was dead." A few days later, Porcher's cousin and aunt died under the same circumstances. Thus began "that fatal fever which ravaged Pineville for several years and drove away most of the inhabitants." The summers of 1834 and 1836 were "dreadful." Pineville, which once had sixty houses, was virtually abandoned. Porcher claimed that all the pineland villages were prone to sporadic outbreaks of a virulent fever that eventually drove away most of the inhabitants. Ironically, by congregating together in the pineland villages to avoid malaria on the rice plantations, the planters may have unwittingly created breeding places for the yellow fever vector and communities dense and susceptible enough to spread the virus.[71] During the 1830s, construction of the South Carolina Rail-Road offered yellow fever a quicker passage into the interior. The railroad ran from Charleston to Hamburg on the Savannah River across from Augusta, Georgia. In 1839, yellow fever broke out in Augusta, and some observers claimed that the fever had come from Charleston via the train.[72]

In addition to questioning the healthiness of the pineland villages, Porcher believed that retreating to them in the summers posed long-term dangers. He claimed that whites who stayed on the rice plantations all year, many of them overseers, often remained in good health for many years. People who avoided the plantations during the warm months might escape fevers for a long time, but "at a price that was often fatal." If they were subsequently exposed to fever, it was more likely to be mortal than if they had remained in the rice lands, where permanent residents rarely suffered more than "a simple and teasing intermittent." Porcher's phrase "simple and teasing" greatly under-states the reality, but full-time adult residents of the swamp lands would have acquired some immunity to the malaria parasites through repeated infection. Conversely, people who sought to avoid malaria by migrating would, if suc-cessful, lose their immunity or, if very young, never gain it. Porcher claimed to have known people who had been perfectly healthy until they began spend-ing their summers in the pinelands.[73] Even Samuel Dubose, who viewed the

---

[71] Stoney, "Memoirs of Frederick Augustus Porcher," 149, 164, 204; Porcher, "Craven County," 162–167; *Marriage and Death Notices from the Southern Patriot, 1815–1830*, comp. by Teresa E. Wilson and Janice L. Grimes (Easley, SC, 1982), 52–53; Benjamin B. Strobel, *An Essay on the Subject of Yellow Fever Intended to Prove its Transmissibility* (Charleston, 1840), 187–188.

[72] A medical committee investigating the epidemic insisted that the disease had broken out before the Charleston passengers had arrived and that it had originated locally. They did not know that infected mosquitoes could also travel by train. The disease could also have arrived by riverboat up the Savannah. Samuel M. Derrick, *Centennial History of the South Carolina Railroad* (Spartanburg, SC: Reprint Co., 1975, c. 1930), 126; F.M. Robertson, *A Report of the Origin and Cause of the Late Epidemic in Augusta, Georgia* (1839), 1–10.

[73] Porcher, "Craven County," 160–161, 163.

villages positively, made the same claim: "[I]t was observed with surprise, and it still remains a mystery, that overseers and negroes and others who lived entirely in the swamp enjoyed more health than those who lived on the uplands."[74] Porcher and Dubose were observing the effects of acquired immunity or resistance in those who remained in the malarial areas. They surely exaggerated the healthiness of the swamplands for the permanent residents, however. Writing in the same decade, Frederick Law Olmsted stated that many a seasoned overseer contracted an intermittent that, though rarely fatal in itself, "shatters the constitution, and renders them peculiarly liable to pneumonia, or other complaints which are fatal."[75]

ISLAND REFUGES

The comparative healthiness of the sea (or barrier) islands was appreciated by the time of the Revolutionary War. British soldiers remained healthy while camped on Long Island (now Isle of Palms) in the early summer of 1776. Some patriot officers convalesced from fevers in the ocean air at Kiawah and Edisto islands south of Charleston.[76] Planters on Edisto Island began to seek refuge from fevers on the nearby sea bays soon after the Revolution. They discovered, according to Isaac Auld, that spending the summers on the island's sandy sea bays helped protect their families from fevers and made them milder when contracted. In the Beaufort area, planters headed for places like Bay Point, Hilton Head, and Bluffton. Planters from the lower Santee went to South Island, where there was a village large enough to attract the services of a minister. Waccamaw and Georgetown area planters went to the beaches at Pawley's Island, Magnolia Beach, or North Island. These places were only a few miles from their plantations but separated from them by broad areas of salt marsh. The most popular of the seaside retreats was Sullivan's Island at the entrance to Charleston harbor. [77]

In the 1790s, many people who lived in or near Charleston began to see Sullivan's as a safe refuge from yellow and other fevers. Elite families were soon resorting to the island, building or renting homes, and spending weeks or months there. During the epidemic of 1799, planter John Ball reported that many people had "flocked down to Sullivan's Island." He refused to join them because he believed it was dangerous to "change the air" and he was "not fond

---

[74] Dubose, *Reminiscences of St. Stephens Parish, Craven County*, 81.

[75] Olmsted, *Seaboard Slave States*, 474. Overseers on the Manigault plantation at Gowrie often suffered from fevers. See letters in Clifton, *Life and Labor on Argyle Island*.

[76] Francis, Lord Rawdon to Francis, 10th Earl of Huntingdon, July 3, 1776, *Report of the Manuscripts of Reginald Rawdon Hastings, Esq.* 4 vols. (London, 1934), 3:177; NGP, 11: 564–565, 577, 593, 614, 624–628, 652, 663, 682–683, 695, 12: 573; "Letters of Colonel Lewis Morris to Miss Ann Elliott," *SCHM* 41 (1939), 10, 131–135.

[77] Ramsay, *History of South Carolina*, 2: 281 Hetty Heyward to Mother, Nov. 8, 1817, Heyward and Ferguson FP, COCSC; Easterby, *South Carolina Rice Plantation*, 9, 119–121; Waring, *Medicine in South Carolina, 1825–1900*, 38–39.

of water." Others also feared the voyage to the island or disliked the society. One woman recalled her distaste at mixing with the "uncouth" islanders, who were "not the pleasantest people in the world." But neither fear of drowning nor of mixing with social inferiors stopped the annual migration.[78] In 1817, British visitor Francis Hall reported that in summer, every Charleston family who could afford it fled to "a barren sand-bank in the harbour, called Sullivan's Island, containing one well, and a few palmettos: here they dwell in miserable wooden tenements, trembling in every storm, lest (as very frequently happens,) their hiding places should be blown from over their heads or deluged by an inundation."[79]

When William Robertson of Beaufort heard in August 1817 that some cases of yellow fever had appeared in Charleston, he became alarmed about his son who was there, apparently attending school. Robertson had made arrangements to have the boy removed to the country but urged that he be sent to Sullivan's Island if "the danger becomes very great." A nurse that Hetty Heyward's mother sent from Beaufort to Charleston in 1817 to help her as she approached childbirth went directly to the island because yellow fever was in the city.[80] In 1827, lawyer-planter James Louis Petigru bought a summer house on Sullivan's Island. Every summer thereafter, he moved his family there.[81]

Sullivan's Island also became a refuge for strangers. By 1800, local physicians were advising the unacclimated to move there during the sickly months.[82] When naturalist Francois Michaux arrived in Charleston in October 1801, yellow fever was raging. Friends advised him to go to the island, where some inhabitants had established boarding houses for visitors. He was told that foreigners arriving from Europe or other parts of North America who went "immediately to reside on the island" were safe from yellow fever. Michaux ignored the advice because he did not want to stay "in such a dull and melancholy abode." He remained in town and got the fever.[83]

The island's reputation as a completely safe refuge did not last long in some quarters. As early as 1805, William James Ball heard a rumor that the yellow fever had broken out on Sullivan's Island that summer but declared he could "scarcely give credit" to the claim.[84] In September 1807, the *Charleston*

---

[78] John Ball Sr., to John Ball, Jr., Oct. 12, 1799, Ball FP, 11/516/10, SCHS; Mary Inglis Hering, to Mrs. Henry Middleton, Jan. 8, 1800, 43/0034, SCHS; A. Izard to Mrs. Manigault, June 15, 1815, Manigault FP, SCL.

[79] Francis Hall, *Travels in Canada and the United States, in 1816 and 1817* (Boston, 1818), 244–245.

[80] William Robertson to Waring, Aug. 13, 1817, Waring Papers, SCHS; Hetty Heyward to Mother, Sept. 13, 18, 1817, Heyward and Ferguson FP, COCSC.

[81] *Life, Letters and Speeches of James Louis Petigru: The Union Man of South Carolina* (Washington, DC: W. H. Lowdermilk and Co., 1920), 75–77.

[82] John L. E. W. Shecut, *Shecut's Medical and Philosophical Essays* (Charleston, 1819), 167–168.

[83] Michaux, *Travels*, 118–119; Ramsay, *Diseases of South Carolina*, 25–27.

[84] William James Ball to John Ball, Dec. 10, 1805, William James Ball Family Correspondence, 1134/02/02, SCHS.

Times reported the deaths of six people who had retreated to the island. The newspaper did not state a cause of death but noted that all but one was a stranger. Newspapers reported deaths on the island during subsequent epidemics but usually listed them as due to the "prevailing fever," a common euphemism for yellow fever.[85] In 1813, the Deas family suffered from fevers on the island, leading Anne Deas to declare that the fever was pursuing her family: "[W]e find those places liable to it which others have thought secure." In 1824, Emilia Bennett, whose family retreated to the island, reported that some families had "suffered exceedingly." A man nearby had lost four daughters, his sister, and two servants in about two weeks. Many other families had lost two or three members.[86] Thomas Simons agreed that yellow fever had attacked the island "with dreadful malignancy." Some victims probably contracted it in Charleston, but many had become ill weeks after coming to the island and must have gotten the disease there. Among other reasons for the disease, Simons blamed "the imprudence of people living there under the full confidence of their exemption." He did not explain how overconfidence could cause the disease.[87] In 1858, a city council report concluded that the disease had "always prevailed on Sullivan's Island, when it was epidemic in Charleston."[88] How perceptions had changed.

[85] *Marriage and Death Notices from the (Charleston) Times*, comp. by Brent Holcomb (Baltimore: Genealogical Publishing Co., 1979), 176–179, 320; *Marriage and Death Notices from the Southern Patriot, 1815–1830*, comp. by Teresa E. Wilson and Janice L. Grimes (Easley, SC, 1982), 54, 121, 124, 164; *Marriage and Death Notices from the (Charleston, South Carolina) Mercury, 1822–1832*, comp. by Brent Holcomb (Columbia, SC: SCMAR, 2001), 70, 75, 148.

[86] A. I. Deas, to Mrs. Manigault, Aug. 13, Oct. 8, 10, 1813, M. I. Manigault to Mrs. Joseph Allen Smith, Oct. 24, 1813, Manigault FP, SCL; ALS, Emilia Bennett to Samuel Andrew Law, Oct. 12, 1824, SCL.

[87] Thomas Y. Simons, "Observations on the Yellow Fever, as it occurs in Charleston, South Carolina," *Carolina Journal of Medicine, Science, and Agriculture* 1 (1825), 3; MSM, Oct.–Nov. 1831.

[88] *Report of the Committee of the City Council of Charleston, upon the Epidemic Yellow Fever* (Charleston, 1859), 16; Bennet Dowler, "The Yellow Fever in Charleston in 1858," *New Orleans Medical and Surgical Journal* 16 (1859), 596; Waring, *Medicine in South Carolina, 1825–1900*, 31, 33, notes.

14

Melancholy

> There is one thing wherein I find the people here generally like those of the West Indies, they are so well persuaded that what they do is well as to be very angry when their mistakes are shewn to them and they will find cunning arguments to oppose truth itself.
>
> Francis Le Jau, 1709

> Ill fares the land, to hastening ills a prey,
> Where wealth accumulates and men decay.
>
> Oliver Goldsmith, *The Deserted Village*, 1770

Visitors during the late colonial period marveled at the glittering lowcountry mansions. During the antebellum period, the luster began to fade. An air of gloomy melancholy settled over a region that once seemed as bright with promise as the flowering of azaleas in a lowcountry spring. Defenders of the plantation system captured the mood best. Edmund Ruffin of Virginia expressed it well while on a visit in 1843: "The mansion houses of different plantations are numerous, and evidently the situations were beautiful in past time. But now almost every place is deserted as a residence and there is in all such places a melancholy appearance of abandonment and decay."[1] Why were the mansions no longer beautiful? Why were so many of them deserted, decaying, and melancholy? Ruffin thought much of the problem was due to poor agricultural methods, and that certainly played a part. In the 1850s, Frederick A. Porcher identified another reason – the planters' migrations to avoid disease:

It is this forced emigration which has given our best plantations an air of incompleteness and comparative discomfort; for there were few inducements to bestow labour upon improvements which could never be enjoyed in summer.... In truth, I have never witnessed a scene that is so truly melancholy as a low country plantation.... the stately

---

[1] *Agriculture, Geology, and Society in Antebellum South Carolina: the Private Diary of Edmund Ruffin, 1843*, ed. by William M. Mathew (Athens & London: The University of Georgia Press, 1992), 92.

mansion is shut up and sheds a peculiar gloom over a prospect which nature intended should have been one of unalloyed delight. It was not so in the last century, then the plantation was in truth the planter's home.[2]

Porcher's nostalgia arose from his belief that the seasonal migrations to escape the ubiquitous fevers of summer and fall had begun after the Revolutionary War. His chronology was wrong. They had begun at least thirty years before. By the early nineteenth century, the fever migration season had grown to at least five or six months. Many planters also spent the winter holiday season in Charleston. For those who could afford it, and trusted their plantations to overseers, life on the plantation might last only a few weeks in the spring and a few weeks in the late fall – if they came at all. To spend a large part of their income to maintain houses they rarely lived in would have been economically irrational, as Porcher maintained. Some South Carolina planters lived in beautiful mansions during the antebellum period, but they built most of them further west, in Georgia, Alabama, Mississippi, and other southern states.

The seasonal migrations of the lowcountry planters turned them into one of the oddest elites in mainland America, if not in history. Whereas most American and European landowners spent the summer and harvest season on their estates, rich lowcountry planters deserted theirs. Those who could afford it spent long periods in the North, Britain, or Europe. In their absenteeism they resembled West Indian planters, who spent much of their time in Europe or retreated to highland locations on their islands. For both regions, absenteeism had negative effects on long-term economic development. Like the planters of Barbados, those of Carolina (and later the South) were renowned for their refinement and hospitality to strangers, or at least for boasting of their refinement and hospitality.[3] The lowcountry elite – like the West Indian sugar planters – had less appealing characteristics. Some observers accused them of being lazy, anti-intellectual sots whose main pursuits were acquiring land and slaves, gambling, drinking, and horse racing. Alexander Garden famously complained that the gentlemen planters were "absolutely above every occupation but eating, drinking, lolling, smoking and sleeping, which five modes of action constitute the essence of their life and existence."[4] He discreetly ignored sex. One can debate how much merit Garden's charges held. Fevers, exacerbated by heat and high alcohol consumption, surely produced much languid and eccentric behavior. Garden himself complained of being unable to pursue

[2] Samuel Gaillard Stoney, ed., "The Memoirs of Frederick Augustus Porcher," *SCHM* 44 (1943), 135–136.
[3] David Watts, *The West Indies: Patterns of Development, Culture, and Environmental Change since 1492* (Cambridge: Cambridge University Press, 1987), 354; Jack P. Greene, *Imperatives, Behaviors, and Identities: Essays in Early American Cultural History* (Charlottesville: The University Press of Virginia, 1992), 54.
[4] James E. Smith, *A Selection of the Correspondence of Linnaeus and Other Naturalists* 2 vols. (New York: Arno Press, 1978), 1: 520; Frederick Law Olmsted, *A Journey in the Seaboard Slave States* (New York, 1856), 500–502, 523.

his beloved natural history for months because of the fevers and heat. Fevers rendered Henry Laurens unable to attend to his business for long periods of time. In the spring of 1766, he noted that he had been "seized by a fever in September which hung about me till February and though I was not always very ill yet the disorder made me exceedingly dronish. I had an aversion to business of every sort."⁵ If the energetic Laurens was rendered dronish by a fever one can imagine how fevers affected those made of stuff less stern. In the planters' defense, let it be said that many people believed that drinking punch or wine would help prevent or cure fevers, and even today some people accuse the inhabitants of tropical regions of being physically and intellectually lazy, when their lethargy is due to disease and heat. Culturally, Charleston during the eighteenth and early nineteenth centuries may not have been a Boston, but neither was it an intellectual Sahara. Throughout the period, it harbored an intellectually active corps within its elite. The same can be said of other parts of the South during the antebellum period.⁶

The problem with the lowcountry elite was not a lack of culture but the fact that they developed a culture of denial. Perhaps all people live to some extent in a state of denial, but in defense of their source of income, lowcountry planters – like their West Indian counterparts – honed denial to a high art. They had a perverse tendency to deny inconvenient evidence right before their eyes. An example is the large mixed-race population that elite males helped produce but wrote about as if some evil force had dropped it from the skies. On the subject of disease, as on those of slavery and race, they were often supremely impervious to logic, and the three subjects were intertwined in their thinking.⁷ The earliest rice planters may not have known the dangers they were courting in their quest for prosperity. But by the mid-eighteenth century at least, the elite knew that the world they inhabited was an extremely deadly place. Their private writings, their migrations, and their quarantine laws leave no doubt of that. In 1773, a troubled Henry Laurens wrote that it promised to be a year of "superabundant importation of negroes" and that meant a danger

---

⁵ *HLP*, 4: 26, 94, 431; *HLP*, 5: 119. See also, *HLP* 6: 112; 7: 125; 7: 384; "Letters from Henry Laurens," *SCHM* 24 (1923), 11.

⁶ On cultural and intellectual life in the pre–Civil War South, see *Intellectual Life in Antebellum Charleston*, ed. by Michael O'Brien and David Moltke-Hansen (Knoxville: The University of Tennessee Press, 1986); Michael O'Brien, *Conjectures of Order: Intellectual Life and the American South, 1810–1860* (Chapel Hill: University of North Carolina Press, 2004); Elizabeth Fox-Genovese and Eugene D. Genovese, *The Mind of the Master Class: History and Faith in the Southern Slaveholders' World* (New York: Cambridge University Press, 2005); Lester D. Stephens, *Science, Race, and Religion in the American South: John Bachman and the Charleston Circle of Naturalists* (Chapel Hill: University of North Carolina Press, 2000); Robert Weir, *Colonial South Carolina: A History* (Columbia: University of South Carolina Press, 1997).

⁷ Johann Martin Bolzius, "Reliable Answers to Some Questions Submitted Concerning the Land Carolina," *The William and Mary Quarterly*, Third Series, 14 (1957), 235; Mark M. Smith, *How Race is Made: Slavery, Segregation, and the Senses* (Chapel Hill: University of North Carolina Press, 2006).

of "dreadful" contagious diseases.[8] He knew that his source of wealth was also a major source of the region's sickliness. Many late colonial observers also observed the connection between slavery, rice, and disease.

Insofar as the elite publicly conceded the health dangers of the region, however, they tended to blame the climate, topography, Providence, and individual imprudence, not the economic system. But they knew *where* the danger lay, and from the mid-eighteenth century, if not before, they chose to avoid it as much as possible. They also knew that their workers, black and white, could not escape. Yet paradoxically, the elite were able to rationalize away many of the dangers of the plantation system. This involved contradictory, sometimes perverse, ideas and behavior. They argued that slavery was necessary because whites could not work effectively in the feverish lowlands. But by leaving behind white overseers and managers to run their plantations and businesses in their absence, the elite partially undermined that claim, as they did by declaring that whites could and did "earn" immunities to fevers by residing there. If the latter was true, then African slavery was not necessary, only convenient and profitable. Indeed, after emancipation, New South boosters declared that whites could, after all, work successfully in lowcountry fields, and some went so far as to claim that the emancipated blacks were doomed to extinction by disease.[9]

Around 1800, Charleston's doctors reframed yellow fever as the apparently less threatening "strangers' disease." They proclaimed that yellow fever was a minor problem that rarely endangered white natives of the city. It affected mainly newcomers, who could avoid the danger by taking proper precautions. Unfortunately, new arrivals were often ignorant of the danger or were not warned of it in time, because announcing the presence of yellow fever had adverse effects on commerce. Most doctors also denied that yellow fever was a contagious or imported disease, thus helping free shipping from bothersome quarantine regulations and fuel epidemics. To be sure, doctors did make positive contributions to the region's health. They used herbal remedies – often learned from Indian or African folk medicine – that relieved some suffering, such as the vermifuge pinkroot and Peruvian bark. They also promoted inoculation and vaccination for smallpox, which greatly reduced the ravages of that disease.

These were positive developments. No one, however, was well served by selective denials of the region's unhealthiness. Certainly not the Africans forced to labor in the rice fields or the white immigrants lured to their deaths by inadequate warnings and misleading assurances. In the end, the denials did not even benefit the planting and mercantile elites. The economy declined anyway.

---

[8] Elizabeth Donnan, ed., *Documents Illustrative of the Slave Trade to America* 4 vols. (Washington, DC: Carnegie Institution of Washington, 1930–35), 4: 458.

[9] Jeffrey Robert Young, *Domesticating Slavery: The Master Class in Georgia and South Carolina, 1670–1837* (Chapel Hill and London: University of North Carolina Press, 1999), 181–184; William Dusinberre, *Them Dark Days: Slavery in The American Rice Swamps* (Athens: University of Georgia Press, 2004), 50–55, 70–75, 80.

Between the Revolution and the late nineteenth century, South Carolina was transformed from being the richest of the thirteen colonies to one of the poorest of the states. Charleston and the lowcountry became renowned for not only poverty and sickliness but a perverse denial or distortion of reality. White immigrants were repelled by the sickly reputation of the area as much as by the slave economy and the lack of opportunities it provided for whites. After the 1820s, most immigrants avoided it altogether and many of those that did not suffered high mortality or moved on to healthier locales.

It is true that disease sometimes aided the white population, or elements of it. As in other parts of America, Old World diseases rapidly reduced the numbers of Native Americans, weakening their power to resist white encroachment. Fevers helped secure American independence by felling large numbers of British soldiers during the Southern campaign of 1780–1781. The migrations of the elite planters, at least when they went to larger cities in the North or to Europe, gave some of them a cosmopolitan sophistication most Americans lacked, especially during the colonial period. Their presence in Charleston for long periods of time gave that city many of the fine houses and other buildings that attract tourists today. But blacks and poor whites that could not migrate to escape disease paid a high price. Even the migrating elites did not entirely escape. Many who had acquired some immunity to malarial fevers lost it during their absences. If they returned too soon to their plantations, or left them too late, they were more vulnerable than if they had remained all their lives. The planter elite were as susceptible to yellow fever as any stranger unless they had survived the disease. Certainty about immunity was impossible. Moreover, the planters' migrations helped spread malaria to the city and yellow fever to the country.

The danger of fevers contributed to the common elite practice of sending children to the North or Europe to be educated. The custom was partly a response to the lack of local educational opportunities, but it was also a means of protecting children from lowcountry diseases. Over time, the two goals reinforced one another and had long-term adverse effects on education. The planter elite that dominated state government supported public education in a parsimonious fashion. A tradition of poor funding of education developed, spread throughout the South, and proved lasting. South Carolina's public education system remains among the weakest in the United States. Southern states have generally lagged behind the rest of the nation educationally. In 1856, Frederick Law Olmsted bemoaned the poor state of education in South Carolina and predicted harshly but with some accuracy that "one hundred years' hence, the men whose wealth and talent will rule South Carolina, will be, in large part, the descendants of those now living in poverty, ignorance, and the vices of stupid and imbecile minds."[10]

The region's sickliness and sickly reputation contributed to its educational weaknesses in another way. From an early period, the lowcountry had

[10] Olmsted, *Seaboard Slave States*, 523.

difficulty attracting and retaining qualified teachers. They were often poorly paid, and if they did not die, many decided that the remuneration was not worth the risk and left or turned to other work. Most rural parish schools did not stay in operation for long, and the difficulties of getting and keeping teachers was part of the reason. The teachers in the first "free schools," mostly Anglican clergymen, were often ill, died, or left citing ill health, and disease continued to deter qualified teachers. These problems, combined with the elite's migratory habits, hurt higher education as well. It came later to the low-country than to most of British North America. Despite the region's wealth, efforts to establish a college got nowhere until after the Revolution. This was partly due to the low density of the white population, the slow penetration of the backcountry, and finally the Revolution itself. By then, the elite practice of sending children to healthier locales for education had become ingrained in many families. The College of Charleston, ostensibly founded in 1770, did not open until 1789. Many problems contributed to its subsequent difficulties, but disease, especially yellow fever, greatly disrupted the institution. The college sometimes closed down for months during epidemics. In 1836, it closed down entirely due to a lack of students and money. It reopened in 1838, but with city support as the first municipal college in the country, and from then to the late twentieth century, the student body and faculty were largely local in makeup. When it became a state college in 1969, it had only about 300 students, most of them locals. Today, the campus has more than 12,000 students from all over the United States and many foreign nations. But the lowcountry is now a much improved place, epidemiologically speaking.[11]

   Disease also influenced the religious makeup of South Carolina and ulti-mately the South. It contributed to the failure of the Anglican Church to win more converts in the lowcountry and beyond. As the established church in Carolina from 1706 to 1778, it had many advantages over its rivals. By the late colonial period, however, it had largely lost the battle for the colony's soul. Disease was not the only reason, of course. The colonial population included many Dissenters from the beginning, and the colony received a large infusion of non-Anglicans during the mid-eighteenth century, with the migra-tion of Germans, Swiss, Welsh, and Scots-Irish into the backcountry. Many things worked against the Anglican missionaries who came to Carolina after

[11] Weir, *Colonial South Carolina*, 248–252; Walter J. Fraser, *Charleston! Charleston! The History of a Southern City* (Columbia: University of South Carolina Press, 1989), 30, 39, 214–215, 236–237, 349; Peter Coclanis, *The Shadow of a Dream: Economic Life and Death in the South Carolina Low Country, 1670–1920* (New York and Oxford: Oxford University Press, 1989), 55–56, 145, 149; Coclanis, "Tracking the Economic Divergence of the North and the South," *Southern Cultures* 6.4 (2000), 82–103; Walter Edgar, *South Carolina: A History* (Columbia: University of South Carolina Press, 1998), 174–176, 297–300; James L. MacLeod, "A Catalogue of References to Education in the 'South Carolina Gazettes,' 1731 to 1770, and Commentary," Ed. D. dissertation, Mississippi State University, 1972, 15–16, 19–20, 31, 58, 68–69, 195–197; J. H. Easterby, *A History of the College of Charleston, Founded 1770* (Charleston, 1935), 46–48, 55–63, 75, 83, 88–95, 136.

1702: inadequate compensation and job security, combined with obstreperous, independent-minded parishioners. But disease greatly exacerbated the problem. Too many of the Anglican clergy, who had to be ordained in the mother country, were constantly sick, dying soon after arrival, or leaving for posts in more salubrious locations. Those who remained often left for long periods for health reasons. Many parish churches had no incumbent for years. The clergy who remained could barely serve the lowcountry parishes, much less proselytize beyond. The turnover also strengthened the parish vestries in relation to the ministers. Dissenting denominations, especially Baptists, were more successful than Anglicans in attracting converts, partly because they could recruit clergy more easily and quickly in America. In the absence of Anglican clergy, many people turned readily to Dissenters for religious services. From the late eighteenth century, the seasonal migrations of the planters led to the closing of many Anglican (or Episcopalian) churches during the summer, for lack of a congregation. These closings, combined with the evangelical revivals of the late colonial and early national periods, weakened the loyalty of people who did not join the elite migrations. By the early nineteenth century, Baptists, Methodists, and Presbyterians had become the dominant churches.[12] This trend continued, with the Baptists gradually outpacing all the rest. In a 2001 survey, Baptists comprised 43 percent and Methodists 14 percent of the state's population. Two percent claimed affiliation with the Episcopal Church, considerably less than most other denominations. Most southern states followed a similar pattern.[13]

The lowcountry's diseases and reputation for unhealthiness contributed to its relative demographic and political decline during the nineteenth century. The population of South Carolina and Charleston grew rapidly until the Revolution, mainly through immigration. Charleston's growth rate averaged 3.3 percent a year between 1670 and 1776. Between 1700 and 1775, only Philadelphia grew faster. It continued to grow rapidly between 1770 and 1800, nearly doubling, despite the upheavals and losses of the Revolutionary War. During the nineteenth century, however, the population grew much more slowly than that of rival cities. Charleston's population doubled between 1800

---

12 Bradford J. Wood, "'A Constant Attendance on God's Alter': Death, Disease, and the Anglican Church in Colonial South Carolina, 1706–1750," *SCHM* 100 (1999), 204–220; Edgar, *South Carolina*, 181–183, 293; Patricia U. Bonomi, *Under the Cope of Heaven: Religion, Society, and Politics in Colonial America* (New York: Oxford University Press, 2003), 31–32; Thomas J. Little, "The Origins of Southern Evangelicalism: Revivalism in South Carolina, 1700–1740," *Church History*, Dec. 2006, 1–36; Thomas Kidd, ed. *The Great Awakening: the Roots of Evangelical Christianity in Colonial America* (New Haven, CT: Yale University Press, 2007), chapters 6, 16; John B. Boles, *The Great Revival: Beginnings of the Bible Belt* (Knoxville: University Press of Kentucky, 1996).

13 Episcopalians were also less numerous than Roman Catholics and "no religion," tied at 7 percent. Among other faiths, self-proclaimed "Christians" comprised 6 percent, Presbyterians 5 percent, and Pentecostals/Charismatics 3 percent. Barry A. Kosmin, Egon Mayer, and Ariela Keysar, American Religious Identification Survey, Graduate Center of the City University of New York, 2001, 41, http//www.gc.cuny.edu.

and 1860, which may seem like a lot. But in the same period, New York grew thirteen times larger, Baltimore eight times larger, Philadelphia and Boston seven times larger. The city and the region's relative economic decline contributed to its slow demographic increase, but epidemiological factors were also important. In the 1830s and 1850s, both decades of severe yellow fever epidemics, the population of Charleston actually declined. Charleston, the fourth largest city in the United States in 1790, dropped to twenty-second place by 1860 and to sixty-eighth place by 1900. The population of South Carolina grew much more slowly than that of states in the North and Border South. The relative demographic decline of city, region, and state was partly due to out-migration. Hundreds of thousands of South Carolinians moved west to exploit the virgin cotton lands of Georgia, Alabama, Mississippi, and beyond, bringing along the diseases that helped forge a sense of southern distinctiveness.[14]

The relatively slow growth of population in antebellum South Carolina was not only due to out-migration. The state received a tiny number of immigrants compared to states further north. In 1860, less than 4 percent of South Carolina's citizens had been born outside its borders. In the North, the proportion was about 25 percent and in the Border South about 16 percent. Many things contributed to this result, including slavery, but disease was one of them, by "sweeping off" many strangers and discouraging others from coming. In a state with a black slave majority, the slow growth of the white population had dangerous political consequences. It increased white paranoia and weakened the state politically in Congress. It sharpened a sense of declining political and economic power that helped boost the nullification and secession movements. In other words, had South Carolina been a healthier place, it might have been politically less radical. The large number of South Carolinians who migrated to other southern states after 1820 also carried some of their radicalism with them, along with their diseases.[15]

As this book has argued, lowcountry diseases were not a natural result of the region's climate and topography. Human action – voluntary and forced migration and alterations of the environment – made the region unhealthy.

---

[14] About 200,000 whites and 170,000 blacks moved west from South Carolina between 1820 and 1860. Tommy Rogers, "The Great Population Exodus from South Carolina," *SCHM* 68 (1967), 14–21; James David Miller, *South by Southwest: Planter Emigration and Identity in the Slave South* (Charlottesville: University of Virginia Press, 2002); Alfred G. Smith, *Economic Readjustment of an Old Cotton State: South Carolina, 1820–1860* (Columbia: University of South Carolina, 1958), 25–26; Emma Hart, *Building Charleston: Town and Society in the Eighteenth-Century British Atlantic World* (Charlottesville: University of Virginia Press, 2009).

[15] Peter Coclanis, *The Shadow of a Dream: Economic Life and Death in the South Carolina Low Country, 1670–1920* (New York and Oxford: Oxford University Press, 1989), 64–65, 112–115; Fraser, *Charleston!*, 241; James Haw, "'The Problem of South Carolina' Re-examined," *SCHM* 107 (2006), 9–11; Rogers, "The Great Population Exodus"; Miller, *South by Southwest*; Manish Sinha, *The Counter Revolution of Slavery: Politics and Ideology in Antebellum South Carolina* (Chapel Hill and London: University of North Carolina Press, 2000).

It is now, as it once was, a relatively healthy place. Climate and topography mattered, of course. They helped make the region markedly unhealthy once *falciparum* malaria, yellow fever, and other "tropical" diseases made the trip from the Old World. But these diseases may not have come and would not have flourished as they did had not the European settlers established an economy that exploited African slave labor to cultivate rice and later indigo. Francis Le Jau sensed the root of the problem, even if he did not understand all the connections between the lowcountry economic system and its disease environment: "This would be a pleasant place if men were but willing to make themselves easy and improve the fruitful soil where anything grows without much trouble ... but they all aim at riches which are hard to be got and they neglect the peace of their conscience and life."[16]

For Le Jau as for so many others, the planters' pursuit of riches proved deadly. For ten years, he was plagued by fevers, fluxes, and other diseases. His misery and that of his colleagues was aggravated by his parishioners' failure to provide promised material and spiritual supports they had been led to expect: "As their fine promises come to nothing some of us have neither houses nor churches. My house is well enough but my church that was begun six years ago is not like to be so soon finished. A trifle would do it but nobody minds it. Several of my brethren are under greater inconveniences than I." In August 1716, Le Jau was attacked with a fever and digestive disorder that confined him to his bed for months. In March 1717, he reported that he expected to die soon, as his body was "worn out with labour in this sickly and desolate country." When Le Jau came to Carolina in 1706, he had described it as a potential paradise. After ten years, he had reframed it as a "sickly and desolate country." He died a few months later, in September, the lowcountry's cruelest month.[17] When he died, South Carolina was poised through slavery and rice cultivation to become the richest of the British North American colonies. In the process, even the wealthy elite paid a high price in illness and death. Like Le Jau, most of the population experienced pestilence without prosperity. It is not too much to say that they also suffered from the perversity of those whose determination to maintain a profitable economic system produced denials about its human costs. South Carolina, the South, and the nation still suffer from that denial.

---

[16] Klingberg, *Le Jau*, 28–29.
[17] Klingberg, *Le Jau*, 138–139, 199–205; Society to Vestry of St. James, Goose Creek, Aug. 14, 1717, SPG Letter Books, A:12, 173; Thomas Hasell, Sept. 20, 1717, SPG Letter Books, A: 12, 83–85.

Select Bibliography of Manuscript Sources

Unpublished Manuscripts

Bedfordshire Record Office, Bedford, UK

Rugeley Family Papers, X 311/155

Boston Public Library, Boston, MA

Benjamin Lincoln Papers, (microfilm, reels 2 and 3, I-II)

British Library, London, UK

Auckland Papers, vol. 5, Add. Mss. 34416
Henry Bouquet Collection, Add. 21631
Liverpool Papers, Add. Mss. 38214
Strachey Collection, Genealogical Papers, MSS EUR F127/478a, Box 1

Charleston County Library, Charleston SC

City of Charleston, Health Department, Death Records, 1819–1868

College of Charleston Library, Charleston, SC

Heyward and Ferguson Family Papers, 1806–1923
Letters of John Vaughan to Philip Tidyman, 1801–1802, Mss. 34/135
Papers of the Society for the Propagation of the Gospel, London (microfilm, East Ardsley,
    Yorkshire, Micro Methods, distr. by Microform Academic Publishers, c. 1964)
Records in the British Public Record Office Relating to South Carolina (microfilm)
Vanderhorst Family Papers, 1787–1838

Edinburgh University, Special Collections, UK

Letters of Alexander Garden to Charles Alston, La. III.375/42–45
Letter of Lionel Chalmers to Robert Whytt, 1763, Dc. 4.98/1, ff. 230–231

*National Archives of Scotland, formerly Scottish Record
Office, Edinburgh, UK*

Murray of Murraywhat Muniments   SRO/GD219
Steuart of Dalgleish Muniments   SRO/GD38/2/9/15

*National Archives of United Kingdom, formerly Public Record
Office, Kew, UK*

Colonial Office (CO)   5/176, 5/519
Public Record Office (PRO)   30/11, 30/55
War Office (WO)   34/35, 34/47

Royal College of Physicians, Edinburgh, UK

William Cullen Manuscripts

South Carolina Department of Archives and History, Columbia, SC

Journals of His Majesty's Council in South Carolina
Journals of the Commons House of Assembly of South Carolina
Journals of the Upper House of Assembly of South Carolina
Letters of William Dunlop to James Montgomerie. Photocopies of originals in Scottish
    Record Office, Edinburgh, UK
Nicholas Trott, "The Temporary Laws of South Carolina." 1707

South Carolina Historical Society, Charleston, SC

Baker Family Papers
Ball Family Papers
Deas Commonplace Book, 1749
Henry A. Middleton Papers
Joshua B. Whitridge Papers
Manigault Papers
Peletiah Webster Journal, 1765
Pinckney Family Papers
Thomas Porcher Ravenel Papers
Richard Hutson Letterbook
Richard Hutson Papers
Robert Raper Letterbook
Roger Pinckney Correspondence
William James Ball Family Correspondence

South Caroliniana Library, Columbia

Cox-Chesnut Family Papers
James Glen Papers
James Grant Manuscripts
Louis Malone Ayers Papers
Manigault Family Papers

Oliver Hart Papers and Diary
Philip Porcher Account Book, Typescript
Ralph Izard Papers
William Blanding Papers
Williams-Chesnut-Manning Families papers

University of Aberdeen Archives, Aberdeen, Scotland, UK

Ogilvie-Forbes of Boyndlie Papers

Waring Historical Library, Medical University of South Carolina, Charleston, SC

Medical Society of South Carolina, Minutes, 1789–1860

Published Manuscripts

Brunhouse, Robert L., ed. *David Ramsay, 1749–1815: Selections from His Writings*. Transactions of the American Philosophical Society, N.S. 55, Part 4. Philadelphia: American Philosophical Society, 1965.

Collections of the South Carolina Historical Society, 5 vols. (Charleston, 1897).

Donnan, Elizabeth, ed. *Documents Illustrative of the Slave Trade to America*. 4 vols. Washington, DC: Carnegie Institution of Washington, 1930–1935.

The Fulham Papers in the Lambeth Palace Library; American Colonial Section Calendar and Indexes. Comp. by William W. Manross. Oxford: Clarendon Press, 1965.

Great Britain, Colonial Office. *Documents of the American Revolution*. Edited by K. G. Davies. 21 vols. Shannon: Irish University Press, c. 1972–c. 1981.

Great Britain, Historical Manuscripts Commission. *Report on American Manuscripts in the Royal Institution of Great Britain*. 4 vols. Boston: Gregg Press, 1972. Reprint of London edition, 1904–1909.

Greene, Nathanael. *The Papers of General Nathanael Greene*. 11 vols. Edited by Dennis M. Conrad. Chapel Hill and London: The University of North Carolina Press, 2000.

Journal of the Commons House of Assembly of South Carolina. Edited by J. H. Easterby. 14 vols. Columbia: Historical Commission of South Carolina, 1951–

Klingberg, Frank J., ed. *Carolina Chronicle: The Papers of Commissary Gideon Johnston, 1710–1716*. Berkeley and Los Angeles: University of California Press, 1946.

The Carolina Chronicle of Francis Le Jau, 1706–1717. Berkeley and Los Angeles: University of California Press, 1956.

Laurens, Henry. *The Papers of Henry Laurens*. 16 vols. Edited by Philip M. Hamer. Columbia: University of South Carolina Press, 1968–

Smith, James E., ed. *A Selection of the Correspondence of Linnaeus and Other Naturalists*. 2 vols. New York: Arno Press, 1978.

Statutes at Large of South Carolina. 22 vols. Columbia, 1836–1898.

Index

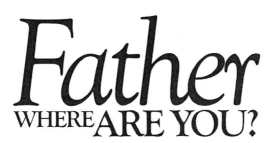

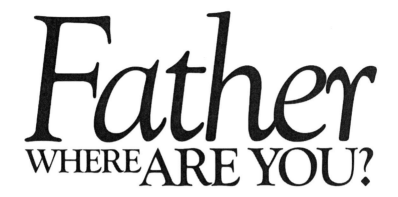

Father
WHERE ARE YOU?

STEFAN DRIESS

Father, Where Are You?

Copyright © 2014 by Stefan Driess.

Published using KWS services. www.kingdomwritingsolutions.org

Cover painting by Oliver Pengilley

No part of this book shall be reproduced or transmitted in any form or by any means, electronic or mechanical, including photocopying, recording, or by any information retrieval system without written permission from the publisher. All photographs are from the authors private collection.

Published by Stefan Driess - Grace-Production
Altensalzer Str. 5, 08541 Neuensalz, Germany
127 Manchester Road, Manchester M28 3JT UK

ISBN 978-3-944760-03-2

Endorsements

This unforgettable tale of one man's journey from being an orphan to being a son is sure to inspire, amuse, move, and enlighten you. If you are asking, 'father, where are you?' this is the book for you.

Dr. Mark Stibbe, bestselling author, script doctor, and CEO of Kingdom Writing Solutions

I have known Stefan for a decade now and he has always surprised me with his ability to love and accept others right where they are. In reading this book, I can see how only God could have healed the boy and raised this kind of man. This book shows Stefan's journey naturally and spiritually.

You will cry with the little boy and flinch at the angry man, while gaining insight into spiritual warfare.

Stefan is now a great prophet and an even greater father. I love to see him with his children, he is so present and engaged. His children know the love, protection, opportunity and spiritual identity that Stefan did not know growing up. God has truly fathered Stefan; he is not just healed, he has been made whole.

Reading this book will cause you to fall in love with God again. This is a "But God" book, meaning only God can show up and bring this type of life change.

God is shown as faithful, powerful and caring and that is how I see Stefan.

Dr. Sharon Stone, President and Founder of Christian International Europe

To Giancarlo Elia
The father who adopted me

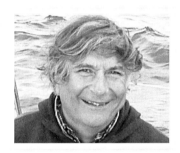

Thank you Dad for showing me the love of the father

Contents

Acknowledgements

I would like to thank my wife, Louise who has supported me on this journey and released me to work away from home all around the world.

I would also like to thank all the people in Germany who work closely and support me: Kathleen and Daniel, Ralph and Doreen, Stefan and Ramona and Christian and Christina. Without them I would not have been able to take the time to write this and other books.

Thank you so much to Ollie Pengilley for the great cover design.

I would also especially like to thank Dr. Mark Stibbe who helped me bring my story and my heart to English speaking readers.

Most of all I would like to thank God my Father. Without him there would be no story.

Foreword

I married late in life and I never had children. I never felt any particular desire to be a father and my life was quite fulfilled by God's presence and by His gifts of a loving wife, intense ministry and before that a successful career as a lawyer.

Then one day I met Stefan.

He was standing in a line of people waiting to receive prayer at the end of a seminar. When I laid my hands on him and started praying, I felt as if I was in the presence of a dear friend or a close relative, finally reunited after a very long separation.

A month or so later, while Stefan was staying with us for a short visit, suddenly my heart was filled with love for this young man - the intense love of a father for his precious son.

When that happened, I knew very little about him, but I knew for sure that a lifelong relationship was being established.

Neither of us was looking for it or expecting it, but that relationship was in God's plans and purposes for both of us: He wanted me to have a real son and Stefan to have a real father.

At that time I had no idea how to be a father and I had to learn, much faster than normal. However, I had a good model in my own father. Unlike Stefan, I had very good, loving and caring parents, who were my best friends and confidants, especially my father. I had an even better model in God the Father, who took good care of both Stefan and me when we had to learn what it means to be a godly father and a godly son. We started an adventure together and it is not over yet, not until I will end my own race.

Stefan's book is not simply a memoir, or a testimony. It is the diary of a journey - a quest that has reached its goal and yet it is still continuing. With God there is always more. Stefan's story is a story of God's amazing grace but also of the honest, human, sincere, down-to-earth, humble response to that grace. There is no attempt to hide weaknesses and failures or to over-spiritualise events and experiences, although many of them are more in the realm of God's supernatural intervention than just everyday occurrences.

Probably one of the most important turning points in contemporary Christianity has been the rediscovery of God as a loving Father. It did not happen by itself but it was part of God's plan for our age. Through the message of God's love and Fatherhood, countless men and women have found a new meaning in their lives and have found faith or rekindled a fire that was close to being extinguished. I have no doubt that Stefan's and my experiences are well within this plan. However, in Stefan's case I see something different. He received a lot from God but he did not remain in a receiving attitude, as many often do. He understood that the love of God has to be received because it has to be given to all those who are around us and this is what Stefan does, in his family, with his friends, with me, in his ministry and through this book.

It has been my joy and the source of tremendous blessings to become a father to Stefan, but at the same time I received a lot from him, not least two super grandchildren, and I learnt more, I understood better, I matured and I grew in love with God and man, just because I was given such a son.

Giancarlo Elia

Preface

Dear reader,

I have written this book because I have a longing in my heart for other people to know the truth about Jesus.

This is urgent because the truth about Jesus has too often been misrepresented by the church and by others - including at one time by me too.

People need to know the true truth about God that he is a loving Father who longs to know us, protect us, guide us and make our lives fulfilled.

I understand that others see the spiritual world in a different way. And I can understand that some people don't believe that there is a spiritual world at all.

But as for me, I have had to write about the things that have happened to me even if some of them will sound like part of a supernatural movie. I know that evil exists and that good also exists and there is a spiritual battle going on - a battle around your destiny and mine. That's why you deserve to hear the truth, whatever you do with it.

When this book was first released in Germany, I was overwhelmed by the emails and the general feedback from people whose lives had been touched and transformed.

Clearly there is a great deal of spiritual hunger in the world today. More and more there is a cry in the hearts and eyes of many people,

'Father where are you?'

'Why am I here?'

'Is there someone out there who loves me?'

This may be a painful cry but it is one that starts a journey to discover your true identity.

This journey almost cost me my life but I found the answer in a place I least expected.

Today I am grateful for my life and my journey even though it has not always been easy.

I want to encourage you.

There is somebody who cares for you and has a great plan for your life.

So even though at times you may think I'm crazy, please continue reading to the very end.

I believe you can find the answer and truth for yourself.

There is a God and he is so different from what you thought.

There is a way to know him too.

So why not join the journey?

I challenge you, there is more than we can see or understand.

Are you ready to face it?

Stefan Driess

Chapter 1

Where is my Father?

'I don't want this bastard!'

I was only a boy when I heard these terrible words. I can't tell you exactly how old I was. But the man shouting was my father. He was drunk and he was referring to me.

I'll never forget it.

Today I can still hear the question that I later asked my mother.

'What's a bastard?'

'It's someone who doesn't have a father,' she answered, before adding, 'but you do have a father.'

A Family Portrait

My father, Ludwig Driess, had married my mother Beate towards the end of the war. They had met in what was formerly known as Czechoslovakia which is where my mother had lived. They had married quickly.

From then on it had been tough for my mother. Marrying a German meant that she was no longer accepted in her own country. Then in post-war Germany she was rejected as a foreigner. This must have been devastating. No wonder I heard her crying from time to time when I was little.

I began my life in the town of Bad Bergzabern in the state of Rheinland Pfalz. On the surface of it you'd think that it would have been relatively easy growing up in a provincial town rather than a big city - none of the problems associated with urban crime and addiction there, after all.

But growing up doesn't just happen outdoors. It happens inside a home too.

And my home life wasn't easy.

When I was born, my older brother already had a daughter so I immediately became an uncle without any choice in the matter or any consciousness of the fact.

How strange it must have been for my brother's little daughter as she looked at a newly born child and heard her father say,

'Look, that's your uncle!'

I was the sixth child to be born to my parents. They had had twin girls but both had tragically died shortly after they were born. In addition to my older brother, I also had two sisters. So there were four of us in all.

When I was three months old, my oldest sister gave birth to twins. This helped my mother out of an embarrassing situation. Since she was 45 years old when I was born, she was nervous about taking me out on the streets. When my sister had twins, my sister used to take me out with them. Needless to say, many people thought that we were triplets.

Since I was the youngest, I was often given preferential treatment. I was extremely happy with this arrangement even though it didn't do my character development any good. I was very spoilt and I cannot remember ever being refused what I wanted, after working on my mother long enough. My favourite and most used phrase was 'I want.'

So I was unbearably selfish.

My mother, on the other hand, was soft and kind. She expressed her love for me by always giving me what I wanted, regardless of the sacrifice.

Sacrifice is in fact a word that could really sum up the whole of my mother's life. When she was a child she had to look after her family because her father died when she was little and her mother had to go out to work. There were ten of them so this was a big responsibility. From a very early age my mother's life had consisted of hard work and unceasing commitment to others.

There were many times that I could tell she missed her homeland. Bedtime was one of those occasions. My mother would come into my bedroom and pray with me and then sing me to sleep with Czech songs.

It was hard for my mother to feel like she belonged. But then I had those feelings too. As I grew older, I often felt as if I was somehow different from my brothers and sisters. Their whole manner seemed different from mine. 'Maybe my parents just found me somewhere,' I used to think. 'Maybe I'm adopted.'

Something wasn't right.

I just couldn't put my finger on it.

A Catholic Childhood

Church was very much a part of my childhood because my family was Roman Catholic. I did have one or two positive experiences. I remember one occasion when the priest gave me a picture. We were very poor by German standards so he gave it to me for free. All the other children had to pay for theirs. This made a huge impression on me. It made me feel special, at least for a little while.

I will never forget that.

On the down side, going to church didn't seem to impact our lives very deeply. Like many other Catholics we only went to Sunday services on an occasional basis. I used to wonder why the church was full at Christmas but not at any other time of the year. I also got angry when Christmas fun had to be put on hold until after we'd attended the Holy Mass (the Catholic Christmas service). I had presents waiting for me back home because everyone was generous even if it meant getting in debt. Even the younger of my two sisters, with whom I often argued, gave me a gift. These presents seemed far more interesting to me than the baby in a manger and I couldn't wait for the service to end.

What made it more difficult was the fact that going to church at Christmas didn't seem to change many peoples' lives for the better. In fact, later I was to learn that Christmas has the highest number of suicides.

Clearly something wasn't quite right.

People would go into a sacred building and become different while they were there. But then their reverent behaviour would disappear the moment they were outside the church and back home.

So church didn't change the people who went.

It certainly didn't change my family.

Life started to get more challenging when I reached the age when I had to go to church more. This was because I was approaching the time when I would be able to take Holy Communion and go through Confirmation - big events in the Catholic Church and ones with which I had to comply.

I had no real problem with this actually. Even though I didn't really understand what it was all about I allowed myself to go through the motions because everyone else did. And besides, I received a lot of presents.

And as you can probably tell by now, I was certainly up for that!

Some time after I was confirmed I decided to become an altar server. In those days, altar servers were young men. Their job was to assist the priest during the service and with other church duties as well. All my friends were becoming servers so I thought I would join in too. The good thing about this was we received a bit of money whenever we helped at weddings or infant baptisms. The people would be so happy that they'd gladly give us a few tips.

Clearly working for God brought its rewards!

I'll never forget my first service though. It was an absolute disaster. We were all standing with the priest in front of the altar. After the consecration of the host (the wafer), we knelt down.

Servers in those days had to wear long red tunics fastened to a pair of braces.

When I stood up again I forget to take care not to stand on my tunic.

The result was mortifying.

I got up in front of the whole congregation but my tunic remained on the floor.

I was exposed.

There was a great deal of laughter but I was really embarrassed.

I never wanted to see any of these people ever again.

For a long time I kept seeing a picture of them standing before me laughing. Although, having said that, I had never heard people laugh so much in church before.

That wasn't such a bad thing.

Asking Questions

As an altar server I would often look at the Cross on the altar.

'It's a real shame they killed him,' I used to think. 'This Jesus was a really good guy.'

Then I would sigh.

'That's the way the world is. Anything good gets destroyed.'

On one occasion I was looking up at the Cross as I sat in church.

'Why did they crucify him?' I asked myself. 'They say it's because of my sins. Okay, but what use is that to me today?'

That question wasn't answered.

Over my parent's bed there hung a picture of Jesus as the Good Shepherd. He had left ninety nine sheep in order to look for one that had become lost.

This made me ask myself more questions.

'Why would anyone in their right mind leave their entire flock without protection while they went and looked for just one stubborn sheep that had wandered off? Who would look after the ones that were left behind?'

Even though I was asking questions, this didn't mean I was cynical about Jesus, let alone dismissive of him. In some ways I thought that his behaviour was really radical and different from the norm.

'This Jesus must have been a mega guy,' I would think. 'It's a shame he's not alive today!'

So I would often just stand and stare at this picture, curious about Jesus' behaviour, but at the same time impressed. The lost sheep spoke to me too. Deep down, I identified with it.

And then there was an intuition I often had - a sense that someone was with me, someone I couldn't see with my eyes but whose presence I definitely felt. What was that all about?

Losing Connection

I served in the church for about four years in all. As far as I was concerned this couldn't do me any harm. When I used to reflect on what I was doing for God I would pat myself on the back. 'What you're doing is really good,' I would think. 'You're on the good side - on God's side, and Jesus.'

But then other interests started to take over. I began escaping into the make-believe world of the movies, of TV and comics. I'd dream of being a Superhero who would save the world from certain destruction. In my fantasy I would be idolised by everyone for being ready to sacrifice my life for the planet.

But none of this was real.

'Superheroes don't exist,' I would think. 'At least, I don't know any.'

Thus it was that my time at church came to an end. Having become disillusioned with the gap between people's beliefs and behaviour, I broke away. I continued to believe in God but I wasn't prepared to live the way people preached but didn't practice. If going to church was the way to know God, count me out. There was nothing attractive about that. The sermons were mostly boring and often incomprehensible. The young people that went seemed like wimps to me. They looked like weak people who couldn't cope with their lives and needed church as a crutch. I didn't. And I didn't want to pretend that I did and become a hypocrite in the process.

It didn't help that I was molested sexually as a teenager by a religious education teacher either. I was hitch hiking at the time. What made it worse was the fact that this man was a friend of the family.

That didn't exactly increase my desire to be involved with church nor did it strengthen my faith in God.

Church therefore became irrelevant.

My idea of a Christian became someone who carried a thick book under their arm containing songs they knew by heart. They would be dressed in old fashioned and cheap clothes and wear a carefully etched, martyred expression on their faces.

'God's just for people like this,' I'd say to myself, 'for people preparing for death. They're just too weak to enjoy life and they forbid anything which is fun.'

So I wasn't exactly singing 'Hallelujah' in those days.

'When I'm old,' I would think, 'then maybe I'll go to church to collect some brownie points.'

I had already worked out that if everything they said about God was true, then I'd rather not find out that I had been wrong when it was too late.

Yes, I would turn back to God when I was old.

That way I could still have a fun-packed life and go to heaven when I died.

So this was my theology.

'God is sitting on his throne in heaven, far away from the world. He doesn't care about us anymore because we have messed up big time. He's just waiting up there for Judgment Day when he can pay everyone back for ignoring him and breaking his commandments. In the meantime, all he does is come down very occasionally from his throne to give us a great big clout for not being good enough.'

As you can see from that magnificent creed my many questions had not really been answered.

'Does God exist?'

'Is there really a heaven and a hell?'

For a little while longer I had a basic respect for God but this was borne out of a fear of punishment rather than anything else.

In the years to come these questions would reach a furious intensity during the biggest battle of my life.

Longing to be Popular

My parents were not well off financially. In fact by German standards you could have said we were border-line poor. This meant that my mother had to economize wherever she could. This was embarrassing sometimes. I had to wear clothes that were old and not the latest fashion. Like the house we lived in, they were worn out. In fact, our house was so old and bare that it had an earth privy! This wasn't exactly conducive for inviting school friends home.

I wanted so badly to be popular. I was searching for love and recognition. When I saw what others had I wanted it too and stubbornly set about getting it. I knew how to manipulate other people to get my own way. I would do that to my mother even if it meant she got in debt buying me what I wanted.

So it was that I was the first of my school friends to have a Super 8 movie projector.

I was now the centre of attention.

That was all that mattered.

The cost was irrelevant.

My older sister was much later to say to me, 'you were really terrible when you were young. Everything had to be done your way. Everyone had to dance to your tune. You were a proper little tyrant.'

She was right.

What made matters worse was that after a good start in my first few years I started to lose focus at school.

The turning point came when I overheard something my class teacher said to my mother.

The teacher in question was someone I liked and respected. He was my favourite teacher, in fact, and something of a father figure.

I stood next to both of them and listened to him saying something about my school performance and my lack of ability in one particular subject.

'If there's no improvement,' he said, 'there'll be problems.'

These negative words cut me to the core.

I was gutted.

Why had he not spoken to me first about this? Why did he have to go straight to my mother? I had trusted him. Now I felt so betrayed. Maybe it was true. Maybe I was a failure.

After this I lost my motivation. I only went to school because I had to. I hardly learned anything and I got through every year by cheating, right up to the time of my school-leaving exams.

Searching for a Father

The words of the teacher had had a profoundly destructive effect. I had been looking for a father figure at the time and I thought that he was it. I only ever saw my own father when he came home from work and then all he wanted was peace and quiet. He would just sit at the kitchen table and read the newspaper and drink wine. On Sundays he would go off to the pub. If ever I had questions he would say, 'ask your mother.'

I so needed a father, desperately.

It made such an impact on me when on one occasion I was allowed to go to the pub with my father. I sat with him while I drank coca cola. It was wonderful. I felt like a grown-up.

But this show of interest was very rare.

I don't have a single memory of him taking me in his arms and saying, 'I love you son,' or 'I'm proud of you.' He didn't seem capable of that. We hardly spoke to each other. He was like a stranger in my own home. I didn't know anything about him at all - who his family were, or details about his childhood. He only occasionally mentioned the war.

Then one day everything changed for the worse.

My mother told me that the man I had always regarded as my father wasn't in fact my father at all.

That was why I felt different!

That was why he would call me a 'bastard' when he was drunk.

My mother told me that my real father was an Italian man who had returned to his own country shortly after I was born. She was already married to my stepfather when she met him. Times had been very difficult for her as a foreigner in Germany and her husband's family had rejected her. She was also treated very badly by her husband himself, especially on the frequent occasions when he was drunk. It was during this very tough time when she felt like no one loved her that she met my real father and the rest is history. She had three children at the time but now I was on the way.

'Come back to Italy with me,' my father had said to her.

'I can't.'

'Why can't you?'

'I don't want to leave my three children with a father who's a drunk.'

And so my father returned to Italy, promising to write to her and one day come back to fetch her. My father did write but his letters never reached her. My older brother and sisters had known about the affair and were afraid that mother would leave them. So they destroyed the letters and she never knew they had even arrived.

There is something terribly sad about that.

The way my mother spoke about him, I realise now that she must have really loved him.

But when she didn't receive his letters, she assumed that he no longer loved her.

And my father must have thought from the lack of replies that she no longer loved him either.

So now everything began to become clear to me. This was why I felt so different from my siblings. This was why I really didn't belong in the family. This was why I lost my temper more quickly than the others.

At the same time I felt cheated. All my life my family had allowed me to believe a lie. My stepfather had not hidden the fact that he wanted nothing to do with me especially when I was younger.

'When you were little,' my mother said, 'he didn't want you. But now he's glad that he's got you.'

HE DIDN'T WANT YOU!

Those words haunted me.

Later I was to learn the full force of this rejection and hatred from my stepfather. When my mother was pregnant, he had tried to kill me by kicking her in the stomach.

Others had suggested she should have an abortion. But my mother refused. She said something that I'm not sure she fully understood at the time.

'If God wants this child to be born, then there is a reason for its life.'

Someone was evidently watching over me.

But I was so angry.

That day, when I discovered that my stepfather had tried to murder me before I was born, a seed of hatred was planted in the soil of my heart.

Once again I had been let down by someone I trusted.

I had trusted this man whom I had called 'father.'

But he had tried to kill me!

And now I really did feel like a 'bastard.'

Chapter 2

A Growing Hatred

Several years before I became a teenager I discovered karate.

I had been looking for something to meet my growing need for a sense of value. Lacking a father's affirmation and direction, I looked for a sense of worth elsewhere. I wanted to be noticed. I wanted to be cool like those who didn't conform to the rules around my school.

Although I was tall I was also thin so my physique was not exactly helpful towards me gaining the respect of others. However, I had come to realize that physical strength was essential for acceptance. So I decided to learn karate. I had watched a training session and had decided immediately that I was going to learn.

'I'm going to be the best at this martial art, and as quickly as possible,' I said to myself. 'When I'm the best, people will admire me.'

I was around about the age of eleven or twelve when I began training. In no time at all I was training with the older students. In fact I was the only one of my age in the group. I spent hours and hours training.

My hero was Bruce Lee, the king of Kung Fu. I idolised him. I read books about him, watched movies with him in, and dreamed of being as famous as him.

Bruce Lee was my god.

The only thing was I didn't want to die as young as he had.

He was only about thirty when he died.

A Substitute Father

My karate teacher was kind to me and always instilled in me a feeling that I was special.

He used to invite the students round to his house to watch karate films. We would often chat together on the way home after training. He appreciated my skills and praised me for them. That meant a lot to me.

I never missed a karate lesson and I trained every day. Quite quickly I became the best in my age group. Even when I joined the age group above, I was one of the best there as well. There was no stopping me.

I just kept on practicing and practicing, even trying out various moves on the other children on my street.

It wasn't long before my karate skills began to win me the recognition I was craving for. At the same time they equipped me for protecting myself. So you could say that I killed two birds with one stone.

The man I wanted to be most like - other than of course Bruce Lee - was my karate instructor.

'I want to be like him when I'm older,' I'd think.

I was even more motivated to follow in his footsteps when I saw his girlfriend.

She was very pretty.

I guess I'd never had an older male role model like this before.

You could say he was a substitute father figure.

Over the next two years or so I invested all my time in karate. I dreamed of taking part in tournaments and becoming the German champion. I was well on the way to that too.

Then my ambitions were shattered.

The karate teacher closed the school down.

The substitute father figure who had meant so much to me moved out of my life - and at the same time that my mother told me that my real father was an Italian man.

These two events hit me hard.

I felt so betrayed and deceived.

Living Life My Way

Up until the age of fifteen I hadn't drunk alcohol or smoked because my life had been karate and I needed to be fit and strong. But now I was devastated. It seemed that every time something started to go right for me and I was beginning to enjoy life, someone would pull the rug from underneath my feet and everything I had enjoyed would be whisked away.

Was God responsible for all of this?

If so I made up my mind to hate him.

I also made the decision to live life in the way I liked.

'People couldn't care less about me anyway,' I thought. 'My own family has lied to me for so long. Now I'm going to do what I want.'

'You're only young once.'

'I WANT TO LIVE!'

So it was that I began to go to pubs and discos with friends. I felt great there. I was doing things that only adults were normally allowed to do. There was no one to tell me what to do any more. I had lied to my parents about where I was. They thought I was having a sleepover at a friend's house. So they couldn't lecture me either.

That gave me a real sense of satisfaction.

The Red Devils

It was when I was sixteen years old that I started on the road to football hooliganism.

Having been denied the fulfilment of my dreams of being a karate champion, I now turned my attention to football.

Up until then I hadn't known much about football. I hadn't been very good at playing so I didn't give it much time. Since others were so much better than me there was no chance of finding recognition and worth that way.

But it's one thing to find value playing football.

It's quite another finding value watching it.

A visit with a few friends to Kaiserslautern to the Betzenberg (now the Fritz Walter stadium) soon changed my perspective. The atmosphere in the stadium was amazing. I had never felt anything like it. There were thousands of people there, all united in their support of the same team. And the noise was incredible. It was electric. I felt as if I was part of a huge family, experiencing a unity that I'd never known and a passion that I'd never even begun to sense anywhere else. Never had I heard such anthems before or wanted so much to join in:

'Olé! Olé! Olé! Olé! Kaiserslautern FC!'

'Marble, stone and iron may break, but our Betze won't!'

The sound of men singing resounded around the famous stadium where the 'Red Devils' (FC Kaiserslautern's first team) played in front of thousands of fans.

I was hooked.

The atmosphere of the place was magnetic.

It drew me back again and again.

My friends and I stood in the west wing of the stadium - the area where the most loyal and radical fans went. We wore the club's red and white colours and sang with all our might the songs that we were now beginning to learn by heart. We sang songs deriding the opposing teams and shouted insults at their supporters. We weren't exactly polite.

The crowd was like an ocean whose powerful currents sucked you into the depths.

I couldn't resist it. It was intoxicating.

After a while I couldn't help noticing that there were different groups among the crowd as a whole. In particular there was one group that was known for fighting for their team and their town no matter what. Members of this group were not afraid to use violence in defending their club and district either, whether that was with opposing fans or with the police. These guys were genuine football hooligans.

I quickly discovered that there were different levels in this group - a kind of hierarchy with the most radical supporters at the top.

The 'Hell's Devils' were the dominant power at that time but there were others such as 'Red Front,' 'Red-and-White-Army,' and 'Mighty Devils.'

Each group had their own name and identity. Even when all the groups joined forces to attack opposing supporters, fighting and rioting would sometimes break out between them, when they had no one else to fight against.

This sense of a group identity appealed to me. I could see that it gave people a sense of belonging and its leaders a level of respect and recognition.

These were things I longed for too.

So I became involved in the founding and leading of a new group and 'the Red Devils' were born.

The Black Hole

It now became important to assert ourselves. We were a new group and we needed to be seen and respected. This meant going to games where it was usual for hooligans to start fighting. We had to be there when fights broke out.

So for several years I went with the Red Devils to matches both in Germany and abroad. We thought of ourselves as true fans. In a sense this was strange because there came a point when the matches themselves were of secondary importance. What mattered were the fights. They were the focus.

For me these matches were a means by which I could channel and expel all my anger and aggression. It was like an addiction. In fact, addiction isn't a bad word for it. I was regularly getting drunk and high on drugs so that I was free from inhibitions whenever I entered a stadium.

This meant that I was more fearless and crazy than I would have been otherwise.

It also meant that I maintained my position in the group and the respect of the others.

With alcohol and drugs as my friends, we began to think this lifestyle was awesome. We were living our lives the way we wanted. We were rebelling against anything or anyone that tried to mould us. We saw ourselves as strong. We weren't going to conform to any rules.

I lived for the weekends and for football matches. I survived the apprenticeship I was doing because I had a kind boss who turned a blind eye to some of my bad behaviour.

I stole.

I cheated.

I was desperately trying to fill the emptiness inside.

But it was no good. It was like drinking sea water. The more I drank, the thirstier I became.

I was hopelessly deceived.

The black hole inside me was just getting bigger and bigger.

The Road to Destruction

I had two dreams during my teenage years which were like vivid pictures of the life I was leading.

In the first I found myself falling into a deep, black hole. I fell down and down and screamed for help. But the hole had no bottom. I just kept on falling.

In the second I was on a narrow path with high walls on either side. When I was half way down the path, the tall walls on both sides started to press in slowly towards me. I couldn't escape either forwards or backwards because the path was too long both ways and I wouldn't be able to make it out before I was crushed.

I pushed against both the walls, desperately trying to hold them apart, but to no avail. I knew that it was hopeless. It was just a matter of time before I would be pulverised.

At the time I was frightened by these dreams but I didn't see them for what they were - warnings about what would happen to me if I kept on living as I was.

Then there was the music I was listening to at the time. I didn't realise it but these two were like a warning about the destructive path I was on.

One song was nearly always on my lips, 'Highway to Hell,' by AC/DC. As the song says, I was 'livin' easy, lovin' free', 'taking everything in my stride', on a highway with 'no speed limit', 'no stop signs', and nobody was going to slow me down. The problem was, like the song says, I was going down, all the way down, because I was on the highway to hell.

Those words should have woken me up, but they didn't.

I was living in a world of delusion - a demonic world in which I was being blinded to the reality of my situation.

I was listening to music that was filled and fuelled by a hate like mine. If I'd thought about it, I might have seen it. The band name AC/DC stands for Anti-Christ/Death of Christ (although this is only known in occult circles).

Accelerating to Disaster

As I increased in speed on the highway so my hatred intensified.

As I continued as one of the leaders of the Red Devils, I didn't even bother watching the games any more at the stadiums. Instead I would spend the entire match at the stadium bars drinking beer with skinheads and members of other clubs and groups. Drinking was mandatory for me. I had to be drunk if I was going to pick a fight with the police or with opposing supporters. I wouldn't have had the courage had I been sober.

And so a seething hatred began to grow and grow inside my heart. It was like a poison creeping through every part of my soul, taking possession of me and controlling everything I did.

I had looked for love, wanted to be loved, but I'd not found anyone who had been able to give me what I needed.

One by one my criminal offences began to mount up. My financial difficulties mounted up with them as I had to pay more and more fines and lawyer's fees.

The walls were pressing in all around me.

Death was encroaching.

In fact, death was getting nearer and nearer.

On one occasion someone held a revolver to my head and was getting ready to shoot me.

On another a guy hit me with a wheel spanner and I ended up unconscious in hospital. The doctors didn't know if I was going to regain consciousness or not. If I did, they couldn't be sure there wouldn't be brain damage.

When I came round, I discharged myself from hospital and went straight to the pub where our club met and started drinking in my blood-stained clothes. A few days later I had to go back into hospital because splinters from my cheek bone had trapped a nerve and half my face was paralysed.

But for now I was enjoying the attention and the respect of people at the bar.

I was oblivious of the devastating power at work over and in my life.

But the clues were there, had I had the eyes to see.

In the room above the bar we had drawn a huge picture of the devil on the wall. He would always be watching over us as we gathered there to plan future fights. The owner of the pub had allowed it because he was a member of the Red Devils.

So there were signs.

My dreams were speaking to me.

The songs I was listening to were calling out to me.

The picture in the pub was staring at me in the face.

But I was on the highway.

I may have been asking what I was here for and what the purpose of living was all about.

But no one could give me an answer.

I was pressing my foot down on the accelerator, picking up

speed in the downward trajectory I was on.

And I had no idea what I was about to run into.

Chapter 3

We'll Get Your Soul

It is probably not surprising, given that I was careering out of control down the highway to hell, that I became more and more fascinated with the occult.

The word 'occult' comes from a Latin word meaning 'hidden' or 'secret.' The occult is an umbrella term that points to the concealed spiritual world and the practices that people use to access it.

Ever since I was a child I was aware of being in touch with this unseen dimension to life. Sometimes I dreamed about things which subsequently came true. At others I had this sense that there was some kind of evil presence near me. If you had asked me what that was I wouldn't have been able to tell you.

Perhaps the most disturbing moments were when I heard a voice telling me, 'your parents don't love you! Your parents don't want you.' I was absolutely convinced that these voices were real and that I wasn't imagining things. I was in touch with invisible realities. The only problem was that they weren't comforting me, they were tormenting me.

The communication from these spirit beings was therefore not one which gave me any peace. They terrified me. The overall message seemed to be 'we'll get your soul!'

I was in contact with the unseen world. But that world was a very dark world.

One time when I was involved in a séance, we asked the spirit we had contacted to tell us his name. The glass on the table moved in various directions and spelled out S-A-T-A-N.

No wonder my experiences filled me with fear.

The Writing on the Wall

And yet, even having discovered the source of the voices that I was hearing, I was not only shocked. I was intrigued. So much so, in fact, that far from putting the brakes on my quest for the unseen world, I pushed my foot down hard on the accelerator.

It had all started when a colleague at work told me how to make contact with spirits. At first I laughed. Yet what she said tapped into the deep fascination that I had had in my life since childhood. I had always been interested in the supernatural, in the invisible world beyond this material world.

When I had been a child, this invisible dimension had from time to time intruded in my daily life.

I remember an incident involving a brother and sister who had become friends of mine.

'I'm in contact with my dead grandmother,' the sister had claimed.

She was always full of tales of the unexplainable, tales which at times were like horror stories.

On one occasion I saw strangely written letters on the wall of her house.

'What do those letters mean?' I asked her.

'Those are the letters I need to make contact with my dead grandmother,' she replied.

'My grandmother appeared to me once,' she continued. 'Since then I've been able to talk to her. She even gives me information about the future.'

Then on another occasion she started to give a prediction about my future. 'When you're sixteen years old,' she said, 'you'll have a moped accident. The moped will be a write-off. But you'll be okay.'

Those words came true. I really did write off my moped in an accident. And indeed I wasn't hurt.

But this didn't mean everything that she said came true. Later I was to learn that she had given another prediction about me to my sister.

'Your brother is going to die when he's twenty two.'

'Whatever you do, don't tell him,' my sister had replied.

My Dead Grandfather

At this stage in my life I thought that there was nothing wrong in being fascinated by this unseen world. I had been open to the supernatural as a child and now that I was older I was even more interested. I saw no harm in visiting a fortune teller, for example. I once entered a caravan owned by an old gypsy fortune teller. There were lots of pictures of Christian saints in the place.

'There can't be anything wrong with this,' I thought as she laid out the cards in front of me. 'If there was she certainly wouldn't have all these pictures in here. There are even ones of Jesus and Mary. How bad can this be?'

So I was deceived into thinking that my interest in the occult world was just harmless fun. I had no idea that this kind of activity is dangerous and spiritually harmful. It was only years later that I would discover in the Bible that God warns us against doing such things.

But at the time I was ignorant.

I was hooked.

I was fascinated by the hidden world.

And I wasn't alone in that. One of my sisters often used to tell us that she could see our dead grandfather. She also said that she could hear footsteps and voices in the house. Sometimes I heard these footsteps too. They came from upstairs. When I went to have a look, there was no one there.

When I was about twelve or thirteen years old, I made the decision to find out whether there was any truth and substance to these mysterious occurrences.

I was lying in the room in which my grandfather had died.

'Right,' I thought, 'if this really is my grandfather who is making these strange noises then I want to see him.'

My sister who had given most of the reports about my dead grandfather's activities was in the same room but she had fallen asleep. To be honest, I hadn't really believed her.

But when I said in my heart, 'I want to see him,' something strange happened. The face of an old man suddenly appeared on the ceiling.

I was frightened and woke my sister.

We found it really hard getting back to sleep after that.

'Whose face was it?' I kept thinking.

I couldn't remember my grandfather very well because I'd been a small boy when he had died. But when I looked at photos of him I realised that the face I had seen had been his.

The First Seance

While the society in which we grew up played down the reality of such experiences - claiming that they are simply exciting fantasies, a world of scary make believe - I became more and more convinced they were far from imaginary. I was constantly aware of a dark and threatening presence in our lives. But this just made me more interested. And so I became fascinated by stories of UFOs, witches, sorcerers - anything that had anything to do with the occult.

My interest started to grow more serious when I spoke to a colleague at work.

'You can make contact with spirits,' she said. 'I learned how to do this at a Spanish convent school.'

I was curious.

'How?' I asked.

'Through what are called 'moving the glass séances,' she replied.

For a long time I had been on the lookout for new experiences which would satisfy the emptiness I felt in my heart. I had tried drugs, alcohol, and sex. These had provided only temporary relief. Afterwards, the feeling of emptiness seemed even greater. Perhaps this was what I was looking for.

Yes,' I thought. 'I'll give it a try.'

That evening I called some of my family together. I laid out the alphabet in a circle on the table, exactly as the woman at work had described.

I placed two slips of paper in the middle.

On one, the word 'NO' was written.

On the other, 'YES.'

I then placed a glass in the centre and everyone touched it lightly with their fingertips.

And then we called a spirit.

The suspense was enormous.

The glass suddenly started to move.

And that night I changed gear on the Highway to Hell.

I was picking up speed.

Becoming a Medium

I became so addicted that I often would contact spirits on a daily basis. It was exciting to learn more about the world beyond, about life after death, about the future. There was something intoxicating about it all.

It made me feel like I was someone special.

When we contacted these spirits, they always used the names of saints, angels or dead people when they introduced themselves.

Sometimes we even communicated with dead relatives. What amazed me was the way in which these spirits knew the exact details about our family members.

This made me believe more and more that I was dealing with a dimension of life that was real.

Sometimes I would ask myself whether I was imagining it all.

'Maybe there's some kind of telepathic power that allows us to move the glass by the power of our thoughts.'

But then I'd realize that couldn't be it.

'If it's just telepathy then how come these spirits had information about people at the table only they could have known? And if it was us pushing the glass, how come it moved so directly and smoothly over the table to the letters, as if it was moved by an invisible hand?'

I knew that what we were experiencing wasn't made up or manipulated. Had it been a purely human phenomenon the glass would have moved to and fro in a jerky motion because everyone would have had different ideas where it should go. It would have been immediately noticeable.

The glass was therefore moved by another force.

But what was that force?

This sense of mystery drove my friends and me deeper and

deeper into the occult. We spent hours conversing with these spirits. As we did, I became a medium without even realizing it. It seemed to be far easier for others to make contact with spirits when I was present. I was becoming a channel for them without noticing.

The Ticking Bomb

I tried to justify what I was doing by making it clear that we were only to contact good spirits. I knew there were bad spirits. No one needed to tell me that. I had often experienced an evil presence in my life so I only wanted to communicate with good spirits. That was the aim anyway.

And so we went out of our way to ensure that dark spirits were kept at bay.

We laid a cross on the table, with pictures and statues of saints and angels.

'These will protect us against evil spirits,' we thought.

But we had no idea what we were dealing with.

If we had all been asked, 'how many of you want to move the glass?' we would all have raised our hands.

If we had been asked, 'how many of you want to press a nuclear missile trigger?' Not one of us would.

We didn't realise we were playing with fire.

And I didn't know that I had pressed the switch myself, initiating a chain of destructive events in my life.

I didn't realise that the demonic powers that were involved would demand a payment in the future.

I had forgotten that the spirit who had identified himself as S-A-T-A-N had promised, 'we'll get your soul.'

For me it was now even a bit of a game.

I learned how to provoke and torment bad spirits and I would annoy them by mentioning God's name, which they didn't like at all.

'Okay, you call yourself Satan,' I would say, 'but God is more powerful than you.'

I didn't know what I was really saying nor did I actually believe it at the time.

But the effects were powerful. The glass started moving faster and faster on the table until it slid towards me. I leaned sideways as it flew past me.

The next time I conducted a séance the spirits threatened not to communicate with me anymore if I mentioned these things again.

That got me thinking.

'Why are these evil spirits so afraid of God if he doesn't exist?'

'Why do they get so angry when I mention his name?'

I was becoming more and more confused.

On the one hand I was impressed that these spirits were real.

On the other I was puzzled by their aversion to God.

My Guardian Spirit

During this time a spirit appeared who informed me that he was my 'guardian spirit' and that it was his task to protect me.

'You've got a big challenge there!' I thought.

The spirit told me his name was 'Don Bosco.'

My sister explained that in the Catholic Church, Don Bosco is the patron saint of endangered youth.

Nobody needed to tell me that I fell into that category.

One day I decided to address my guardian spirit directly.

'Would it be possible for me to see you?' I asked.

He replied that I only had to give my permission.

So I did.

He promised to come to me that evening. All I had to do was wait. He would come into my room.

That night I lay on my bed with intense anticipation. Maybe this was the night that I would find out once and for all what lay behind all that I had been experiencing.

But then doubts crept in.

'Come on Stefan,' I thought. 'You surely don't really believe that anyone will come. This is all just a game. Forget the whole thing.'

It was at that moment - just I was trying to convince myself - a figure appeared at the end of my bed.

I saw a white body - arms, hands, legs and the upper torso.

I saw the head and then the outline of the whole body.

I rubbed my eyes.

'You're overtired,' I thought.

'You're imagining things.'

But however hard I rubbed my eyes, every time I opened them the figure was still there.

I decided to conduct a test.

I waved to it.

The figure waved back.

With that I dived underneath the bedclothes.

It was then that I understood for the first time that this unseen world really does exist. I knew that now, without a shadow of a doubt.

When I at last plucked up the courage to come out, the figure had gone.

'What was that?' I thought.

As soon after that as I could, I held a séance. I made contact with the spirit world and asked Don Bosco if it was he that I had seen and, if it was, why he had disappeared.

He told me that it had been him and that he had only left because I had been scared. But the less I was frightened and the more I allowed him to visit, the better I would see him and at some stage even hear him.

Once I again I felt special.

Only very strong mediums were allowed this kind of direct communication with spirits.

Clearly I was unique.

And clearly this was a good spirit.

Don Bosco had appeared in white.

'White means good, right?'

So I resolved to see more of him.

My contact with him through séances increased.

His appearances in a spiritual but bodily form grew more frequent.

He had told me he was my guardian spirit.

'He's here to protect me, right?'

What could possibly go wrong?

Chapter 4

You're Gonna Die!

'You will die of cancer.'

These words came from a spirit during a séance.

They were directed at a Turkish girl who was taking part.

Everyone was shocked.

Up until then, the spirits had never said anything like this.

This was wholly different.

What was going on?

From then on, terrifying incidents began to increase. One of my nieces called Silvia, three months younger than me, experienced one of them. She was in the kitchen preparing dinner while her twin sister Petra was standing watching her, not saying a word. Silvia was talking to her and glancing at her from time to time. But her sister was not replying.

When Silvia saw her sister a bit later she asked, 'why didn't you answer me when I was talking to you earlier in the kitchen?'

'I wasn't in the kitchen,' Petra replied. 'I swear I was upstairs in my bedroom the whole time you were cooking. I was with my friends. You can ask them.'

Hearing this, Silvia was terrified.

Later she was to tell me that there had been something dark and lifeless about her sister when she had been just standing there, watching her cook.

These sorts of frightening episodes began to become more common. Poltergeist manifestations began to take place. Objects began to move. Some were thrown about without being touched.

Could all this be real?

It seemed like the stuff of Hollywood movies.

Surely things like this only occur in horror films.

The Last Temptation

One day I was driving my car and I heard a voice. 'If you serve me and bow down to me, I'll give you women, power and wealth - everything you want.' It was as clear as if someone had been sitting next to me.

Even at that time, I knew that the devil or something evil was speaking to me. I knew that the devil, spiritual darkness, whatever you want to call them, was real. That might sound crazy, but it's true. Satan was offering to give me everything I had craved - the things that I thought would fill the deep void in my soul. I was being given the opportunity to satisfy my deepest longings. Yet something held me back from saying yes. I knew instinctively that if I accepted that I'd be giving my life to Satan. That would mean the end for me.

Later on in my life I met people who had said yes to this kind of offer and who had dedicated their lives to Satan.

One young man who had dedicated his life to Satan during a ritual told me that he had been offered exactly the same things. The only thing was that Satan had lied. He had not kept his side of the bargain. We shouldn't be surprised at that. Jesus once said that Satan has been a liar since the beginning. His chief tactic is deception.

When this young man asked me if Jesus would forgive him I answered, 'of course.'

My friend recognized that he had been deceived and that he was now standing at the edge of an abyss. After he renounced his vow to Satan he was set free after a time of intensive ministry.

None of this I knew at the time, however.

That was still a long way off in the future.

For now I had heard Satan's voice, offering me everything I had hungered after.

But I had not said yes.

I had not yielded to his temptations.

Losing Control

In spite of that I continued to long for more knowledge of the supernatural and for more experiences of the occult world. I was fascinated, addicted even. I was on a search for the unknown in the hope that in some miraculous way I would find something that would fill the terrible emptiness in my life.

In actual fact, my quest was successful. I did manage to fill my life with supernatural realities. But these forces and powers were dark, demonic and destructive. Far from satisfying and fulfilling me, they drove me to the very edge of despair, and even to the point of death.

From this time on I began to contact the spirit world more frequently and dramatically. In the process I was often overcome by that same terror that had gripped me when the spirit had threatened the Turkish girl in a séance, or when Silvia had seen a spirit manifest in the form of her twin sister.

Sometimes I was so overpowered by these evil spirits that I lost control of my actions altogether. I became aggressive, knocking people about. All I could hear was an inner command.

'Kill! Kill! Kill!'

To be honest with you, if police, onlookers or friends hadn't stopped me I'm sure I was capable of committing murder while I was in that state.

But it didn't stop there. These spirits began to affect more and more situations in my life. I heard voices - sometimes internal, sometimes audible - and under their influence I was driven to actions over which I had no control.

The dreadful sense of fear began to intensify. When I was in my bedroom, I felt as if I was not alone. There were various spirits there. They inhabited my room whether or not I had called them. They were no longer bothered whether I had invited them, or whether I wanted them there.

I was now living in a permanent state of terror.

This, allied to my loss of self-control, began to take its toll.

I was in a desperate place.

I was totally out of control.

I had reached a dead end on the highway to hell.

And now that I was there, I considered a new thought - 'perhaps the only way out of this chaos is to kill myself.'

The dead end was just that - a place to end it all in death.

I Can't Go On

In a last frail attempt to get my life back I decided to cut off all contact with the spirit world and forget the whole experience.

I gave up séances immediately.

I ignored the voices and apparitions and just hoped that everything in time would sort itself out.

But I couldn't have been more deluded.

As soon as I started to resist the spirits, they showed their true colours and I now realised that the angel of light was a grotesque master of deception.

My now heightened levels of spiritual perception opened the door to a bombardment of hideous faces and terrifying manifestations. I was scared that I was going mad. There was no one I could talk to. I was convinced that I was going to end up in a mental hospital and that thought filled me with dread.

There was no going back.

I had invited the spirits into my life and now I couldn't get rid of them. I had installed them in the hard drive of my soul and I couldn't un-install them.

Everything now began to implode around me.

My life descended into chaos.

Inside I broke down completely.

I was mentally shot and physically burned out.

I was tortured by the thought that there was no way out.

Having tried to get rid of the spirits and failed, I decided to end my life.

I was so full of hatred, especially for myself. I blamed myself for everything I had done and for how far I had sunk. I blamed God. I blamed my family. I blamed my society. I especially blamed my girlfriend, who had just ditched me, leaving me in a desperate state. She had broken up with me after a long relationship, saying that she didn't see any future in our being together.

I was just twenty two years old.

I wanted to die.

Ending it All

Thoughts of suicide began to fill my head. It gave me some

satisfaction to think of the people I'd be hurting if I ended my life, although that was offset by my fear that there was nothing after death, or that even worse horrors were waiting for me.

I was drunk the first time I tried to kill myself. I had decided to do it publicly, in a disco where I knew my ex-girlfriend and other friends would be present. I slashed at my arms but in my inebriated state I couldn't find the right place. In the end I was restrained and persuaded to stop.

But then a little later I reached the stage where I didn't care at all what came after death, or whether people wanted to try and stop me.

I was no longer seeking attention or sympathy.

I had now had enough and all I wanted to do was sink into an ocean of nothingness.

It was then that I came up with my final plan.

I would go to a vineyard outside the village where my girlfriend lived.

There I would end it all.

And so it was that I found myself running along the track that led deeper and deeper into the vineyard. 'You are finally on the path to where it will all finish,' I thought. 'This is where it's going to end.'

I knew exactly what I was going to do.

This time I was determined.

I had always wanted to live but I had never found real life - fulfilling life.

It was time to bring the curtain down on my life of lies.

Nobody wanted me. So I wouldn't be missed.

'I'll show you all!' I thought.

In my mind I pictured my mother and my ex-girlfriend crying at my graveside, blaming themselves for my death.

For a moment I wept.

No one likes the thought of dying.

But my life was desperate and I could no longer cope with the speed at which I was accelerating out of control.

And the voice that had shouted 'Kill! Kill! Kill!' when I had been harming others now began to turn inwards, 'Kill yourself! Kill yourself! Kill yourself!'

This is Your Life

As I raced to the end of the track, I resigned myself to the fact that this was now final. I despised myself. I had never wanted to become like my stepfather but now here I was even worse than him.

'Was THAT my life?' I asked myself.

Suddenly my life began to unfold in front of my eyes like the scenes of a film. In a few seconds the two decades of my life flashed before me. These weren't pleasant or happy memories. I didn't see any episodes at church during Christmas or Easter. I didn't see the time that I bought a homeless man something to eat to ease my troubled conscience. I didn't see the one and only time I went to confession. No, all I saw were the unpleasant and unhappy memories.

I remembered the times when I had lied to others, stolen, beaten people almost to death.

I saw moments when I had been despicable to those who loved me, when I had hurt them terribly.

Suddenly the tears began to fall.

I wept bitterly.

'Is this all I have accomplished in twenty two years?' I cried.

'Is this all I have to show for myself?'

I sat down on the ground and leaned back against a pile of wood in the vineyard.

I couldn't have felt emptier.

The tears now began to cascade down my face.

And in those tears there was something remarkable.

I hadn't cried in a long time. In the Red Devils, my philosophy had been, 'the strongest survive. Feelings are for weaklings. I won't ever let myself get hurt.'

The few times I had cried were when I had been drunk and my girlfriend had said she wanted to split up because I had treated her so badly. Oh yes, I had shed tears then.

But apart from that, I had not wept in years.

Now all that changed as I sat at the end of the path in the vineyard.

I had lost all my self-respect.

I was a loser.

I was appalled by the fact that there seemed to be nothing good about my life.

Now I was so desperate that I was prepared to do anything.

I had experienced what it was like to black out - to get to the place where through drugs and drink I had lost all consciousness of what I had done, even shameful things.

Now it was time to enter the ultimate black out.

Someone was holding up my past and saying, 'this is your life.'

I saw a demon laughing at me and heard a voice say, 'I told you we would get your soul.'

Satan was mocking me.

You Shall Live!

Suddenly, from somewhere deep within, defiance began to arise.

To this day I don't know why but I stood to my feet.

I looked up at the night sky.

And I began to cry out.

'God, if you exist and you love me, please do something! I don't know if there's a place called hell or whether I'll end up there if I commit suicide. But I just don't care anymore. If you are real, do something now!'

I can't say there was any real faith behind my words.

But I do know that I was desperate.

From the depths of my soul came one last cry for help, one last attempt to find a way out of the darkness and chaos.

As I finished speaking, a strong wind suddenly began to whirl all around me.

I heard a scream as the demon who had mocked me fled from the scene.

A power that I had never felt before began to fill my entire body.

I was overwhelmed by an intense and beautiful feeling of love and peace.

It was so profound and it was so pure.

And at that moment I realised, 'this is what I've been searching for all my life.'

Nothing I had ever experienced before had come close to making me feel so satisfied, accepted and hopeful.

It was glorious.

I wanted it to go on forever.

In the end, I have no idea how long this experience lasted. All I knew was that something miraculous had happened inside my heart.

My mind was trying to tell me, 'Stefan, nothing has changed. Go on, kill yourself.'

But my heart was filled with hope for the future and a will to live.

In my heart I heard a new voice, a gentle voice, a reassuring voice - a voice I had never heard before, a voice that was the furthest remove from all those hurtful words I had heard which had questioned my right to exist:

'You shall live! You shall live! You shall live!'

'Who is this?' I thought.

'Who is speaking to me?'

'Can this really be happening?'

Chapter 5

Life and Death

That night, leaning against a pile of wood in a vineyard, my life changed.

I knew that.

I had cried out to God and he had answered.

But this gave rise to some big questions.

Who is this God?

What is he like?

Is he an old man sitting up in heaven, swinging his hammer every time we do something wrong?

Or is he an old-fashioned spoil sport, an ancient killjoy, determined to prevent us from having fun?

So I prayed.

'God, I don't know if it was you, but when I cried out to you, something happened. Please show me how to find you!'

The Number of the Beast

Some time after this I was in the car with my girlfriend. We had made up and were back together again. Somehow I just couldn't let go.

As we drove along I suddenly had this strong feeling that we should go home. On arriving I saw to my horror that an emergency doctor was there. As I entered the living room my mother, who was struggling for breath, looked at me and cried, 'Stefan, I won't be coming back!'

Not coming back! What was she talking about?

'Of course she'll come back,' I thought. 'She's often been ill and recovered.'

But I wasn't convinced.

Something in my heart said, 'she's right.'

My mother was taken by ambulance to the nearest hospital where she was transferred to intensive care. She had suffered a heart attack and needed constant monitoring. My sister Marianne lived next door to the hospital so I was round there a lot from then on, whenever I went to visit mum.

Like many people, who turn to God only in a crisis, I thought now was the time to pray. Maybe he could help my mother get better. So I took an old Bible down from my sister's bookshelf and just opened it. The pages fell open and I started to read a verse from the Book of Revelation (the last book in the Bible, about the end of the world).

And the number of the beast is 666!

Those words hit me like an express train.

It was using words I knew from one of my favourite songs, 'The Number of the Beast,' by Iron Maiden. We had used the image of the devil on the album cover as the symbol for the Red Devils. So these words were very familiar.

Yet I didn't understand them.

So I asked my sister. 'Do you know what this means?'

'No,' she replied. 'I've had that Bible in the cupboard for so long that I haven't read it. I haven't a clue what it means. But if you're really interested we can phone someone who would know and we can ask them.'

My sister told me about a really nice man who had moved with his family into a house where she had once lived. He and his family held weekly meetings in their home where they prayed and read the Bible.

Keen to make a good impression on God, I phoned the man.

'It can't do any harm,' I thought.

The man answered in a kind voice. He tried to explain the verse to me. At the end of the conversation he said that it would be a good idea for us to meet because there was so much more in the Bible to talk about.

In my head I said 'never!'

But out of my mouth came the words, 'okay, you come over.' And a date was fixed for him to visit me with his wife.

'This must count in my favour with God,' I thought.

Drawn not Driven

The closer the date came, the more my stomach churned. I was ready for anything except discussions about religion. So I decided to invent an excuse.

I went to my sister.

'Marianne,' I said, 'there are two people coming over later to talk about God. You speak to them. I'm going to the hospital to visit mum.'

Surely there was no better reason for missing a meeting?

And in any case, my sister was more religious than me.

'She'll enjoy it,' I thought.

But when the couple arrived, the wife was very persistent.

'Where is Stefan?' she asked. 'It's very important that we speak to him. Please take us to him.'

And so they came to the hospital!

'We'd like you to spend some time with us,' they said. 'We have something very important to talk to you about.'

Again my first thought was 'never!' But because they were so warm I wasn't able to say it. So I thought, 'okay, I'll go with them and listen to them for a while. Then they'll be happy and when they've gone, I'll be happy too.'

So that's what happened.

The man started to explain why Jesus had died for me. He told me that Jesus had been raised from the dead and that he is alive, so that meant I could experience his love and receive his friendship today.

I'll never forget that.

And I'll never forget how his eyes shone as he spoke about Jesus.

It was as if he had known him for a long time.

'This man has something I haven't got,' I thought. 'What is it?'

It was as if this couple had discovered the best thing that anyone could find and he spoke as if it was only a matter of time before it would be mine too.

There was no pressure, no manipulation.

This wasn't like what I had experienced before, especially from Jehovah's Witnesses.

This man spoke with such love.

I felt drawn, not driven.

I wanted what he had.

O Happy Day!

Then the man said something that clinched it.

He mentioned that Jesus is alive and that he still heals people today.

'Healing?' I thought. 'That's what my mother needs. Will this Jesus be able to help her?'

In my heart I started to bargain with Jesus.

'Jesus, I'll come to you and make you happy. In exchange you can heal my mother and make me happy. Things can't get any worse. I'll give this Jesus a try.'

'What must I do?' I asked the man.

'Say a prayer after me in which you ask Jesus to forgive you for all the things you've done wrong and invite him to come into your life to be your Lord and to guide you.'

I nodded.

'That's good,' he said. 'Before you say this prayer, we want to meet with you again in the next couple of days and bring a few others to join us in praying for you.'

The day they returned they brought two others. I was surprised that it needed four adults to pray with me.

However, it transpired later that the couple had been listening very carefully as I had narrated the story of my life and had concluded that I had opened a door of my soul to demonic powers through my involvement with the occult. They suspected that these powers were in control of my life but that I wasn't aware of it. They knew that there was going to be a confrontation between the forces of light and darkness when they prayed for me.

I'm so glad they didn't tell me that at the time.

I wouldn't have understood it then.

I certainly do now.

After a few minutes of getting to know each other, I sat on a chair and they began to pray for me. One of them led me through the prayer that the man had told me about. I said the words after him.

'Jesus, I'm sorry for everything wrong that I've thought, said and done in my life. Please forgive me. Come into my life and lead and guide me in everything I do, now and in the future, I pray.'

'Now God has something for you,' one of them then said. 'He's called the Holy Spirit. You need him and you need his power if you are to live the way God wants you to.'

They then explained to me that the God of the Bible is three in one - three persons in one being. They shared that the Holy Spirit is the third person of God and that he is the most wonderful person whose power is available to everyone who puts their trust in Jesus. Jesus has gone back to the Father in heaven but has given us the Holy Spirit until he returns.

'When you receive the Holy Spirit in your life,' they said, 'you'll be able to understand the Bible better and draw closer to God. You'll also be able to pray in a special language which he gives, like the first Christians did after the Holy Spirit came upon them two thousand years ago.'

Of course all this was very strange to me.

It may be to you too.

But I knew I could trust these people and no one needed to tell me that I could live a good life in my own strength. I needed God's help.

'If it's free, I want it!' I said.

'Okay,' one of them said. 'We'll lay hands on you, just as they did in the Bible, and then you can ask God the Father to give you his Holy Spirit. We will begin praying in the special language which he has given us. When you hear us doing that, you can join in to.'

And then it happened.

To begin with I was a little shocked by the strange sounds that were coming from their lips. I was a bit uneasy. For a moment I thought they were sorcerers or magicians.

But then I began to sense this wonderful presence in and around my body.

A feeling of peace began to bring calm to my mind.

That same presence I had sensed in the vineyard was back. It was flooding the reservoir of my soul. It was so pure, so deep, so glorious, so intense.

Then, just as I thought it was going to overwhelm me, I suddenly sensed there was something within me trying to stand in the way of this heavenly love.

It was resisting.

But its resistance was futile.

The power of this Holy Spirit was greater and stronger than any unholy spirit.

The forces of darkness that I had so foolishly invited into my life were beginning to retreat.

Their time had come.

It was the moment for them to leave.

As they did, I felt an indescribable pressure in my head.

Then I experienced an equally indescribable peace.

The demonic spirits had gone.

Later, my sister - who was present during this time of prayer but not yet a believer - told me that she saw a dark cloud leaving my head and disappearing through the window.

And then the special prayer language I'd been told about began to flow for several minutes, much to everyone's surprise - mine included.

When I got up from the chair I was a changed man, a brand new person. The deep hatred I had felt for so long had gone. The Father's love had started to fill the places which hatred had occupied. For the first time in my life I felt that I was capable of really loving others. It was as if the burdens of decades had been lifted. It was amazing.

From Death to Life

From that day on, I had no doubt at all. Jesus is alive! I had met the Resurrected One. Just as everyone in the Bible was changed when they encountered him, so was I.

I walked through the streets like a dreamer.

I wanted to embrace every person on the planet.

At night I would lie in bed and pray for hours in the new language my heavenly Father had given me. Every time I spoke to God I would sense his presence and his love. I knew that the Holy Spirit was with me and would never leave me.

Everything was different.

Before I had felt despair, now I felt hope.

Before I had felt hatred, now I felt love.

I had found what I had been searching for when I prayed a very simple prayer:

'Jesus, if you can do anything with my wrecked life, then please do it. I surrender it all to you.'

Praying that, I found love - unconditional love - and I never wanted to lose it. For twenty two years I had been wandering on this earth like a living corpse. I had almost died as a result. But the

day I handed my life over to my Father in heaven, I started to live
- really live.

Everything around me was so new, so alive.

Suddenly I became aware for the first time how unutterably
beautiful God's creation is.

I had been blind, but now I could see.

I had been deaf, but now I could hear.

One night as I lay in bed I was overwhelmed by the Father's love
and forgiveness. 'I had no idea it was so wonderful to know you,' I cried.
'All these years I never knew you were so real, that I could actually
experience you.'

Whenever I spoke to my Father in prayer like this, there was
nothing religious about it. I didn't pray set or pre-formulated
prayers. I just spoke to him naturally, heart to heart, as a son speaks
to his Dad.

As I got to know this perfect Father better, I became convinced
of this one thing. I would now live only for him.

No matter what happened, I would never go back to my old life.

I had chosen life. I was not going to choose death again.

I had never known my earthly father, but now I had at last found
my heavenly Father.

As I wept and thought about my heavenly Father's love, I
suddenly heard a gentle voice in my heart:

'Stefan, there are still so many who are held prisoner by darkness
and loneliness, just as you were. Go and tell them what I've done for
them and that I love them. Tell them that I am alive and that I have
not forgotten them or this world.'

I realise now that my Father in heaven was at that moment
calling me to go and tell others how to get free in the same way I

had. He had a plan for my life. My heavenly Father had a future and a hope for me.

An Overwhelming Comfort

One week after I had surrendered my life to God, my mother died. She died at exactly 8pm when most of the family were sitting in a free church and for the first time doing a Bible study together.

To this day I can remember something my mother once shared with me.

'Stefan, I am praying that all of my children will come back to God and go to church again.'

At that time I had laughed to myself. 'Church is for the old and the weak. It's not for me.' At that time I had no idea that having a living relationship with the Father and being a part of his family, the church, are integral to each other.

Today, my sister and all three of her children are believers. Two of the children have been to Bible School to train and prepare for the work God wants them to do.

I am convinced that one day my mother's wish will come true and that every member of my family will be a committed follower of Jesus Christ.

Just before she died, my mother gave her life to Jesus. She had always been more open to God than most people are, all through her life.

An hour before she died, my mother was connected up to machines in the intensive care ward. She was unable to speak to my sister and me.

As we were sitting there praying, I looked up.

Suddenly I saw something I'll never forget.

Jesus was at the head of my mother's bed.

He was tenderly stroking her hair.

Before I was able to say anything to my sister, she said,

'Jesus is here!'

She couldn't see him but she could sense his presence. The atmosphere had changed in the room.

'I know,' I replied. 'I can see him.'

There he was - the one who had died for me, saved my life, and loved me like no other.

I lost myself in his wonderful eyes as he looked at me.

Waves of comfort broke upon my soul - comfort from another world.

As Jesus gazed at me, his eyes spoke to my heart.

'Everything will be all right.'

One hour later my mother died.

Chapter 6

Defeating the Darkness

Now that my mother had died I was living alone at home with my stepfather who was now an invalid. One of my nieces moved in to help. That was a God-send. The truth is that even though I was twenty two I had been spoiled by my mother and everything had always been done for me. Now I had to grow up quickly and learn how to run a house and manage the finances. For this I was really going to have to depend on my heavenly Father.

It was few days after the funeral that our doorbell rang. A debt collector was standing there.

'I am here to collect 230GBP for unpaid car insurance.'

I was horrified. I didn't have that amount of money. All I had were debts - quite a lot of them.

'I'll be back at noon tomorrow. If you don't pay up, your car will be taken off the road.'

I was desperate.

'Lord Jesus, you know I have no money,' I cried. 'Please help me.'

The next morning I visited a pastor who had heard about what God had done in my life. We spoke all morning. The moment eventually came to leave and the pastor offered to drive me back. I gratefully accepted.

When we arrived at my house, the pastor stopped me as I opened the door of the car.

'Stefan, do you need money?' he asked.

Embarrassed, I didn't answer.

'Do you need money?' he repeated. 'I believe the Lord has spoken to me,' he continued, 'and told me to give you some money.'

I was shocked. But I was also filled with joy.

'I do,' I replied, 'the debt collector is coming soon to collect 230GBP for unpaid car insurance. I don't have anything to give him.'

Later the debt collector returned.

I was waiting in joyful anticipation with the cash.

I don't suppose he had ever met anyone who was so happy to see him!

I had learned to trust in Jesus.

He hadn't let me down.

Everything will be All Right

The early days of being a Christian were not easy but I learned a vital lesson during this challenging season. In fact, it was during this time that my heavenly Father taught me a lesson that I would never forget.

One night I was lying in bed thinking about all the problems and pressures in my life. As I did, I suddenly saw in my mind's eye a huge mountain. Next to the mountain there was the tiny outline of a person, so tiny in fact that I could hardly see him. Then the Holy Spirit spoke to me.

'Look at Jesus!'

Then I understood. The small figure standing next to the great mountain was Jesus.

As I looked at him, he quickly started to grow bigger and bigger until the mountain shrank and then disappeared altogether.

The Lord taught me an unforgettable truth that night.

If I concentrate my attention on the mountain (that is, my problem), then my unbelief will grow and I will limit in my heart what God is capable of doing.

But if I focus on Jesus and his possibilities instead, it really doesn't matter how large my problem is, my faith will grow and the difficulty will decrease and eventually disappear.

So from now on I decided to focus on the greatness of Jesus rather than my difficulties.

Jesus had reassured me at my mother's bedside in the hospital, 'everything will be all right.'

All I had to do was believe in him and trust in his promises.

So this is what I started to do.

And as I did, miracles began to occur.

Perhaps the most amazing was to do with my stepfather, who was by now getting weaker and weaker.

One week before he passed away he gave his life to Jesus.

He was the very last person I would have expected to turn to the Lord. He had always considered that the church and the sacraments were enough to secure his salvation. But as he faced death, he came to see that it is Jesus alone who can lead us into an eternal friendship with God our Father.

Back to the Red Devils

After my life-changing experience of the reality of God, I rather naively thought that everyone would not only want to know about God but also want to experience him.

When I spoke to some of the lads in the Red Devils I was sure they would be interested.

'Listen to me everyone. This is what we've been looking for. Jesus is the answer.'

But their only response was to laugh at me. They thought I was on a religious trip and a rumour started that I was walking around in sandals, as Jesus had done.

One day I spoke to a guy called Thomas, a member of the Red Devils. Thomas had some mental problems and had recently been in trouble at a pub, having fired a shotgun through the pub window. I shared with him what Jesus had done on the Cross. I could see that he was moved but the pressure of looking good in front of his peers was too great.

'Stefan,' he said, 'this business with Jesus is probably all right for you. But it's not for me.'

Those were the last words I heard him speak.

A while later he shot himself.

Just before he did, I was told that he had been looking for me.

Another friend of mine in the Red Devils was sent to prison for eight years. When I found out I wrote a letter to him explaining what had happened to me and what he needed to do if he was to give his life to Jesus.

He wrote back to say that he had prayed the prayer and accepted Jesus.

I was overjoyed.

However, a few weeks later he wrote another letter.

'Stefan, I can't manage it here, being a Christian. The devil rules in this place.'

I was sad yet I do believe that the prayer he prayed was not in vain.

A while after I left the Red Devils the group broke up. The Red Devils were now history. For me, that way of life was a thing of the past.

I Don't Fight Anymore

My biggest concern now that I was a Christian was always how I would react if I was attacked again.

I didn't have long to wait before finding the answer.

I used to go quite often to the disco to tell those who knew me about Jesus. One evening I bumped into a girl who was the girlfriend of one of the lads in the Red Devils. She had problems with her boyfriend so I sat down at a table with her and told her about my new-found friend, Jesus.

'He never lets you down,' I said.

After speaking for a while, she said she wanted to go home. I offered to escort her to her car. When we reached the vehicle someone suddenly jumped on me from behind, knocking me to the ground, kicking me two or three times.

I leapt to my feet.

I looked my assailant in the eyes and clenched my fist, ready to hit back.

Before I had become a Christian it would have been normal for me to retaliate immediately and aggressively, sometimes using objects that were ready to hand. On one occasion I almost killed one of our lads because of a minor disagreement. I had taken a full coke bottle and hurled it at him. The bottle had smashed against the wall and fragments of glass had ricocheted onto his face, cutting it in a number of places, leaving him covered in blood. Had the bottle hit him directly on the head, he would probably have been killed.

So I was ready and poised for violence.

But this time I reacted differently.

Standing in front of my aggressor, a peace began to well up inside me, drowning out the rage that used to take control of me. I was totally disarmed by it. My anger and aggression disappeared in a heartbeat as I heard a gentle voice in my head say, 'you won't be fighting this way anymore.'

I unclenched my fist.

I looked at my aggressor.

'I don't fight anymore,' I said.

And with that I turned and walked away to my car.

To turn your back on your attacker is one thing.

To just leave him standing there is quite another.

But as I walked away he didn't run after me and knock me down again. He just let me get into my car.

As soon as I was inside, I started to complain to God.

'Why wouldn't you let me hit him?'

'I love him,' I sensed God reply.

'But no one would have done that to me before I gave my life to you. Is that the thanks I get for being on your side?'

'I love him.'

'Okay, okay, but he started the fight. Didn't I have the right to defend myself?'

'I love him.'

'Okay God, I forgive him.'

That night I felt like a true winner.

Jesus had proved to me that he would help me to win any challenge if I let him take care of things his way.

My way wasn't effective.

I would never fight this way again.

Cheap Imitations

The first time I saw a video of a well-known preacher praying for the sick I was so moved I wept. So many of the people he prayed for told how Jesus had healed them. Some of them had been sick for years.

As I watched, a longing began to burn in my heart.

'I want to do that too. I want to experience what it's like to help sick people in this way. I can't go on living as I am. There has to be more.'

So I made a pact with Jesus. I would step out in faith the following Sunday morning in church and do what I had seen the preacher doing. He would speak to me like he had spoken to the preacher on the video and the sick would be healed.

That was the plan, anyway.

By the time Sunday arrived I had watched the video a number of times, memorizing the phrases the preacher used, studying the way he behaved.

The man received supernatural knowledge about the medical conditions of people in the congregation, name those out loud, and then declare that people were healed of them.

Afterwards people would come to the front and testify to the fact that they were no longer sick.

As I prepared to take a step of faith, I felt no audible voice, no sudden illumination, no lightning bolt of revelation, no sensations in my body - nothing!

I walked nervously to the front and asked one of the leaders if I could say something and he said yes. But what was I supposed to say? I didn't have a clue.

I told the people to close their eyes and then began to remind them about what Jesus had done for them on the Cross, how he had suffered for them but then been raised from the dead so that he is alive today.

No one knew that I was repeating what I'd heard the preacher say on the video.

I even tried imitating the way he spoke.

I started to move my body like he did.

If it worked for him, surely it would work for me.

But nothing happened.

Then I began to try another approach.

'There is someone here,' I said - 'that's quite good,' I thought, 'the preacher said that too' - 'there's someone here, you are a Christian, and you have suicidal thoughts. God says today that you shall live.'

I paused.

No response.

'There is also someone with pain in the right shoulder. You can feel the warmth of the Holy Spirit coming over you right now. The pain is disappearing.'

No response.

No one knew that the man on the video had said these things.

I made a few more comments, waiting for a reaction from somebody in the congregation.

I didn't feel a thing.

I had just obeyed what I sensed God had called me to do.

The seconds that followed felt like an eternity.

Then a young woman began to weep.

'Oh Jesus, please forgive me for thinking of killing myself,' she cried. 'Forgive me.'

Others also began to respond.

But where was the person with the pain in their shoulder?

There had been no response to that word.

Was that from God or from me?

Did I make a mistake?

I was still asking myself such questions when a leader came up to me after the service and said, 'Stefan, that was really good but next time just be yourself.'

That Sunday morning I went home full of self-doubt.

'Who do you think you are? Did you really think you could do what that preacher did? Just remember where you've come from; you're not holy enough to do that.'

It was six months later when a man from church came up to me.

'Do you remember that Sunday?' he asked.

'Which Sunday are you talking about?'

'The one when you went up to the front and said that there was someone with a pain in their shoulder.'

'I remember.'

'Well, it was me,' he said. 'As you spoke those words I felt this warmth in my shoulder. From that moment on the pain was gone.'

At that moment I was torn between gratitude that the man had told me he had been healed and strangling him for waiting six months to tell me.

But if I had, I would have needed another miracle!

That day I learned two key lessons about ministering to others.

First, trusting in God doesn't involve our feelings. Faith is not about feelings. It's about choosing to believe what you can't yet see.

Second, we shouldn't imitate the way other Christians speak and act. Our heavenly Father wants us to be priceless originals not cheap imitations.

Look out World!

These lessons would stand me in good stead as I went to Altensteig (a town in the black forest area of Germany) to take part in what is called a School of Discipleship. Jesus had disciples. Disciples are essentially people who learn. I wanted to learn. It was only a few months after I had become a Christian in the summer of 1989 and I was determined to learn as much as I could about Jesus and his call on my life.

I had been drawn to this School of Discipleship because it was run by an organization called YWAM (Youth with a Mission). I had just read a book by YWAM's founder, Loren Cunningham, and it had inspired me. I wanted now to join with many other enthusiastic young people and find out how God wanted me to serve him for the rest of my life.

There were just two problems.

The first was that the school cost a lot of money.

The second was that it was now very late to register.

But I had learned to focus on Jesus not the mountain (the problem), so I decided to trust him.

Not long afterwards I was accepted and I had most of the money, thanks mainly to people in my church who had decided they wanted to invest in my future.

The people in the Free Church really believed in me and gave me such encouragement.

So I went off to the Training Centre where I was to learn more about the life and teaching of Jesus.

I didn't realize I still had a long way to go. I had only been a believer for three months.

All I did know was that Jesus had told me, 'go and tell everyone I send you to about my love and that I am alive.'

Arriving at the YWAM School I was shown to my quarters and introduced to my roommates. I was shocked. They were the kind of people I wouldn't have been seen dead with in my former life. There was a banker, a young guy still very dependent on his mother, and a motorcyclist (the one I liked the most).

After a few days I was glad to find someone else in the school who smoked. Smoking was not allowed. But we sneaked out thinking we were really clever and that no one would know. However, we must have stunk to high heaven of cigarettes so I'm not sure we were ever as clever as we thought.

As I settled into the life of the community, the new regime was a shock to my system. It was really a bit like living in a monastery. Every day we had prayer, worship, singing, lessons, more prayer, Bible study, and work time.

Everyone seemed so holy.

It felt like I was the only one full of faults.

Defeating the Darkness

After fifteen months of feeling a failure - and living a secret life of moral compromise with the girlfriend I had at that time - I began to grow cold spiritually. I no longer wanted to pray or read the Bible. The sense of God's peace and presence had gone. I continued to go to all the meetings in church but inside I felt empty.

Things began to turn when I realised that my girlfriend did not want to go in God's direction. This pushed me to the point of decision. We were effectively living in two different worlds. I therefore knelt down and prayed, committing this relationship to my heavenly Father, confessing my weaknesses and fears, telling him that I wanted to do his will.

When I had finished I felt peace in my heart again.

I had looked to my girlfriend to meet my needs.

Now I was looking to my Father again.

Shortly after, the relationship ended.

One morning I was sitting in the house of a dear friend, after a long night out. I was feeling totally frustrated about all my failures. My friend listened to me as he was walking up and down the kitchen with his newborn son on his arm.

All of a sudden a thought came into my head.

'Why don't you take the baby and throw it out of the window?'

I was appalled.

That just wasn't me at all.

I loved this friend and I was thrilled that he and his wife now had a child.

What was wrong with me?

I was still troubled when some time later I went to a seminar on deliverance from evil in our church.

Surely Christians can't be troubled by evil, can they?

When I gave my life to Jesus I had been set free from a dark and negative spirit of hatred.

Surely I wasn't being afflicted by such things any more.

As the woman began to teach the seminar, I felt an inner resistance to what she was saying about how Jesus set people free from spiritually dark forces. I didn't want her to come anywhere near me. Whenever she spoke about how evil tries to destroy our lives by holding us in bondage, I felt as if she was looking right into my soul. She was talking about things that I had actually experienced.

During question time after her talk I mentioned that a Christian I knew had had this dreadful thought about throwing someone else's baby out of a kitchen window.

After the seminar I confessed to the woman that it had been me. She told me that there was still some spiritually dark forces trying to influence and destroy my life and that it would be a good idea for us to pray.

That gave me hope.

We met in my sister's flat a few days later and this woman and one of our church leaders started to minister to me in prayer.

When the two asked God to release me from every trace of darkness, I felt as if something was taking over my entire body. I collapsed to the floor and my body rolled about uncontrollably. My head shook to and fro with unnatural speed. I heard voices in my head, a scream 'they want him to die.' I knew instantly that this referred to my family.

The lady commanded whatever was attacking me to leave me but it was stubborn. I kept hearing the scream, 'No, he belongs to me. They wanted him to die. I'm not going.' My body continued to be thrown about on the floor.

Then the voice inside my head shouted, 'take the television and throw it at her!'

I resisted inwardly and said no.

At the same time the lady, who had no idea what was going on inside me, said, 'I forbid you in the name of Jesus to take the television. Leave him and go.'

My sister, who had come into the room because of all the noise, fled when she saw what was happening.

Again and again the two of them kept commanding the darkness to leave.

Eventually a deep and audible voice came out of me.

'No, I will not go. He belongs to me. Stop it. I can't bear to hear that name anymore.'

And then the darkness left.

And the presence of God - as strong as a fire - filled the room.

Everyone sensed it.

It swept through my whole body, purging me from everything unclean.

When I got up from the floor that afternoon I was filled with the presence of the Holy Spirit and my body was shaking all over.

Everyone was amazed at what had happened.

Light had come.

Darkness had been defeated.

I was free from destructive influences.

Jesus was my Victor!

And it was now time to get back on track with his plan for my life.

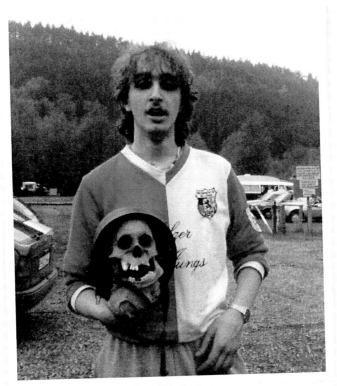

Stefan Driess aged 20, with his 'friend' called Dead

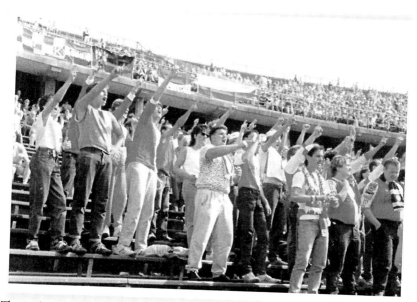

The Red Devils supporting their club

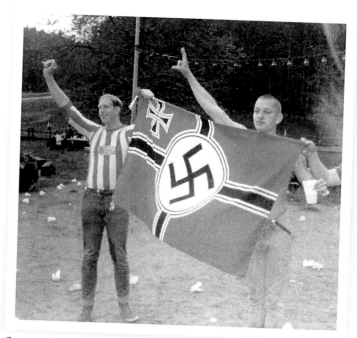

Some right-wing club supporters Stefan associated with

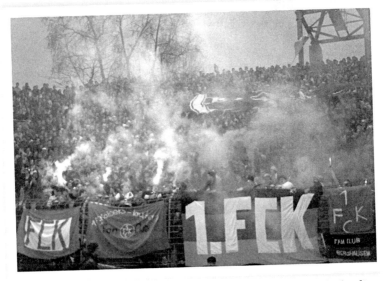

The club stadium set alight by hooligans

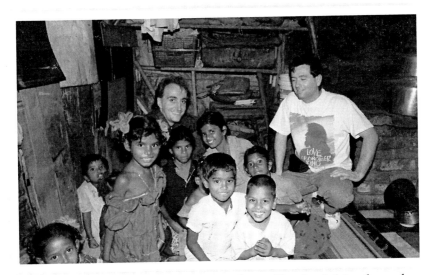

Transformed by Jesus – Stefan Driess in the slums of Bombay helping the needy children

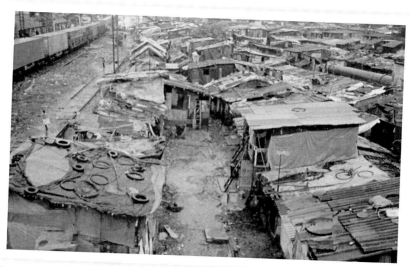

Extreme poverty in the slums

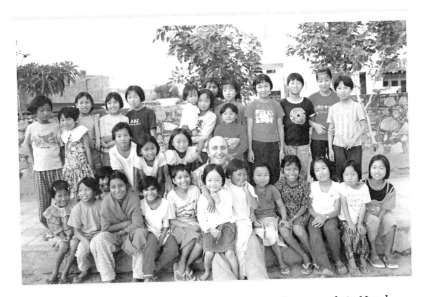

Stefan, with the help of others, saved these girls from the sex trade in Nepal

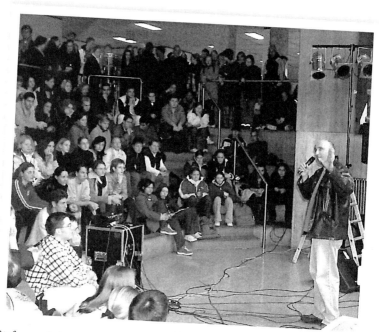

Stefan explaining to German school children how knowing God as Father changed his life

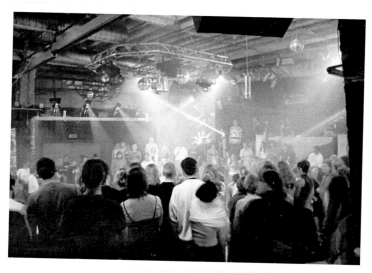

Hundreds of young people came to know God through the GOD ZONE a disco run by Stefan and his team

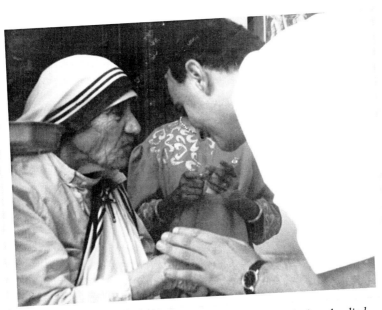

Stefan meeting Mother Teresa in Calcutta a few months before she died

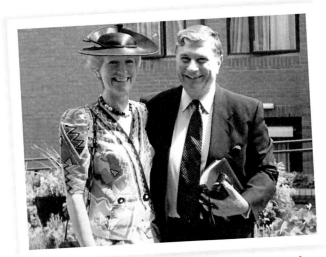

Giancarlo & Catharine Elia, Stefan's God given adopted parents

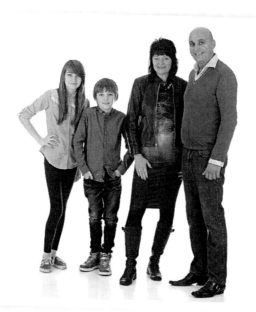

The Driess family in 2013 – Grace, John David, Louise, Stefan

Chapter 7

The Death of Self

'Go back to Youth with a Mission.' That's what I sensed my heavenly Father saying as I prayed for new direction. 'Go back to Altensteig. Get back into the plan I have for you.'

I wanted that with all my heart. Having earlier quit the training school and run away from my true destiny, it was now time to get back on track.

So in the spring of 1991 I returned to the Bible School, free from the demonic spirits that had plagued me, free from my addiction to things like alcohol and cigarettes too.

I knew now that there were no shortcuts. I had to stay on track, living every day in obedience to my heavenly Father, recognizing that running away is always a step backwards and never a step forwards.

I still had problems comparing myself with other students. But little by little my loving Father began to shape me more and more into the person he wanted me to be.

There is so much I could tell you about my time at the Discipleship Training School - like the fact that I had wanted to preach right from the start but was given the joy of cleaning the toilets and helping in the kitchen instead; or the time when I organized a men's night for fun which turned into a complete fiasco; or the ups and downs I went through, the teachers and fellow students with whom I crossed swords when I didn't get my own way; about my apology to the course director for the stolen cassette tapes.

It was truly a time of transformation and preparation.

My Father was getting me ready for his future plans for me.

A Season of Restitution

I had finished the School of Discipleship and joined YWAM's School of Evangelism (a school designed to train people to share the Good News of Jesus in different ways) when one day, during a prayer time, I sensed God say to me, 'take a sheet of paper and write down what I show you.'

God began to remind me of the people I had treated badly. He prompted me to write letters asking their forgiveness. I did this and with each letter I wrote I experienced a deeper freedom. It was very humbling, especially the letters to the people who should really have said sorry to me. But that wasn't the point. God wanted me to take responsibility for my own actions. I had the choice whether to forgive or not. Even though it was difficult, I decided to forgive.

A while later I watched a video where a well-known preacher whom I greatly respect spoke on the power of restitution. He recounted things from his own life and the lives of those with whom he worked. I felt the Holy Spirit speak to my heart saying, 'this is for you!'

To begin with I wasn't that enthusiastic about what the preacher was saying because he was telling stories about how people gave things back and repaid money they had stolen. 'Oh no, not that as well,' I thought.

A time followed in which I decided to put various things right. I went to the police and told them everything I had done. I admitted being in the possession of drugs and dealing with them. I went into shops where I had stolen things and confessed what I had done or gave them the money back where possible. Naturally people were astonished.

One day I walked into a large supermarket and was taken to the manager's office. He asked me what I wanted.

'I have become a Christian and I would now like to pay for the 100 DM worth of goods that I stole here.'

The man got up from his chair, closed the door.

'What do you mean, you have become a Christian? I am a Christian too – although my wife more so than me because she has more time – but what do you mean when you say you've become a Christian?'

I explained to him that there is more to being a Christian than just the name. I told him that I had met Jesus and that he had changed my life.

We chatted a while and then I paid my debts and even received a receipt with the words, 'for theft.'

I had to confess to my former boss that I had stolen thousands of Marks from him during the time I had worked for him. He was surprised by my letter but he thanked me for my honesty and even released me from the debt. His letter ended with the request that I stay in touch with him if possible so that he could see how I got on.

Another time when I was at the Police Drug Department I confessed that I had lied during a court case and this confession gave them the evidence against me which they had wanted for years.

'Good,' the police investigator said, 'then give us the names of the other people involved and then we'll see what we can do for you.'

'No, I can't do that,' I replied, 'these people are responsible for their own actions. I am here for what I have done wrong. God has forgiven me and now I want to sort some things out.'

'Well, we can't do anything for you then,' the policeman said. 'You will probably go to prison.'

I left the police station feeling a bit scared.

'Jesus, even if I have to go to prison there will be a purpose in it. I trust you!' I prayed.

A few weeks later a letter arrived from the public prosecutor saying that the case against me had been dropped.

'Thank you, Jesus!' I exclaimed.

The Prince of Cheese

There were eight of us in the School of Evangelism and we lived in a former guest house in the town centre. From this base we were sent out on mission trips all over the world. It was a very special season of my life.

Once again my Father had put me in a room with not exactly my favourite kinds of people. They were so different from me. But I was beginning to get used to this. Youth with a Mission attracted young people from many different countries, cultures and social backgrounds. The nations were not just on my doorstep. They were in my room!

This diversity meant that we just had to learn to get on with each other, allowing the Holy Spirit to address character issues in us as we learned to be God's family, living in community together.

This process of character development happened most dramatically when we were on outreaches in other countries.

I remember one time when we were in Yugoslavia we assembled for a time of intensive prayer. As we reached a high point in our praying we began to proclaim the verse of a well known Christian song. At this stage in my life I didn't speak any English but I very quickly picked up the chorus: 'Jesus, Prince of Peace! Jesus, Prince of Peace!'

The words had been chanted many times and so I thought to myself, 'right, I've got it now.'

I repeated it in my mind while others were proclaiming it with their mouths.

Then it was my turn.

I was ready.

The pump was primed.

I took a deep breath.

I shouted with great determination.

'Jesus, Prince of Cheese!'

At that moment it was as if the whole world had suddenly ground to a halt. Some tried to be polite and cover up their laughter. But then everyone burst into hysterics.

I was mortified.

The wonderful atmosphere of prayer had gone.

Everyone was laughing.

No one could focus on praying any more.

Later a member of the team came up to me.

'Don't worry about it Stefan, Jesus is the Prince of Cheese as well!'

As he walked away smiling, I cannot honestly say that my thoughts towards him were good!

I Can Kill You!

In the same country we had meetings every night in the town of Skopje. There were about one hundred people at these meetings and the team was made up of people from all over the world - from Sweden, Norway, Germany and America. Each night we told them how through Jesus they could get to know their loving Father in heaven.

The Swedes had their own band with them and an evangelist who often walked up and down the platform during the meetings, shouting loudly.

I'll never forget the way his eyes shone as he called out to the audience, 'Buddha is dead! Mohammed is dead! JESUS IS ALIVE!'

'That's really bold,' I thought. 'There are very many Muslims in this city.'

One evening after a meeting I went up to a man who was still sitting in the audience.

'Did you like what you have just heard about Jesus?' I asked.

'I don't believe in Jesus,' he replied. 'I have telepathic powers.'

From here he went on to boast about all the things he could do with his 'powers'.

I kept drawing his attention to the power of Jesus.

'I can kill you with the power of my thoughts,' he said.

This was too far.

He had challenged the power of my Lord.

Plus he had stepped on my pride a little.

'You can't do anything to me,' I said. 'Jesus is much stronger than you. He protects me.'

Then I added, 'shall we see who is the stronger? You try and kill me with your power. I'll pray in the name of Jesus.'

I could sense some of the people standing nearby thinking 'this guy is crazy.' Their faces were etched with a mixture of fear and dismay. However, I was convinced that my Lord is stronger and that he would never fail me.

'Okay, let's do it,' the man said.

He stared at me with intense concentration, giving me what in occult circles is called 'the evil eye' - a look of intense focus designed to cause injury and even death.

As I looked into his eyes, I saw his pupils turn red. Redder and redder they became. I could feel power coming from him.

I began to pray.

'In the name of Jesus I speak to the one who has power over this man. You have no power over me! Jesus is stronger!'

I repeated this statement two or three times as his eyes became redder and redder.

Suddenly he leaped to his feet and began to run.

'Stop it!' he shouted. 'I can't stand it!'

Once again Jesus had proved that he is Almighty and that we have nothing to fear if we are in relationship with him.

That night I slept particularly well.

Praying with Authority

During this time in Yugoslavia we saw a lot of young people becoming receptive to the message of Jesus. Many of them became Christians and several home meetings began. It was so wonderful to show others the way to a new beginning with God.

After one evening meeting my friend Paul and I went back to the campsite to rest. The camping place was next to a lake. There was a large open-air disco on the other side of the lake. That was a problem; at night the loud thumping of the beat was carried across the lake to the campsite, often robbing us of our sleep.

We had hardly slept the night before so Paul and I decided to speak to God about it in prayer. We felt that no one should be allowed to rob the hard-working children of God of their sleep.

From our shore we looked over the lake to the other side where the disco was and pointing towards it we made a proclamation together, using the authority that we have in the name of Jesus.

'That disco will close down!'

A couple of days later we went on an outreach to Albania. After about a fortnight we returned to our campsite. We were surprised to notice that it was very quiet. There was no music.

What had happened?

One of the locals told us that the day after we left for Albania the police had closed the disco down.

'Why?' we asked.

'I don't know,' they replied.

This taught us a vital lesson about the power of our words.

Plus we now got to sleep well!

The Dying Man

Another time we were on an outreach to Romania. I was with my team in a gypsy village with the local pastor and his helpers. We wanted to go on an outreach but it was cancelled because there was too much snow. However I felt an urgency to continue so I asked my team leader if I could go anyway. She gave me permission and I set off with the village pastor, a few of his helpers, a translator and a girl from our team.

Usually the pastor went on foot with his team every week (no matter what the weather), He would visit a handful of believers in a house 25km (approximately 15 miles) away. However, because he was looking after comfortable western Europeans we went by train that day, and he paid for it. This made me feel quite ashamed.

We arrived at 9pm and the house was full of visitors waiting expectantly.

I spoke from the Book of Hebrews where it says, 'Jesus Christ is the same yesterday and today and forever!'(Hebrews 13:8)

It wasn't a great sermon and it only lasted a few minutes. When it had ended I called the sick to come forward so that they could experience the reality of what I had preached. Quite a lot came forward. We were praying for them when my translator suddenly interrupted me.

'Stefan, a man has fallen over at the back.'

'So what,' I thought. 'That often happens when great men of God are ministering.' I had heard before of people falling to the ground under the power of God.

'You must take a look at him,' my interpreter said.

I went over to the man and what I saw made my blood run cold. He was clearly dying!

I had preached my first sermon - a sermon about how God still heals today - and now a man had fallen over and was about to die.

Fantastic!

As I bent over him, every trace of faith seemed to leave me.

The faith that had been turned up to a level of +10 during my sermon fell within seconds to a level of –10!

Fear gripped me as I saw the man taking his last breath.

I could only think of praying one thing.

'Jesus, please don't let him die – not while I'm here.'

The gypsies from the village were standing around me with anticipation. They had just heard me preach boldly that Jesus heals. Now I wished I was anywhere else in the world but here.

Suddenly a phrase flashed through my head - 'a spirit of death.' Without really knowing what I was doing, I said, 'in the name of Jesus, you spirit of death, get out!'

I had hardly spoken this when the dying man took a deep breath and then his throat rattled even more!

'Oh no, what have I done now?' I thought.

To gain a bit of time, I sent a few people with the man to an adjoining room to pray for him. My only thoughts were now about how to get out of there alive.

The atmosphere had now become quite tense. So far nobody had been healed.

The only thing that people knew for sure was that the old man was now dying.

Someone brought an old woman to me who could hardly walk. I placed my hands on her just as the first Christians did.

I prayed for her twice, and each time when I asked if the pain had gone she answered, 'no.' I laid my hands on her bad knees for the third time and said, 'Jesus, please heal her.'

In my mind I had already made the decision, 'if I ever get out of this place alive, I will never again pray for the sick.'

No sooner had I thought this something began to stir all around me. The people were discussing loudly with one another, with looks of astonishment on their faces.

My translator told me what had happened.

While I was praying for the old woman, two women standing nearby had been spontaneously healed from their pain and sickness. One woman had a swollen leg with a lot of fluid in it. As I prayed the fluid disappeared and the leg became quite normal.

What was happening?

I couldn't understand God. I had prayed for the older woman in the middle and he had healed the women on her left and right!

Feeling sorry for the older woman, and to cover my embarrassment, I said to the woman, 'walk in the name of Jesus.' The woman got up and walked about a yard in great pain, then suddenly she turned around with eyes wide open and communicated through nods and smiles that she was healed. She could walk without pain!

Our joy was even greater when a half an hour later the dying man in the adjoining room came and sat with us again.

After these events they did not want to let us go and we shared some truths and principles from the Bible, prayed and sang through the night until six in the morning.

Then we all walked to the next station, feeling tired but happy, to meet up with the rest of our team.

On the way to the station, the old man told us his story. The doctors in the hospital he came from had told him that his heart was in a very bad way and had sent him home to say goodbye to his family. He was told not to exert himself because that would mean certain death.

The man had heard from friends that some Germans were going from village to village, claiming that Jesus healed even today. He believed this and found out where we would be next. Although he knew that every step could be his last he decided to make the trip to the village.

He walked the three kilometres from the station to the village and when we arrived, he had already been waiting in the house since 3pm (we should in fact have arrived at that time). When we finally did arrive his strength left him and he collapsed.

With eyes shining, he said to me, 'I knew that Jesus would heal me.'

That was it!

I understood immediately – the key to his healing had nothing to do with us but with his firm conviction that God would do it.

We walked to the station together and this man who had been at death's door now walked faster than us youngsters.

Three days later I visited the man in his home and had the

privilege of seeing his whole family putting their lives into the loving hand of our Lord Jesus.

The neighbours and everyone who knew him were amazed.

'Whatever has happened to you?' they asked. 'We saw you come home like a corpse. Every step could have cost you your life and now you go shopping and are walking around like a young man! What happened?'

'I met Jesus and he healed me,' he answered.

Learning to Listen

We had been on quite a few outreaches when we found ourselves in Hungary. While we were there I sensed the Father saying to me, 'I don't want you to speak today on the streets. I want you to be in the team and enjoy what I do through the others.' I was quite taken aback. I was even more taken aback when I sensed him add, 'I want you to lay your life on the altar and I will decide what will be done with it.'

I began to weep.

'What, give up preaching and talking about Jesus?'

I loved telling others about Him and preaching his word. After all that I had experienced in Romania, what was this all about?

But no answer came. God wanted me to obey and not discuss.

I don't know how long it took, but after I had struggled with this I went on my knees and said, 'Jesus, I give you everything. Your will be done.'

I shall never forget the following days. We went to the nearby market place as usual. There were a lot of tradesmen there and we knew that they couldn't just walk away when we preached the gospel. They had to carry on with their businesses. So we could preach as much as we liked. Well, the others could. I couldn't.

I stood there and sang a few songs with the others and inside I was fuming. I was so angry I could have cried. Then our leader started to preach. He was a typical communicator of God's truth and because we were very similar in our zeal for God, I had a really hard time not being jealous.

Consequently my heart really wasn't in it.

Over the next few days we went out on missions trips. During that time I sensed that something in me was dying and that my attitude was changing.

I think it was on the third day that I reached the point where I could enjoy the fact that God was using others. I sang and worshipped God with all my heart in the middle of the market place surrounded by drunkards. I could feel the presence of God so strongly that I didn't care about anything else. It was no longer important who addressed the crowd. It was just great being part of it all.

After we had sung and put on an evangelistic sketch, our leader Peter preached again. This time it felt so good to listen to him and I had great peace in my heart.

Suddenly a man interrupted the preaching and began shouting wildly. I saw that Peter was getting flustered. Our translator told us that he was shouting because we were German and because of what the Germans had done to the Hungarian people. No matter what Peter tried, the man would not be pacified.

I could see that Peter was getting cross and thought, 'Oh no, that's all we need – these two to start shouting at each other.'

I started to pray in my heart. A lot of people had gathered around to see what was going on. The man just wouldn't stop shouting at us.

Suddenly the Holy Spirit spoke to my heart, 'go to the microphone and apologize for what the Germans did to these people.'

At first I wondered why I should be the one to apologize. For a start I wasn't a pure German and secondly how could I really know that it was God who had spoken to me?

The only way to find out was to just do what I believed God had said.

While the man was still berating us, I took the microphone in my hand.

'I would like to apologize to you in the name of the German people. I know that Germany did a lot of harm to you and your people, and that one day we will have to answer to God for it.'

I had hardly spoken the first sentence when the man became quiet.

He went away shaking his head and didn't say another word.

He hadn't expected to hear anything like that from a German.

This step of obedience to the Holy Spirit had disarmed him.

That morning my Father in heaven had taught me how important it is to listen to Him and be obedient in every situation.

The Running Man

It was on that day my leader asked me if I would like to preach in the city hall the following Saturday. I told him again that God had told me not to preach but agreed with him to seek God on this through prayer and fasting.

I can't remember how long I fasted, but it certainly wasn't very easy because Hungarian food is so good.

At some stage I began to sense God's permission to preach on Saturday. I had learned my lesson and I joyfully began to prepare. My prayer was that God would show signs and wonders so that many would believe in Him.

In my humble opinion I prepared the best message of my life. I was very nervous; it was the first time I had been asked to speak in such a large hall to so many unbelievers.

But I was raring to go and practised the sermon in my room.

Up until this point I had shared testimonies about what Jesus had done in my life and had also preached to small groups. But this time I had finally made it to a city hall!

Imagining that maybe hundreds would come, I could hardly wait. I recalled the time when I was a new Christian and no one wanted to listen to me or let me preach. So I preached to the vineyards, to snails, to cows, anything. In my spirit I saw myself speaking to hundreds and thousands of people.

Once when I was preaching to some cows in a field and only one of them was looking at me, I ended with an appeal for conversion. All the cows came to the middle of the field and listened attentively, watching me with their big eyes!

Once as I preached to beetles and snails and was disappointed that none of them came forward, I said later to myself, 'Stefan, you made a mistake. You should have gone back again – snails need a bit longer.'

All this may sound crazy to you, but there was a fire burning within me and I had to preach the Gospel, the Good News about Jesus.

Now the time had come. I prayed for all I was worth. My prayer life always seemed to change radically before such events because there was one thing I was conscious of, 'if God doesn't do anything I'll look a fool.'

Saturday came.

We arrived at the hall. There weren't many people there yet. After about 80 people had arrived my leader came to me and said he had heard that nearly all of them were Christians. He asked me if I was still prepared to speak to them.

'Oh no,' I thought, 'my lovely message - all for nothing.'

'I'll manage somehow,' I said. 'Jesus will help me.'

There was no way I was going to miss this opportunity.

So I started to speak just what came into my mind. I spoke about the power of words and our confession. I could feel God's presence very strongly and power flowing from me with every word I spoke.

Later my leader's wife, who had been sitting right at the back during the sermon, told me she had felt power coming over her like waves.

At the end of my message I called the sick to the front for prayer. A man with cardiac asthma came up to me. I prayed for him and then asked if there was something that he normally could not do. He said that he could hardly climb stairs. Immediately I said to him, 'in the name of Jesus, run up and down the stairs in this building.'

He ran off.

We had been praying for the sick for quite a while when I suddenly remembered this man. I asked someone if he knew where the man was and I received the answer.

'He's still running up and down the stairs – he is healed.'

As I went to bed that night, I felt moved and changed by what God had done that day.

I knew, 'what happened there had nothing to do with me.'

I had learned my lesson.

It is not about me.

It is about Jesus.

It's ALL about him, in fact.

'Thank you, Jesus.'

Chapter 8

A Passage to India

'Go to India for me.'

That was the thought that came uninvited into my mind one day while I was speaking to God in prayer. Up until this moment I had had nothing to do with India so I was surprised.

'This can't be God,' I thought. Some years earlier I had sensed a call to Asia. But Asia and India were not connected in my mind. This just highlighted my laziness at school. I didn't realise that India is part of Asia!

So I put the call to India down to a distraction from the devil and I placed the lid firmly down on the thought. But however much I tried to keep the lid on it, the lid kept popping open again.

'Go to India for me,' I kept hearing.

A subsequent conversation with a friend at Bible School seemed to confirm my decision to ignore this thought. He scathingly described India as the dirtiest country in the world, a place where people go to the toilet in the middle of the street.

'Okay,' I thought. 'That wasn't God then.'

But wherever I went and whatever I did, India kept appearing. Whether I opened a newspaper or looked at an advertisement, there it was:

'INDIA!'

Even when I was sitting in the restaurant car of a train bound for Hamburg, two Indians came and sat opposite me, even though the rest of the carriage was empty!

Some time later, God won the battle.

I was back at my home church for the weekend when a businessman walked up to me.

'Stefan, I've heard you may want to go to India.'

I thought, 'oh no, now what?'

'God's told me to buy you the air tickets,' he said.

I was gobsmacked.

'Okay,' I thought, 'you win, God. I'll go to India, sit it out, then I'll return to Germany.'

In the weeks that followed I began to prepare. I was going to have to speak English in India but my English at that time was poor. I could handle rudimentary expressions like, 'my name is Stefan,' or 'I am hungry,' but that was it. And of course I spoke none of the 1600 dialects spoken in the various regions of India. I had an air ticket but I had no money, no idea what I was supposed to do there, and no linguistic skills. I was hardly qualified to be a missionary!

Yet God was calling me there.

So I began to dream a big dream.

'Africa has Reinhard Bonnke. America has Benny Hinn. Germany has Peter Wenz. India is about to have Stefan Driess!'

It was not a very humble dream.

I was naive.

I was proud.

There was work to be done on my character.

Total Surrender

While I had been at Bible School with Youth with a Mission I had met a young lady. We became friends and later got engaged. So when the trip to India became a reality we decided that we would go there together and then get married afterwards. We made preparations for our journey to India, which was planned for November 1992.

At our engagement God gave us both a word from Isaiah 55: 8-9:

For my thoughts are not your thoughts, neither are your ways my ways, says the Lord. For as the heavens are higher than the earth, so are my ways higher than your ways and my thoughts than your thoughts.

Deep in my heart I had an inkling what that meant. It meant that my thoughts and God's thoughts were worlds apart. But I didn't want to admit that. My plans were fixed. My fiancée and I were both committed Christians. Our plans were focused on God. Surely they couldn't be wrong?

There is an old joke that goes like this.

Question: How do you make God laugh?

Answer: Tell him your plans.

That was me. I had my plans thinking they were God's plans. I had forgotten the Bible verse that says, 'many are the plans in a man's heart, but it is the Lord's purpose that will prevail.'

It may come as no surprise then to learn that we ended our engagement and broke up just before the trip.

So it was that a few weeks before my trip to India I found myself on the floor of a friend's flat, utterly distraught, completely broken.

I just didn't understand.

I had given up so much for God - a five year relationship, not to mention my friends in the Red Devils.

Now my dream had burst like a bubble.

Never before had my faith in God been so sorely tested.

If anyone asked me, 'how are you?' it was enough to make me break down in tears.

I was at the end of my tether.

I was a broken man.

What I didn't realise was that my plans had not been God's plans and that coming to this place of total self-emptying was part of God's plan for my life.

How easily we fool ourselves. We glibly say, 'Jesus, my whole life belongs to you,' but the words are shallow. They are not really true until they are tested.

And now my Father was testing me.

What he wanted was for me to die to myself - for me to get to the place where it wasn't about Stefan and his dreams but about Jesus and his purposes.

So from a broken heart I said the words that my loving Father in heaven had been waiting for his child to say.

'Do whatever you want with me.'

One Last Fight

In my mind it was now impossible for me to go to India. I was in turmoil emotionally and in addition my ex-fiancée had decided to fly out to India anyway and was ready to fly.

So I decided to stay at home in Germany.

Once again then I had made a plan, not reckoning on the fact that God's plans and thoughts are so much higher than ours. He had said, 'go to India for me.'

That command pursued me every day and night that followed. Even though my friends were supportive of my decision to stay (because of my emotional state) God was not.

So I began to complain in my prayers.

'Jesus, don't you understand? I can't go to India for you. I'm not even sure that you called me. And the others all say it would be better for me to stay here. My leaders say so, my friends say so and my family says so. And in any case, I can't go for the simple reason that my ex-fiancée and I would be sitting next to each other for eight hours on the plane! I can't go to India for you. Jesus, I'm finished!'

If I was expecting a comforting stroke on my back I was gravely mistaken.

The only reply I sensed from heaven was this:

'Didn't I tell you to go to India for me?'

That was my Father's final word on it.

I knew it.

There was no escaping from it.

In one last desperate attempt to avoid going, I went to my church leaders the day before my departure.

'Have you received a definite 'no' from the Lord about me going?' I asked.

My pastor answered.

'We haven't had a 'yes' and we haven't had a 'no.'

With that I knew my fight was over.

'Will you give me your blessing if I go?' I asked.

They agreed.

So I went home to get ready for my flight to India the very next day.

The following day I spent the longest eight hours of my life sitting next to my ex-fiancée on the plane. We hardly spoke a word to each other. There was barely a moment that I didn't wish I was anywhere else but there.

On the 1st November 1992 I arrived at the airport in Bombay. Even though it was a very difficult and challenging day I kept in mind that I had promised my Father in heaven that I would go to the darkest places for him.

It was now time to come good on that.

My prayer and my passion had been to go to the murkiest places of oppression on the planet, to bring the light of Jesus into the lives of those who were bound and beaten up by the devil.

What follows are words of mine that sum up that longing:

In the coldness of this world, where darkness rules and people are treated like puppets serving their masters (hate, rejection and death) – let me be warmth and light here.

In places where people are wounded, where words strike the hearts of individuals like destructive hammers and then weigh on them like heavy burdens – let me be healing and encouragement here.

Where fear and intimidation dwell, and people hide from the morning – please let me be peace and hope there.

Only to go where you would go, only to knock on the door where you would knock, only to say what you would say, please let me do that.

Let me be an ambassador of your love.

It was time to forget about myself.

It was time to be an emissary of the Father's love.

First Impressions

One of the leaders of Youth with a Mission was waiting at the airport and drove us to our quarters. As we drove through the streets of Bombay, exhausted from the flight, I was bombarded by my first impressions of this vast city, inhabited by fifteen million.

There were countless people living on the streets or in the slums - nine million, as I was later to learn. They had no home and often no roof over their heads. Many of them only had makeshift shelters, consisting of a few sticks driven into the ground with a piece of cloth or plastic attached to the upper end of these.

As we drove, I was overwhelmed by the contrasts and contradictions.

I looked at the street children, their bellies swollen with hunger, begging in front of magnificent villas and palaces, asking passers-by for alms.

I looked at the sick, crippled bodies lying at the edge of the road and the magnificent tourist hotels offering every kind of luxury.

Even the best cameras cannot portray the combination of urine and excrement on the one hand and the colourful and aromatic mixture of spices on the other.

God had made a promise to me.

'When you go to India for me I will show you a piece of hell.'

At the time I had been excited.

Now I was appalled.

There was sickness and poverty everywhere.

The caste system was clearly trapping millions in destitution and despair.

In addition, the belief in reincarnation had caused people to believe that this was the consequence of what they had done in a former life.

Thus cultural and religious lies kept them imprisoned in a mindset that said, 'this is your lot. Accept it. Submit to your karma, your destiny. There is no way out. You will never be free in this life.'

'I'm in India!'

With my mind still a maelstrom of first impressions, we stopped outside the house where I would be living. It was surrounded by small shops. These were not like shops in Europe. A hairdresser lived and worked within an area often not larger than about eight square yards. In the evening he pulled down a blind (if one existed) in front of his shop and slept on a cloth on the floor. The next morning he began the whole cycle all over again.

A few yards away, on the other side of the house, there were rows of self-built, ramshackle wooden huts packed closely together. A family of seven or eight persons would often live together in a few square yards of space and take it in turns to sleep inside the hut.

So the sights were different.

And so were the sounds.

Rickshaw and taxi drivers spent innumerable nights of their lives in their expensively hired vehicles in order to earn a living for their families. The city never seemed to rest. The noise from people and machines alternated with the sounds of the different horns.

In the early morning things were a little quieter. All I could hear then were the dogs and the rats.

With my senses experiencing a relentless bombardment I was glad to go inside the house alone. My ex-fiancée was taken somewhere else. I was told that there would be two other people joining me in the house over the next few days.

I closed the door of my room and lay down on a mattress on the floor.

I slept for several hours.

When I awoke in the evening it really hit me.

'I'm in India!'

Here I was on another Continent, in another world.

I was far from home.

I was hurting inside from all the emotional turmoil of my break-up.

I felt abandoned.

And I was holding my own pity party.

Be a Father to Them

For two days I broke the world record for self-pity before the two new occupants of the house arrived. This enlivened the place a bit, especially as I tried to communicate with them with my masterly attempts at English and my extravagant gesticulations and signs.

After a few weeks of this I began to settle in and my English improved. But what was I supposed to be doing? I knew my heavenly Father wanted me to come to India, but what did he want me to do specifically?

The following Sunday I decided to go to church. One of my house mates, Joshua, had formerly been a Hindu and had converted to Christianity. He said he knew a suitable church for me. In the best way he could, Joshua explained that this was an English speaking congregation.

'This will be good for your English,' he said.

As we arrived at the large building I could see many believers sitting with their Bibles, reading and praying.

'The people are having a Bible study,' Joshua said. 'They always do this before the service begins.'

As I looked around I sensed the Holy Spirit beginning to say, 'this is not the place for you.'

But Lord,' I replied, 'they look so devout and the church is so big. I'm a stranger here. And this is Joshua's church as well.'

There was no answer.

So I turned to Joshua.

'Is there another church nearby?'

'Yes,' he replied. 'But it is very small, with only a few people.'

As soon as he said those words I knew that this was the place God wanted me to be.

So I went to the little church.

The pastor greeted us warmly. He was pleased to have a white person in the service (it was hard for me to conceal that fact!).

During the service a young woman stood up and told of her work among the street children on the streets of Bombay. She described how she, a teacher, had heard God call her to serve these children. She told of their needs, the dangers to which they were exposed, and the fears they faced daily.

She spoke of the terrible abuses they experienced from their family members, corrupt police officers and the people who wielded power in the seedy worlds of prostitution and drug dealing - worlds into which they were tragically being drawn and exploited.

She explained that she had only just started the work and had begun with nothing more than the call she had received from God.

I was impressed by the fire of the Father's love burning in her heart.

I was moved by the tears in her eyes as she spoke about the children.

I was challenged and inspired by her commitment - by her determination to persevere whatever the cost, even to the point of giving her life.

That day I went back to my house in a state of confusion. As I lay on my mattress I could not forget what I had heard in the church. The pictures of the crying children who lived on the streets kept echoing in my mind.

I remembered an experience I had had in Hamburg in the spring of 1992. In a time of worship one morning I had been greatly moved by the presence of God and I'd had a vision which unfolded like a film. I saw children lying on the street crying, alone and fearful. I saw children in their mother's womb, embryos fighting for their lives, and a deep pain went through my heart. For twenty minutes I could only weep. I wept and wept. It wasn't just the pictures that made me cry, but the deep pain I felt - a pain that God later showed me was his pain for the children of this world.

Once more I saw these children before me, this time mixed with the real pictures I had seen during these first weeks.

'Someone must do something! Jesus, somebody must do something!' I cried. With that a new cry began to emerge. 'Why don't I do something?'

A battle began to rage in my heart.

On the one hand I couldn't deny what I had seen and heard and just continue living as though it was nothing. On the other hand I hadn't come here to serve children.

'Children get on my nerves. That's definitely no job for me. After all, I've come here to preach to thousands and become well-known.'

I don't know how long I battled with God.

At some stage I said to him, 'if you want me to help children, then I will.'

With that God spoke very clearly to me.

'If you help these children, then only do it if you are prepared to give your whole life for them. That means you must be prepared to stay here forever if that is my will. It means that you must be willing to invest your life in a handful of children at one of these stations even if no-one knows you and you never become well known.'

That really hit me. I realised that if I now said 'yes' to God, it could mean that I would never return, that no-one would ever hear of me, that I perhaps wouldn't stand before thousands but just in front of a handful of children, and that I might never marry.

I fell on my knees and placed all my wishes and dreams into the hands of God.

I said, 'Lord, I'm afraid and I don't know whether I'll manage it but I'll go to the children if that's want you want. I don't know how I should talk to them because I don't speak their language. I don't know what I should give them, but I'll do it – for you.'

God's answer came straightaway.

'Be a father to them - the father that they have never had. Show them what I am like. Cry with them, laugh with them. Take them in your arms. Show them that I haven't forgotten them.'

On the way to India God had given me a verse from the Bible which said, 'I will close your mouth for a time.' Now I understood what that meant.

Although I did not speak the children's language, there is a language that we all understand - the language of love.

Sleeping with Fleas and Rats

I met with the woman who had spoken at church. Her name was Juliett de Souza. With me on board, our team was made up of a grand total of three people.

Pretty quickly we had to ask God for financial help. He spoke very clearly to us that we should give what we had and He would supply the rest. This meant our abilities, our time and our finances, which weren't very much anyway.

The finances were one of the smallest sacrifices for me because it doesn't hurt so much to give when one doesn't have much.

Several times a week we went to the various train stations in Bombay and visited the children. Many of them live there, because stealing and begging is easier in such places where there are a lot of people.

I very soon made friends with them. They loved having a six foot tall, white climbing frame. They loved pulling my hair out (the results are still visible today - I don't have much hair!).

One day God spoke to me.

'Stefan, I want you to sleep alongside the children on the street.'

'What! Sleep on the street?'

Anyone acquainted with the streets of India will know why I questioned this so emphatically. Rats, dirt, excrement, urine, germs - all were resident there.

Was I really meant to sleep there?

'Yes, for three days,' God replied.

After a bit more resistance I finally agreed. With Juliett translating for me, I told the children that I would sleep where they slept.

They were far more excited about this than I was.

That evening I arrived with my bedclothes. One of the boys we looked after immediately took me to his so-called house. This consisted of various bits of wood which the boys had collected and piled together to provide some shelter. We lay down in a box which we were allowed to share with his chicken.

After a short while it became unbearable because of the high humidity so we decided to sleep outside the box.

The boy enthusiastically brought two wooden boards, which he placed on the left and right of some disused train rails.

'Your bed' he said to me in broken English.

'Wonderful,' I thought.

Hardly had I laid down when I just could not stop scratching myself everywhere.

The children had settled where they were in the dirt and had fallen asleep within seconds.

I couldn't sleep at all but was engaged in a ferocious battle against the fleas.

'Okay, Jesus,' I said. 'I can put up with a lot. But if rats come, I'm going. I've put up with mice and bats. But if there are rats, I shall be off. Indian rats are enormous!'

Laying there on my street bed, I suddenly realised where these children actually live and what dangers they face daily For the first time in my life I was able to thank God with all my heart for what we have in Germany. I thanked him for butter, for water, for a bed – for everything which would have been so welcome at this moment.

Then suddenly I heard it – the familiar sound of rats squeaking.

I saw the eyes of a rat gleaming as it ran to and fro, and my only thought was, 'Lord, if it comes here, I'm going.'

Once again Jesus spoke to me.

'Stefan, you can't even manage to identify with the lives of these children for one night. Can you imagine what it meant for me to leave my Father's glorious presence to come into this world? And not only that, can you imagine what it meant to go to the lowest place of humiliation to identify with your sin, and all of that for you?'

But the rats were coming and they were running in my direction!

I jumped to my feet, prodded the boy sleeping next to me and said, 'see you tomorrow.'

Then I hurried home and the first thing I did was have a shower.

I thanked God for the shower and for the house I had, although I had previously so often complained because the rain came through the roof.

But that didn't matter anymore.

There were millions who didn't have it as good as I did and who had no opportunity to pack their bags and disappear when the rats came.

Even if the poor people and children on the streets of Bombay were forgotten by the world, someone had not forgotten them - their friend Jesus.

I, too, was determined never to forget these children, no matter whatever else happened in my life.

These were the Father's never-to-be-forgotten children.

Chapter 9

The Journey Home

Adjusting to a new culture can take time. It took me six months to acclimatise to Bombay. At the beginning it was almost too much for me. I would stay in my room for hours, overwhelmed by the shock of the new. India was so different from Germany that sometimes I felt lost.

One of the reasons I hid away was because everytime I went out I would be mobbed by beggars. Being white, it was always assumed that I was wealthy. One time I explained to a beggar in what little Hindi I knew that I had no money. The man's reaction was immediate.

'Why are you in this country if you don't have money? You should get out!'

Often I had to learn the hard way, like the time I was walking along the streets of Bombay and I saw an old beggar sitting by the road. I went up to him and, with the help of a translator, shared the Good News about Jesus with him. I then asked, 'may I pray for you?'

The old man looked at me with dark and empty eyes.

'For me, something to eat is like a prayer,' he replied.

I was so ashamed. All I had been interested in was the man's soul when what he needed food. By the time I finally gave him something to eat, I had learned my lesson.

Adjusting to Indian, urban culture was therefore an enormous challenge. I hadn't been as prepared as most missionaries normally are. I didn't know the language and I had gone into parts of Bombay that even the seasoned missionaries didn't know about.

Six months in, however, I was beginning to feel more at home. I had also passed the moment when I could have flown back to Germany using my return air ticket.

I now realised that I was meant to stay longer in a country I hadn't even wanted to visit. Now I had no money and no prospects. If I was going to return to Germany it was going to have to be the result of a divine intervention.

Show me your Glory!

During the testing time that followed I went to a seminar run by one of the leaders of Youth with a Mission. He spoke about the glory of God – by which I mean the radiant, manifest and holy presence of God. Listening to him a hunger began to grow in me. 'Father God,' I prayed, 'I need to experience some of your glory. If I don't, I won't be able to carry on.'

Out of desperation I decided to fast until I saw God's glory. In other words, I went without food as an expression of my hunger for more of God.

After three days I knew that it was time to finish my fast. This was not because I was hungry (I was!) but because I just knew in my heart that God was saying 'stop.'

As I sat in my room on the fourth day, thinking about my time in India, the whole atmosphere in the room suddenly changed.

There was a powerful and intense presence around me.

I knew without any doubt that God had entered the room.

All of a sudden I found myself before a brilliant throne.

Someone was sitting there.

From their knees down to their feet I saw a robe and the normal contours of the lower legs. Above the knees, all I could see was a bright shining light. This light was greater in its purity and translucence than any light we know here.

On one side of the throne was a rainbow, with many coloured lights around the throne and the one sitting on it. I saw colours. I saw red, and yet it wasn't the red we know. The other colours, too, were not the colours we know. Everything was filled with life – every single colour. Even the throne seemed to be filled with the life of the one seated there.

In front of the throne I saw four figures who were serving the one sitting on the throne.

The atmosphere was filled with wonderful music and with an indescribable love and peace.

I sensed someone standing on my left, without seeing him. As soon as he said 'come with me', I knew that it was the Holy Spirit. I just knew it. He was a familiar friend and my escort on this journey into glory.

Like a camera showing a new scene, I was suddenly in a different place. I saw David defeating Goliath. I saw Abraham moving out through faith to the land God had promised him. I saw Paul in his shipwreck.

Everything happened, so it seemed to me, within seconds.

People often ask me what the individual people looked like. I couldn't give an exact description of any of them, but I knew at that moment what I was seeing and who it was.

Then I heard a voice saying, 'everything which happens in faith lasts forever. There is no time here.'

And I understood. Everything we do in faith continues to exist in God's eyes as if it were happening right now even if it happened fifty years ago. These acts of faith are eternal remembrances of His power.

Then I was led to the left, to a different place where I saw a host of angels with golden breastplates, swords and shields in their hands. It was a powerful sight. The atmosphere was charged. I could sense that this army was either waiting for a command, or for something to happen.

Then I saw a flash of light. This flash of light became a person at the front of the army, and then flew off at an indescribable speed. All the angels followed him. During the short time the figure was visible at the head of the army I could see that he was different from the other angels. He radiated a power, majesty and determination beyond description. For one short moment I wondered, 'Who is that?' and the Holy Spirit, still at my side, read my thoughts and answered, 'that is Michael.'

Communication was so fast. Before one had even thought a question properly, the answer came. Thoughts could also be read like a book. Nothing could be hidden any more.

In the meantime I saw that Michael - the Archangel in charge of God's angelic army - had flown over a country with the whole host of angels and that a fierce spiritual battle was taking place there.

The voice spoke to me again, 'God will visit Brazil.'

A short time later I heard from some missionaries in India that God had begun to do wonderful things in Brazil. And He is still working there today.

Then I was standing before the throne again.

'Open your mouth,' the voice commanded me.

I knew that it was the voice of my Lord.

As I opened my mouth I saw a huge hand place a white cube in my mouth. As I began to chew the cube, my tongue swelled up. It became as numb. Then I saw Jesus coming towards me with outstretched arms, carrying a light in His hand. He looked at me seriously, and with an urgent expression in his voice he said, 'carry my light.'

Then I was back in my room.

My heart pounded.

I felt like the Old Testament prophet Isaiah, who said, 'woe is me, for I am unclean' when he had a vision of the glory of God (Isaiah chapter 6).

I knew that I had seen something of God's glory.

It was only a very tiny part but I would not have been able to bear any more.

For two hours I couldn't speak properly.

A great reverence for God came over me.

I looked at the clock and what to me had seemed like only a few minutes had in reality been almost half an hour.

Looking back I have to say that I don't know why I was allowed to experience this. I am nothing special. I am not more gifted than anyone else. But this experience changed my life and gave me strength for the things which were to come. It was the right word at the right moment.

An Unexpected visit

The voices on the other end of the telephone were full of excitement.

'We're coming to visit you in India!' they said.

The voices were those of my two nieces. They had never travelled abroad before.

'Do you seriously mean that?' I replied incredulously.

My two nieces are only three months younger than me. Growing up together they had become sisters to me, and I a brother to them.

'Yes, we do,' they cried.

I was a little nervous, I'll be honest. India was perhaps not the ideal destination for a first trip abroad. But my excitement about having visitors from home was greater than any anxiety I felt. 'They're old enough,' I thought.

'Tell me exactly when you're arriving,' I said, 'and I'll pick you up at the airport.'

Then I thought about my stomach.

'Please be sure to bring me some tins of sausages from back home,' I exclaimed.

Over the coming days I looked forward with keen anticipation for the arrival of my sausages and my nieces (note the order!).

I planned to take them by taxi through the less shocking roads from the airport. I wanted to shield them from the overwhelming poverty as far as I could.

When we met there was a fond reunion accompanied by affectionate hellos. Once I had made sure that the sausages were safely secured we started our journey to the house. In spite of the fact that I had planned a more sanitised route they were still staring out of the window as we drove down the streets and caught up on our news.

And then it happened.

As we were waiting at some traffic lights a woman carrying a sick child came up to our car. She bent down and through the open car window she asked us for some money.

As my nieces saw the sick child in the woman's arms they began to cry. The child's chest was deformed by rickets and his breastbone and ribs protruded in an unnatural way.

The child lay there weak and suffering. His dark eyes seemed dull and full of despair yet he looked at us in a pleading and heart-rending way.

This was too much for the girls.

I had been here several months now, and had seen a lot of suffering, but I hadn't planned for us to be confronted with such need right then. Yet without warning they had seen India's true face – poverty, sickness and despair.

However, this would not be the worst thing they would see during their visit.

They'll Kill You

A few days later we were on our way one evening to visit some friends in the city. All three of us were sitting in one of Bombay's many thousands of rickshaws.

As we were going along the road on which I lived, I suddenly saw a crowd of people. They were all staring in horror at something on the street.

As I looked I saw a man lying in the middle of the road in a pool of blood.

As we drew closer we could see blood spurting out of an artery in his neck.

Our rickshaw-puller moved to the side to avoid the almost lifeless body. Horrified at what I saw, I thought to myself 'someone is bound to take care of him.'

For a split second this reassured me until I suddenly sensed the power of God going through my body.

God spoke to me clearly.

'If you do not turn back and help this man, there is no difference between you and all the other people here.'

I was appalled at this thought and told the rickshaw-puller to turn back. I didn't understand the words he then said but I could tell that he wasn't enthusiastic about the idea. His face was full of fear.

Immediately I began to try to negotiate in my heart with God.

'Lord, I've got the two girls with me. This is their first time in India! If I leave them here in the rickshaw, who will look after them? They don't know the way back. It's dangerous here for white women. They are my family, Lord. What if I get drawn into a fight between rival gangs?'

Clearly I thought God didn't know all this already!

The truth was, however, I was afraid. I had seen with my own eyes how easy it is to lose one's life in this country. In Bombay, if someone wants you dead, he can hire a killer for between twenty five and fifty Euros. He may perhaps pay the same sum to the police and then the matter is settled. So it was hardly surprising that I was afraid.

Yet I knew that God had spoken to me and that he was waiting for my decision.

We had now reached the dying man again.

I jumped out of the rickshaw and told the puller he should wait. As I ran up to the man I saw that in the meantime more people had gathered around him. So far no-one had helped him. I couldn't believe it. Why didn't somebody help him? Not far away a few policemen were standing but they were not paying any attention to what was happening.

When I drew close to the man I saw that his whole body was lying in a pool of blood. His skull was split open and the artery had almost stopped pulsating.

I could see in his eyes that his body was being drained of blood and that the battle between life and death was nearly over. I didn't know what I should do. So hesitantly and unsure of myself I said, 'spirit of death, leave this man alone.'

The moment I said this, he took one more deep breath.

I took the dying man in my arms. His clothes were soaked with blood. As I held him I felt that there was no strength and no life in him. I looked around and shouted, 'why doesn't someone help him?'

I beckoned a rickshaw-puller over, hoping that he would take the man to hospital.

He turned down my request on the grounds that he didn't want his rickshaw getting dirty.

The people standing nearby had by now moved in closer and were staring at us, wondering what this white man was going to do.

The traffic had come to a standstill because I was standing in the middle of the road, holding this man covered in blood in my arms. He can't have been more than thirty and he was clearly dying.

After several minutes, which seemed to me like hours, a man ran up to me agitatedly and waved for a taxi.

'I'm a friend of his,' he said in English.

We tried to lay him on the back seat but his clothes were so wet with blood that he slid off the seat.

His friend jumped into the passenger seat and called to me as I stood at the roadside.

'We'll drive him to hospital.'

As they drove off, I looked down at myself. The white jogging suit I was wearing was covered in blood.

Then I suddenly remembered my nieces. I made my way through the crowd back to the rickshaw. Both girls were still in the rickshaw but were shocked when they saw me approaching with my clothes covered in blood.

We drove straight to their hotel, which was in the same street.

I tried to explain to them what had happened but I was in shock. It had suddenly become more real to me than ever before just how little a human life is worth in our world, and how quickly everything can be over.

As I stood in front of the mirror in the bathroom, I broke down altogether. I wept and wept.

'How can people just stand and watch when someone is being killed?' I cried. 'Why did nobody do something? If something had been done sooner, he might still be alive. Is he perhaps still alive? I won't stay here any longer. These people don't deserve it. Anyone capable of something like this doesn't deserve to hear of your love.'

When I returned home a little later I immediately put my clothes in a large bucket of water and left them overnight. The next day my cleaning lady came. I wasn't at home at the time, but my neighbour told me that the cleaner had left in great haste. When she saw the clothes she thought that I had killed someone. As she ran away she told my neighbour to tell me that she wouldn't be coming back.

Not everyone enjoys cleaning for a murderer.

In the meantime the news had long reached my neighbour that a tall white man had tried to save a dying man's life the previous evening.

'Why did you do that?' she asked fearfully. 'Why did you interfere? They'll kill you!'

Then she began to explain the circumstances surrounding the whole affair.

The young man had just come out of prison. Three years ago he had killed a member of another criminal gang, who were now avenging this murder.

'I don't care about all that,' I said. 'I just saw a dying man, and someone had to do something.'

'They will think you were the one who killed him!' she exclaimed.

'Why do you think no-one helped? People are frightened. If they help, the police arrest the last person who was with him and try to put the blame on him. Or it can happen that the Shiv Sena (the name of the gang he belonged to) think that you did it, and then they will kill you.'

That was all I needed.

From then on I kept hearing the words, 'they'll kill you' in my mind. Even when I went into my room the menacing words did not go away.

'It's fortunate that I have to leave town for a few days,' I thought.

I even considered whether I should come back at all.

But then I pulled myself together. Fear is not from God. It is one of Satan's weapons.

'Okay Jesus,' I said. 'You got me into this. You said I should help this man. Now it's your job to protect me.'

In spite of my words of faith, I was very relieved not to be in town for a few days.

When I came back I heard that on the day after my departure all the shops on our street had been closed. The gang to which the man belonged had gone in a long procession along the street with his coffin. The shop owners had been afraid that there would be fights between the rival gangs.

For a time I too had to battle with this fear until one day normal life was restored.

Some time afterwards God explained why He had allowed me to experience something like this. He wanted to show me how close death can be.

And he wanted to ask me once again, 'are you prepared even to die for me?'

That was a sobering question.

Was I really prepared to go that far?

An Angel's Visit

One day when I was not feeling like one of God's missionaries, and certainly not like one of God's heroes, I started to talk about my frustrations to my heavenly Father. I felt like I was under great pressure and that he wasn't listening to me.

'Father, can you hear me?' I said. 'I need a sign. I need a sign that you are there.'

I knew that the Bible says God is with us and will never leave us but I was having one of my moments again – the ones where my feelings were shouting louder than my faith, louder than the voice of God.

There was no response.

Nothing happened – no writing on a wall, no flash of light, no booming voice, absolutely nothing.

So I finished my prayer time and set off to one of Bombay's many communication centres.

These so-called communication centres are small, rented shops, often smaller than a garage in the West, in which there are several telephones and fax machines. On paying a fixed fee anyone can make a phone call or send a fax.

When I arrived at the communication centre I chatted to the owner, whom I knew quite well. I gave him my fax and while he tried to send it, I gazed through the shop window at the crowded street outside.

I immediately noticed a man walking across the street from the other side, right through the middle of the crowds. I don't know why, but I couldn't stop looking at this man. He was walking directly towards the shop.

The man was dressed in clothes that were strikingly white, at least within this Indian context.

He radiated an atmosphere of peace and harmony.

The man stopped a yard before the shop and looked at me through the window pane.

He looked right into my eyes, smiled, then put his hands together and pointed to the sky.

All this happened within seconds.

While I was still wondering what he wanted from me, our connection was broken by the shop owner's voice. The fax had gone through and I now had to pay for it.

It only took a brief moment, but when I turned back to the window, the man had gone.

I ran out on to the street but he was nowhere to be seen.

That was impossible. He couldn't have gone so far in the brief moment our eye contact was interrupted – not far enough for me not to see him any longer. He would have been especially noticeable with his white clothing.

Then I understood.

He was a messenger from God – an angel.

He had pointed to the sky with a reassuring smile.

The message was clear.

'Your heavenly Father hears your prayers.'

I was so encouraged.

From then on I went to the children several times a week. The children had become part of my life. I had now come to terms with the thought of staying in this country. The greatest miracle of all was that I even felt happy at the thought.

The Time has Come

I don't know exactly when it was but I sensed in my spirit that God was saying it was now time for me to return home to Germany. I was initially shocked at this because I had resigned myself to staying in India for the rest of my life. At the same time it wasn't such a great surprise to me. God had begun to prepare my heart for a number of weeks before this sense of imminent closure began to become more clearly defined. He had been making me ready for my departure.

But once again I put up a fight.

'Go back?' I said to God. 'No, never, that's impossible, Lord. I don't want to go back. This is my country. It has become my home. And apart from that,' I said, playing my trump card, 'I've agreed with the leaders of Youth with a Mission not to fly back before the 15th October.'

My plan had been to go home for three months and then return to India in January.

But God's plans are greater and wiser than ours and his plan was for me to go home for much longer.

In my heart, I knew this and I also knew that when I did I would not see India again for a very long time.

So he was preparing me.

And when I received a call from my home church back in Germany that they would pay for my flight home, the matter was decided. My excuse that I didn't have the money to buy a return ticket was now redundant.

I cushioned the blow of my departure by telling myself that I'd be back in three months but deep down I knew that wasn't true.

I went to my YWAM leader and told him what the Lord had said to me and he was less than enthusiastic about me going. But in the end he gave his blessing, as did the others.

Now the toughest challenge came.

I had to tell Juliett that I was leaving, and of course the children. As I did I promised them that I would come back one day and that I would never forget them.

How could I ever have forgotten them?

That would have been like forgetting part of my heart.

I can still remember how I felt the day I visited the street children for the last time and then drove away in a rickshaw.

All at once my departure became very real to me.

'I'm going. Maybe I won't ever see the children again. Will I ever come back?'

It was as though someone was tearing my heart out.

I couldn't stop seeing the faces of these beloved children in my mind.

I cried and cried.

I had not cried when I had left Germany. What on earth had happened to me in this land that I had come to love the people so much? Why did I now feel like I was leaving my own family, perhaps never to see them again?

With great sorrow I stepped on to a plane at Bombay Airport in September 1993.

During take-off I looked for the last time down at this city, hated by many.

I realised that there was nowhere else in the world that I could call 'home', except Bombay.

But now I was on my way back to Germany, not knowing what awaited me there.

Chapter 10

A Suitable Helper

Returning to Germany was a massive shock to my system. Walking through Frankfurt Airport I was amazed at how quiet and tidy it all was. On the drive home, I'd forgotten how clean and well maintained our motorways are.

Everything felt different.

Sitting on the sofa in a friend's large house, I felt unsure of my bearings. The wealth and splendour of my surroundings overwhelmed me. If I had experienced a seismic shock when I had first seen the poverty of India, I was now experiencing the same kind of thing as I became reacquainted with the affluence of Germany. Now it was Germany which felt like a foreign country.

I therefore found myself missing the distinctive smells of Bombay, the never-ending background noises and the dark-skinned, friendly smiling faces.

I had gone to India purely in obedience to God ten and a half months before. Now I had come back to Germany purely in obedience to God.

I had returned a month and a half earlier than expected, but four and a half months later than I had first planned.

All I could think of was taking my short leave and going back to the land that I loved.

India felt like home.

Germany did not.

What I didn't realise, however, was that my heavenly Father had different plans and these were much better than mine.

Resting in the Father's Love

Not knowing what I was supposed to do, I made the decision to become actively involved in my church. On the one hand it felt good to be back in the church where I had become a believer, surrounded by friends and family. On the other it was an intensive time of profound transformation, wrought by the hand of my loving Father in heaven.

One of the main areas where he was challenging me was in relation to my self-worth. It came as a real surprise to me when I began to see that so much of my relationship with my heavenly Father had been based on performance. If I did enough things for him in ministry, and especially effective things, then I felt loved by him. That was not healthy.

Instead of doing things for God because I was loved by him, I was doing things in order to be loved by him.

Consequently, pretty well everything I had done in ministry had been performance-based.

It had been done for approval rather than from approval.

Now I was at a critical moment. I had nothing to do for him, at least in terms of ministry. I had returned from the mission field in India and I was disoriented. So much of my sense of identity and worth had come from what I had done for him. Now that I was without a ministry my relationship with my heavenly Father began to deteriorate. I didn't understand at this stage in my Christian life that the Father's love for me is not based on what I do for him but simply on who I am in Christ. Put another way, I didn't realise that his love for me was based not on my performance but on my position. As a son of God by adoption, he simply loves me for who I am!

I had believed the lie that says, 'I do, therefore I am.' I had yet to see that the truth is the opposite. 'I am, therefore I do.' I hadn't reached the point where I knew by revelation that my sense of who I am and what I'm worth does not derive from the things I do for God but simply from the fact that I'm his son by adoption and he adores me for who I am.

So it was that over the next few months I began to build a new relationship with him - one based on resting in my position rather than striving to earn love through performance. I was now without a ministry so I was empty-handed. I had nothing tangible to offer the Father in terms of preaching, acts of mercy, praying for others, feeding the poor, and so on. In any case I had deceived myself in the past that these were necessary to secure the Father's affection and affirmation. Now I had nothing that I could offer him. Now I was being called to exchange performance for position and my natural resources for the power of the Holy Spirit.

This was therefore a low point.

I had no daily routine for prayer or Bible study.

I even had to declare myself bankrupt, which my Italian pride didn't like one little bit.

But in this place of spiritual and material bankruptcy, I asked the Father to help me and he, in his kindness, answered my prayer and began to restore our friendship.

In the weeks that followed he started to heal my inner wounds and I began to understand that even though we may sometimes give up on ourselves, he never gives up on us. He invests in us again and again, even when we fail, because he believes in us.

Oh no, I'm in Love!

I eventually found employment in a church in Stuttgart and it was there that I was asked to join a team travelling to Jaipur, in the north of India. It was a fourteen day trip and our task was to assist in establishing a new congregation of Christians.

This was not without its challenges. In the region where we were sharing the Good News about Jesus the temperatures reached 50 degrees centigrade during the day.

There were seminars every day and open-air meetings in the evenings.

One young lady on our team had to be flown home after having been sick in hospital for two weeks.

So there was a big cost to what we were doing but the rewards were amazing. We saw numerous Hindus come to believe in Jesus. The regional TV station came and filmed what was going because so many miracles were being reported. One evening we prayed for a man who was hemiplegic. He was touched by God and as a result was able to move and walk again.

After my return from this mission I was scheduled to travel with some of the teenagers from our church to a seminar in northern Germany. I didn't feel like going. However, because I had promised the young people and because the theme of the seminar was 'bringing Christian values into schools,' I decided to go. We had recently started a work in schools which was now growing fast.

The seminar was conducted by a team from England belonging to the organisation 'PAIS-Project.'

Today this organization has more than 100 full-time workers up and down England and teams all over the world with hundreds of staff.

I was sitting and listening to the leader giving his talk when I suddenly noticed an attractive young lady.

There was something special about her.

Just as I was thinking, 'I'd love to know if she's still single' the leader of the team, Paul Gibbs, gave an example of his distinctive English humour as he introduced the team.

'This is Louise,' he said, pointing to the attractive girl who had caught my attention. 'Louise is still unattached - something she would like to say to all the single men here.'

He winked very conspicuously.

No one could miss it.

The English people in the audience all laughed.

We Germans were amazed at this strange humour.

As I lay in bed that evening I just couldn't stop thinking about Louise.

After about two hours of this I realised what had happened.

'Oh no, Lord,' I cried out. 'I think I've fallen in love! But I don't have time for a relationship. How could it work anyway? She is from England and I still haven't spoken a word to her!'

But it had happened and all my further arguments had no impact whatsoever on either my romantic emotions or my Father in heaven.

A Time of Testing

Sometime later my heavenly Father said to me in his typically loving way, 'would you like your timing or mine?'

'Yours, Lord,' I replied, 'but you'll have to help me.'

A year before this I had had a very special experience during a time of prayer. Two very dear friends of mine from England were praying with me. The moment they laid hands on me it was as though a glorious cloud covered me. There in this cloud Jesus met me. He spoke to me about various things which were to come. Those present heard me speaking to someone but they couldn't see anything themselves and only heard what I said. The room was thick with the powerful presence of God.

After Jesus had shared one or two things with me, he asked me a question.

'Stefan, are you prepared to remain single for me?'

These words were like a sword plunging into my heart. I had often surrendered my life to God, or responded to the altar-call of a preacher to commit everything to the Lord. But this was something different. I began to weep. It was clear to me what saying yes to this would mean.

I had often dreamed of having a wife and children. But now my loving Lord, to whom I had much to be thankful for, stood before me, and was asking me to lay down this dream.

What shocked me most and reduced me to tears was the fact that from the bottom of my heart I wasn't prepared to answer with a loud and immediate 'yes.'

Was there something I loved more than my Lord?

I asked Jesus to give me time to think it through. I knew that if I answered Jesus with a 'yes,' he would take my decision very seriously and that could mean giving up everything.

For some weeks this question was on my mind. I considered the possible consequences of my answer, talked it over with my pastor and close friends, until the day came when I fell on my knees.

'Lord, if it is your will,' I said, 'then it shall be so. But you must give me the strength to remain single.'

As I said these words a supernatural peace flooded my heart. A short time later I was greatly relieved when God spoke to me through different people that he had only wanted to test me. He had wanted to see if my heart was fully surrendered to him in this area of my life.

He then told me that I would remain alone for a short while

until the time came when he would bring the woman He had chosen into my life.

All this had happened before the seminar.

On the day after I had realised I was in love, I took part in Louise's workshop. I sat in the first row and observed the kind of person she was - how she dealt with people, how she expressed herself – and I was thrilled.

'What a woman!' I thought.

As I sat there my notes were filled with declarations of love for her.

What on earth had happened to me?

Louise told me later that she noticed me staring at her and had thought, 'O my God, he's one of those critical Germans and he is bound to ask critical questions later. The way he's staring at me he obviously doesn't agree with what I'm saying.'

If only she had seen my notes!

She said, 'you must have a vision, a goal, in life.'

I wrote, 'my goal is to get to know her.'

She said, 'then you need a promise from the Bible that confirms your goal.'

I wrote, 'God's promise to me is "it is not good for man to be alone!"'

My notes were full of her.

I was in love.

Later I thought how embarrassing it would have been if another seminar participant had asked me for my notes, or had wanted to look at them.

But at that moment I only had eyes for Louise.

Such a Beautiful Woman

The morning workshop came to an end and I still hadn't been able to speak to Louise. Other people were around her continually.

'Lord, this just can't go on. Look at how I'm behaving. I'm not a teenager any more. We are leaving tomorrow. If you don't do something now, I'll forget everything. She is from England so there's no point in it anyway.'

In the dining room I was the first one from our Stuttgart team to sit at a table. Suddenly a man came up to my table, wanting to sit down. I was rather discouraged so I didn't want any company at that moment. But it was obvious that this man wanted to talk. I thought up an excuse.

'I'm sorry,' I said, 'I'm with a group of teenagers here. They are still in another workshop. We want to sit together, so I'm afraid there is no more room.'

The man got up and went to a neighbouring table.

Suddenly Louise entered the dining room. My heart beat faster as she came towards my table. 'Oh no,' I thought, 'she is going to sit at my table and the man I have just sent away is already looking at me. What will he think if I allow her to sit here? He knows which church I come from. He is certain to think, "he won't let me sit there, but a pretty woman can."'

But it was too late now. Louise walked up to my table and sat down. I had to say something. The man was watching and listening.

'Excuse me, but I'm here with some teenagers and we want to sit together.'

'I'm sorry,' Louise said, and got up.

'But I think they would be pleased if they could practise their English. Please stay here.'

The words just shot out of my mouth!

At long last the opportunity had come. We were pretty much alone and had some time to talk to each other. So I invited her for a coffee.

The next day I asked her for her address and telephone number so I could keep in contact with her. She thought I only wanted her address so that I could ask further questions about the work in schools. As I looked at her my heart took over and words once again shot out of my mouth.

'You are such a beautiful woman!'

'Oops,' I thought, 'what was that?'

I started to apologize.

'Please forgive me. I just don't know what the matter is with me. I don't normally say that to women.'

Fortunately we were soon to go home.

On returning I immediately phoned her, although I knew that her team couldn't possibly have arrived home yet, and I spoke on her answering machine.

Louise told me later that the moment she listened to my message, she knew she would become my wife.

A few months prior to these events, one of the students of our Bible School had a dream in which he saw that my wife would come from an English-speaking country. In this dream God showed him several things which were all true of Louise. When he told me this at the time, I only half listened but after I had met her I asked the student to describe the dream to me again. God had wanted to reveal His plans to me months beforehand.

God's ways are good. Very often I had wondered, 'Lord, why do I have to wait so long?' (I was 32 years old when I got married.)

Looking back, however, I have to say that it was very good the way things worked out. Earlier I would not have been capable of conducting a relationship in line with God's standards.

The Lord once said to me, 'Stefan, the partner I have for you is very precious to me. That's why I have to prepare you very thoroughly for her.'

My dear Lord Jesus had to work on me for ten years after my new beginning until I was able to receive His precious gift - my dear wife!

Today I enjoy the gift of marriage and sexuality as never before. We had a lot to learn during the first years of our marriage (that wasn't always easy) and we are still learning.

However, it is wonderful to know that marriage is God's invention and that if we follow his instructions, it becomes better with each passing day.

No matter what others say, I am completely convinced that God still knows best what marriage should be like, because he invented it.

After all, it was he who said, 'it is not good for the man to be alone. I will make a helper suitable for him' (Genesis 2:18).

Chapter 11

An Army of Love

'I think he would understand me,' said the boy. 'I'd like to talk to him.'

These were the words of a young prisoner in Germany whom everyone in his world had now consigned to the trash heap. 'There is no hope for him,' the social workers and lawyers had said. 'He will spend the rest of his life in prison.'

But a social worker whom I'd known in India had phoned and asked me if I would come to the juvenile penal institution where she worked and tell the prisoners about what Jesus had done in my life. I had been working with young people for a while by this stage so I was on the lookout for opportunities to share my story.

As I went to the youth prison I had mixed feelings. I knew from my own past that the last thing young people like this are interested in is God or church. But I wasn't going there to talk about church. I was going there to talk about the wonderful love of Jesus and so I was also excited. I trusted that he would give me the right words - words which would get past the defences of these boys and girls and touch their hearts.

When I arrived, I looked at the high walls that surrounded the building and the bars on the windows. I thanked my Father in heaven that in spite of my criminal past I had never had to experience being imprisoned.

As I saw the young people my heart was filled with love and compassion for them. These were the Father's lost and abused children. I knew something of what they were going through. I had been one once.

'I don't know how many will come to listen to you,' my friend, the social worker, said after the heavy gate closed shut behind me. 'We have left it up to them whether they stay in their cells or come to your meeting.'

In the end all except one of the prisoners came to the meeting. As they came into the room I could read the looks on their faces. They had been told that they were going to listen to someone who had once been a rioter but who now serves God. I could tell what they were thinking by simply looking at their expressions.

'He's crazy.'

'I won't believe a word of it.'

But those attitudes didn't last.

As I began to speak the love and the presence of God filled the room so powerfully that everyone started to listen with rapt attention.

Having spoken for about an hour about what my heavenly Father had done for me, the way he had so lovingly rescued me from a life of darkness and despair, you could have heard a pin drop. They were all so moved that they didn't know how to react or what to say. They knew that being 'cool' - their normal reflex - wasn't the right response.

It was a boy from another country who broke the silence.

'Wow, that's really incredible,' he said. 'My parents tried unsuccessfully to bring me up to be religious. After hearing what you've said today, I'm going to have to think again about this God.'

With that I decided it was time to say a prayer.

I asked Jesus to show himself to every single one of them - to give all of them an experience of his love.

Finally, I gave an invitation for those who wanted to have personal, one-on-one chats with me while everyone else went off for supper.

'I Believe in You'

'He wants to speak with you on his own,' my friend the social worker said excitedly. When I asked who, she replied, 'the boy I was telling you about. He says he thinks you would understand him.'

So it was that I found myself face to face with a very troubled boy whom I will call Sven (not his real name). He had just finished a spell in solitary confinement for trying to smuggle a weapon into prison on his very first day. The time alone had given him a chance to think deeply about his life. He was now keen not to spend more time than was absolutely necessary in prison.

His head was bowed as he told me his story, a story that I'd heard so many times before. He was only fourteen and he seemed younger than the others.

We sat together in a separate room where he started to share, tears pouring down his face.

'I'm scared! My mum threw me out of the house when I was thirteen years old. Her boyfriend beat me continually – he was also in and out of prison. I'm in a gang now and I had needed a weapon for protection. I just won't allow anybody to hurt me again.'

Sven went on to tell that he was terrified he was going to lose his girlfriend, who meant a lot to him.

He talked about his uncertain future, with more court proceedings pending.

He opened up his heart and disclosed his fear and pain to me.

It was as if he had known me all his life.

'I really would like to start again,' he cried.

As he spoke, I felt the grief of Jesus in my heart, his pain at all that this young man had already gone through.

I simply sat and listened to him, with tears in my eyes.

I didn't see a criminal sitting in front of me. I saw a boy who was trying to survive without a father and mother, a young man who once had dreams and joy in his life like other boys, a child abused by Satan just as I had been.

When he finished, I told him again about the love that Jesus had for him. I shared how Jesus had changed my life and that he could do the same for him.

Like a father I put my arm around his shoulders, looked at him and began to speak.

'Sven, I believe in you. You will make it. Everything will be okay.'

His eyes filled again with tears. I knew what he was feeling only too well; I had experienced the comfort and hope that comes when you hear for the first time that somebody believes in you, that somebody out there loves you.

As we prayed together, Sven gave his life into the hands of the one whom I'd been trusting for years.

When I left I knew that there was someone far stronger and bigger than me watching over him.

He was now protected by his heavenly Father.

On that day and during other visits I often had individual talks with the young people - talks which ended in tears and a decision to live for Jesus.

Some of them wrote to me and others still write to me now. For most of them, it was the day when Jesus came to visit them in prison.

Every one of these young people had their own story. Some had been repeatedly raped. Some had run away from home. Others had been brutally beaten up by someone in their own home, such as their mother's boyfriend.

Many were full of hate for their fathers.

One of these fathers had even poured boiling water over their child's arm in a fit of rage, scalding them badly.

Each one of them had their own litany of pain. But they all had one thing in common, the same profound yearning for love that no one can satisfy except the person whom the Bible calls 'our Father.'

He is God.

And as the Bible says, 'God is love.'

He loves these boys and girls.

He's crazy about them.

Marching for the Father

I remember during this time having a very vivid scene play like a movie through my imagination.

I saw a large number of skinheads marching forward like an army.

But they didn't look threatening and violent.

That shocked me because I knew from my time as a hooligan that aggression and hatred always seethed underneath these shaved heads.

In fact Hitler himself once spoke of 'the youth that carry my name.'

When youths march in anger, they are often blinded and deceived by this evil, violent spirit.

But what I was seeing now was very different. This was not an army of hatred. It was an army of love.

As I watched the scene play out, I sensed my heavenly Father beginning to speak to me.

'These are my leaders but they are currently blinded by the enemy. The gift that I gave them to lead was abused by the devil for his destructive purposes. You only see their outward appearance and consequently you're afraid. But I see their broken and deceived hearts.

Even if you forget them, I will not forget them. Go to them and tell them about my love and don't be afraid. The day will come when they will march with conviction for me and nothing will stop them. They will unite in the one goal to honour me. Pray for them and don't curse them.'

Once again I felt the deep pain that God has in his heart for his lost children and I knew one thing for sure: even if we forget them, he will not.

Not Just a Sausage!

My life in recent years has been a learning curve in which I have discovered what it means to be part of the Father's army of love.

Let me give you several examples of how I have had to go through quite a process (and still am), discovering what it really means to show God's love to those who most need it.

I was now working full-time for God. One afternoon in Stuttgart I saw an elderly tramp sitting on a bench. I felt sorry for him and decided to buy him something to eat.

I walked up to him with a sausage and gave it to him with a smile.

He thanked me.

'That's alright,' I said. 'There is someone who loves you and his name is Jesus.'

After a short chat I went on my way.

I had only gone a few yards when God spoke to me.

'Is that all?'

I was surprised.

'What do you mean, "Is that all?"'

'Take this man home with you!'

God's words were so clear that I couldn't have denied them even if I had wanted to.

Immediately I started a silent discussion with God.

'Lord, I can't do that! What will I do with him when I go to work during the day? What if he ransacks my home when I'm not there? Lord, I haven't the time for things like that!'

But God was teaching me a listen about what it really costs to bring transformation to a person - not the price of a sausage, but everything!

And so I took this man with me to my small flat. There I listened to his story. I then told him about the love of Jesus and how valuable he is to him.

A few days later I helped him to obtain help from various authorities in the town.

I am so glad that I listened to the loving Father who was more interested in this man than in my schedule or appointments.

I wanted to give him a sausage. But his heavenly Father wanted to give him a place to sleep and a place to receive love.

He knows exactly what we need!

The favourite shirt

Another time I was in the Bible school in Stuttgart speaking about how important it is to obey the voice of the Holy Spirit whether we understand it or not.

Towards the end of the lesson I sensed God speaking softly to my heart.

'Go to the main station in the city.'

I had just been speaking to the class about obedience. So it felt to me as if God was now testing me as to whether I myself was always willing to obey.

At the end of class I gave the students the task of asking God to speak to them before the next lesson, and then to do whatever God had said.

'It is not important to understand everything,' I added, 'just obey.'

Now it was my turn to obey the loving Father and go to the main station that evening.

To begin with I thought, 'Okay, I'll go sometime this week.'

But God spoke very clearly, 'No, now!'

A few minutes later I was on my way to the main station with a friend called Thomas.

We arrived and marched through the main hall keeping our eyes open, looking out for what God wanted us to do, the person he wanted us to meet.

After we had walked up and down the hall for a while, I suddenly noticed a man sitting at the edge of one of the platforms.

For a moment it seemed as though my whole attention was fixed on him. He was a tramp.

I stood there, tired after a hard day and thought, 'the man doesn't look like an easy customer. I'm really not in the mood to be confronted by a person and his problems.'

We walked on.

As we did, I spoke to Jesus silently in my heart.

'Lord, if this man is the real reason you sent us to the main station then let him be sitting on the bench over there when we come back to this platform.'

We strolled along platform twelve to pray.

When we returned the man was still sitting on the bench.

I had made an agreement with God and now I needed to keep it.

We walked towards the man, who was about thirty five years of age.

I opened the conversation, as I had often done in the past, with the question, 'are you hungry?'

The man looked at us in surprise.

I pulled a twenty Mark note out of my pocket which I had placed there ready.

'Why are you doing this?' asked the man.

'Because there is someone who loves you!'

'What are you talking about? Who?'

'Jesus loves you and he has sent us here to show you that.'

I had hardly spoken the name Jesus when the man became very angry. He held the money out towards me and said very aggressively, 'Keep your money, I don't want it. I don't want anything from your God. I don't need him!'

He continued to berate us while I tried to listen to God.

I stood there feeling rather uncertain. I had only wanted to do a good deed and now this was all I was getting by way of a thank-you. Had it really been God's plan for us to speak to this man? It seemed as if he wanted nothing to do with God. What he wanted became clear when he suddenly said, 'I don't need the money. I'd rather have a shirt!'

A shirt!

That was all I could hear and now I knew what God wanted from me.

'Give him your shirt.'

'My shirt?' I thought. 'But Lord, don't you know that this is my favourite shirt?'

That morning I had stood in front of my wardrobe and was about to put on something different when I suddenly had the strong feeling that I should wear my favourite green shirt from India. That was no problem for me; I liked this shirt a lot! Now here I was being called to give it away and suddenly I understood what God wanted me to do.

'Give away what you love.'

A struggle began inside. I was not very enthusiastic at the thought of taking my shirt off there and then and giving it to this strange man. People from my church might see me without a shirt. 'And after all, Lord,' I added, 'this is my favourite shirt!'

But my loving Father in heaven wasn't interested in my nice shirts. He was interested in giving the man a shirt.

My favourite shirt was the one he had chosen.

So I looked at the man.

'You need a shirt,' I said. 'Here, take this.'

I took off my shirt and passed it to him.

The man stopped his words in midstream and looked at me in disbelief.

'Hey, what are you doing?' he asked. 'You can't be serious!'

'Here, take this shirt. I'm sorry we troubled you. We'll go now and leave you in peace.'

We turned to leave the station but we had hardly begun to walk away when he came after us.

'Wait!' he cried. 'Why did you do that?'

I began to explain that there is someone that loves him and who cares when he is cold or sad, someone who doesn't mind what he looks like or smells like. He is called Jesus.

This time the conversation was quite different. The man told us his sad story, the reason he had ended up on the street and why he was so angry with God.

'Where was God when that happened to my friend? Where was he when all these terrible things happened in my life?'

These are questions that many thousands ask.

I responded to him in the same way I had answered many others who had the same kind of questions.

'I don't understand everything either, but one thing I do know: Jesus loves you, and he wept with you when all these things happened.'

We talked for a while and I explained the only way to find real love.

At the beginning I had felt awkward speaking to this man. I didn't know what to talk about and above all, I didn't know what to do.

But God knew what this man needed. He needed a shirt.

This shirt spoke louder than any words of the existence of a loving God.

Showing the Father's love may have cost me my favourite shirt. But it cost Jesus his life.

What a comparison!

That evening I had the great privilege of being an instrument of the love of the Father.

His message to the man was, 'I haven't forgotten you!'

A Father to the Fatherless

Maybe you find it difficult to believe that God is this kind towards people in prison or on the streets.

If you do I want to show you some verses in the Bible. You can find them in the Old Testament, in Psalm 68:4-6:

> Sing to God, sing in praise of his name,
> extol him who rides on the clouds;
> rejoice before him – his name is the Lord.
> A father to the fatherless, a defender of widows,
> is God in his holy dwelling.
> God sets the lonely in families,
> he leads out the prisoners with singing;
> but the rebellious live in a sun-scorched land.

These words tell us some important truths about God.

First of all, they tell us that he is 'a father to the fatherless.' This is really important in our world today where so many people in every country and on every Continent don't know what it's like to be brought up by a father. To those who have never known a father's love, God says 'I'll be your Dad.' That's a phenomenal message of hope especially for people in prison, most of whom are there because they have never known what it's like to have a positive, older male role model in their lives. Boys and girls need their dads, and when their dads are missing they so often go off the rails and end up in prison. God says here that he has a special place in his heart for the fatherless. He wants to be a Dad to them.

Secondly, these verses tell us that God is a 'defender of widows.' Throughout the Bible we see this. God is full of compassion for those who have lost loved ones and whose lives are full of grief. He has a special love and affection for widows, for those whose husbands have died and whose families are therefore without a father figure.

Thirdly, 'he sets the lonely in families.' God is a Father who wants those who feel isolated and all alone to be embraced within a family. He longs to create new families and to expand existing families, making room for the lost and the unloved so that they can find a place they can call home. All over the world God is doing this right now.

Fourthly, he is a Father who 'leads out the prisoners with singing.' He is a Dad who has a special affection for those in prison and who is constantly at work to help prisoners come to a place where they are no longer bowed down with despair but full of love and hope. He alone can do this by setting them free 'on the inside,' free enough to leave prison with a song in their hearts.

So when I talk about God as the most amazing, loving, heavenly Father - a Father who wants young people in prison or people living on the streets to know the love of his Son, Jesus - this is no pipe dream.

This is not religious rhetoric.

It is reality.

This is the cry of God's heart.

This is who God is.

He wants to be a Father to all the people who, like me, never knew the love of a father and who are looking for a father's love in all the wrong places.

He wants people to know that their hunger for a father's love is not met in the affirmation of gang leaders or in the momentary relief of sexual experiences.

It is met in the One whom Jesus taught us to call 'our Father.'

He wants people to know that their deep need for a family is not met in criminal gangs or in tribes of hooligans.

It is met in becoming part of God's family, in which we find our adopted brothers and sisters in Christ.

This is why God is moving so powerfully on the earth in this generation.

God is creating an army of love in which young men like Sven can play a vital part, sharing the Father's love with the fatherless.

He is working in prisons to set men and women free from their destructive patterns of thinking and behaving and to release a new song from their lips.

This is Dad's army.

It is already marching.

If you listen carefully enough, you can hear the sound of beating drums and stomping feet.

Chapter 12

Finding my Father

As I come to the end of this book I realise that there is so much more I could tell you about how my heavenly Father has completely transformed my life.

I could tell you about how he not only gave me my wonderful wife Louise (to whom I have been married fifteen years) but also two beautiful children, Grace Louisa and John David.

I could tell you about how the revelation of God as a loving father has inspired and encouraged me as I have tried to be a good dad to my children.

I could tell you about my time working on the staff of a church of 2500 members in Stuttgart and how I founded and led a prophetic school there, taught in the Bible School, and oversaw a regional network of house churches.

I could tell you about how I felt called to the UK in 2002 and how I have travelled from there to teach about prophecy and about the Father heart of God.

I could tell you about my current role mentoring people from all sorts of different backgrounds, coaching them to live out Christian values in their spheres of influence.

I could tell you about my role advising churches and Christian groups, and about how I set up and now lead a network in Germany called United for Christ (UFC).

I could tell you about how I founded and now run an online Spiritual Development School (SDS).

I could tell you about how I am currently training to produce and direct short films.

I could tell you about how we have rescued hundreds of children from the mafia in India, setting them free from the sex trade where they can be sold for less than $250.

I could tell you about how I met Mother Theresa two months before she died and how I shared with her about going home to her heavenly Father to receive her reward.

I could tell you how I saw the Father's love shining like bright stars in the eyes of this precious, wonderful and inspirational woman.

I could write so much about all of these things but perhaps they are for another time and another book.

I mention them only to say this: these things point to how my Father in heaven has utterly transformed my life.

They show how the Father can take the most ordinary person and give them an extraordinary purpose.

They are a source of hope for everyone.

God is our Father

But I don't want to end by talking about myself.

I want to finish by coming back to where I began this book, with a focus on fathers.

It won't have escaped your attention that I started out with a severe disadvantage in this regard.

I didn't know my biological father. All I know is that he was an Italian and that by all accounts my mother loved him. But more than that, I am in the dark.

My biological father is a mystery.

My mother eventually married my stepfather but he didn't fill the gap left by my biological dad. He was unable to share his love for me. He was physically present but emotionally absent, like so many fathers today.

During my teenage years my father wound became more and more acute. I was hungry for a father's love. Having lacked a healthy attachment to my own father, I looked for substitute fathers - for father figures who could fill the great void in my heart and be an older male role model to me. The first of these was my karate teacher but there were others too. However, none of them could fill the father-shaped hole in my soul. I had to learn the hard way that you cannot find in human beings what you can only receive from Father God.

And that brings me to the passion, purpose and priority of my life, which is the message of God the Father's love.

You see for many years I thought that Christianity was just another religion - just another dry, formal and oppressive belief system in which God is a distant master and we are dutiful slaves.

But then I met Jesus and everything changed.

I realised that Jesus didn't come to begin a religion. In fact, my reading of the Gospels (the four stories about Jesus in the Bible) suggested that he didn't like religion at all. No, Jesus didn't come to start a religion. He came to restore a relationship - a relationship with the world's greatest and most adoring Father in heaven.

That was a massive paradigm shift.

It was like an earthquake in my soul.

After nearly a quarter of a century of being a Christian I now realise that the primary reason why Jesus came to this earth was not just to rescue us from our sins but to reveal that God is a Father who loves us relentlessly and who is waiting with open arms to welcome us into an intimate relationship.

That has made all the difference in the world.

I may have never known my earthly Father, but I have a heavenly Father.

My earthly father may have disappeared from my life, but my heavenly Father has promised he will never leave me.

I may have had a stepfather who was emotionally absent, but I have a heavenly Father who is interested in absolutely everything in my life, rejoicing with me when I'm happy, weeping with me when I'm sad.

I may have missed out on an earthly father, but in Jesus I have found a perfect Father and in doing so I have found my heart's true home.

The Antidote to Fatherlessness

But this is not just for me. It is for everyone, especially for the millions of people right across the earth who either have never known the unconditional love of a father or who have lost that love.

The Good News is this: in Jesus we can all find the love that we so often look for in all the wrong places.

In Jesus we can find the Father's love, which is the love of all loves.

This is the true message of Christianity.

We all know the alarming damage that is caused by absent, abandoning or abusive fathers today. Our prisons are full of fatherless boys and girls. Our streets are haunted by gangs whose leaders have become a dark and destructive expression of fatherhood to young people. Millions of young people growing up in all the Continents of the world are suffering from fatherlessness. The social consequences of this are indeed catastrophic.

What will turn the tide?

How will this great pandemic come to an end?

It will come to an end as Christians come to understand more and more that God is the Father we have been waiting for, that God is the dad who loves us like no imperfect, earthly father ever could.

It will come to an end as Christians become filled to overflowing with this heavenly Father's love and then start to give that love away to the fatherless, whether on the streets of Europe or in the slums of India.

When people miss out on a father's love they are denied a source of affirmation and inspiration that is essential for life. Denied the affection and direction of a good dad, most people grow up feeling like something is missing in their lives - a sense of being valued and honoured for who they are; a sense of hope and purpose. This then leads people to try and find a sense of self-worth and significance through success in sports, work and studies, or through becoming someone that isn't really them, or through earning lots of money, or through relationships with people whom they think will make up the love deficit left by the fathers for whom they long.

But none of these will ultimately satisfy.

None of these earthly realities can fill the hole in the soul.

Only the love of our heavenly Father can do that.

And I know from working with thousands of people all over the world that this is what everyone needs.

They may be top managers in a business or the poorest of the poor on a city street but they all need the same thing.

Some may call it destiny.

Others may call it enlightenment.

But I call it what Jesus called it - the love of the Father.

No More Orphans

On the night before Jesus died he said something really significant to his disciples. He said, 'I will not leave you as orphans' (John 14:18).

For a long time I was really puzzled by this. Surely Jesus had got it wrong here? Most of the disciples were not orphans. They had dads. Two of them had a father called Zebedee.

But then I realised that Jesus was speaking figuratively not literally. In other words he was using the word 'orphan' in a spiritual not a literal sense.

In the Bible the word 'orphan' means someone who doesn't have a father. They may still have a mother, but if they don't have a father then they are called an orphan.

When Jesus said that he would not leave his disciples as orphans, he was referring to their spiritual state. He was saying that they weren't going to be separated from their heavenly Father any longer. He was going to do something very drastic to make sure that they could be reconciled to the Father and experience his love. In other words, he was going to die on the Cross.

This then is why Jesus came to earth. He understood that every human being is a spiritual orphan. Every one of us is separated from our true Father's love. So when he started preaching at the age of thirty, Jesus constantly spoke about God as a loving Father. He completely subverted the religion of his day by telling everyone that God is not a slave driver but an affectionate Daddy.

That was radical!

On one memorable occasion he told a very moving story about a dad who went to unbelievable lengths to show his wayward and rebellious son just how crazy he was about him.

And to the religious leaders who were listening, this was a real rebuke.

They had turned God into an angry lawmaker who wanted to punish human beings at every opportunity.

But in painting a picture of this forgiving and extravagant dad, Jesus told his audience what the living God is really like. Our truest picture of God is found in his timeless portrayal of the father who sees his rebellious son returning home. That dad's response is to run to his son and hug the hell out of him, kissing him repeatedly and tenderly.

This then is the Good News that authentic Christianity is called to broadcast to a fatherless world.

Religion won't share this message.

But true followers of Jesus will.

We may have all been orphans spiritually. But thanks to Jesus, we can know the one whom he taught us to call 'our Father in heaven.'

We can come home to the world's greatest dad!

We can be adopted into his family.

And in his arms we can find true happiness.

'I'm not Good Enough'

The message that I share when I minister to others today is this: if you are deep down searching for a father's love, you'll only find it in Jesus.

You may look for it in criminal gangs, secret societies or football clubs, but you won't find it there.

You may search for it in toxic relationships with men or dependant relationships on father substitutes, but you won't find it there either.

The only place you're going to find it is in Jesus.

And the only thing that's going to stop you from finding it is the lie that you're not good enough.

If you feel that way, then please consider this.

Who did Jesus like hanging out with most when he was here on the earth two thousand years ago?

Was it the religious people who thought they were good enough?

Or was it the sinners who knew they weren't?

In case you don't already know, I'll tell you. It was the sinners that Jesus loved being with. He constantly had meals with messed up people, banquets with broken people, and feasts with fallen people.

In fact, Jesus had little time for religious people.

He had all the time in the world for those whom the religious leaders of his day had marginalised.

This is why even prostitutes came to his meal table, soaking his feet with their tears.

By being this radical, Jesus was making a statement about his heavenly Father.

He was saying that his Dad in heaven does not believe in exclusion. He believes in embrace.

He doesn't believe in raging at people and delighting in punishing them. He believes in revealing his love.

So if you think that you're not good enough, that's a lie that you've almost certainly been sold by some religious person or people.

But it isn't true.

Jesus came to tell us that God's the Dad we have been looking for in the wrong places, and that he doesn't look at us with angry and disapproving eyes but with immense love and compassion.

If only people knew that God was this good, this kind, this nice, they would run without hesitation into his warm and open arms.

I truly believe that.

Learning from my Children

What a difference it makes when a child grows up knowing that God is a Dad like this. Instead of believing the lie that God is remote and frightening, they grow up believing the truth that God is relational and trustworthy.

For such a child, it is impossible to understand how anyone could reject such a Father.

This is why my daughter Grace one day came home from school with a look of puzzlement on her face.

'Dad,' she said. 'Not everyone at school believes in God!'

Brought up with a picture of what God is really like, she was shocked. How could anyone in their right mind not want to know and love someone this good?

Truly the peoples of the world need a revelation of the Father's love!

I remember an occasion with my other child, my son John, where I received an insight into the Father's love.

One evening I was sitting in a chair by his bedside, watching him as he slept. There was such a look of peace in his face. As I watched, I was filled with joy and affection. I felt such love for him at that moment.

As I sat, a verse from the Bible came to mind.

'He who watches over Israel will neither slumber nor sleep' (Psalm 121:4, New International Version).

The reference here is to God watching over Israel as a father watches over his child.

Another translation of the same verse known as 'The Message' puts it like this:

He won't let you stumble,
your Guardian God won't fall asleep.
Not on your life! Israel's
Guardian will never doze or sleep.

'That's it!' I thought. 'The verse says that God doesn't fall asleep. The reason he's always awake is because he's a dad who watches over his children and he can't keep his eyes off us! He's not distracted by the angels discussing the affairs of the world. He's not turning round to issue orders and decrees. He's looking at us and he's gazing at us with such joy, such love, such focus. He is thinking, 'this is my daughter! This is my son!' And he is revelling in the dreams he has for us.'

That for me was revelation.

It was as if God was saying, 'look at the way you're watching over your son. That's how I am towards you, towards every one of my children.'

That changed me.

God is an adoring Father.

This is what he's saying right now as he looks at you:

'I can't keep my eyes off you. I love you so much.'

A Message for Everyone

My purpose in life is now to share this message of the Father's love all over the world, beginning in my own home and with my own family.

I want everyone to stop believing the lie that God can't wait to punish us. God isn't like that. He is an affectionate, patient and compassionate Father. I want people to know that his arms are as open as his heart. He wants us to enjoy an intimate friendship with him. He is not looking for religious specialists. He is looking for sons and daughters.

Once a person has been captivated by this revelation, they can then transmit the message of the Father's love wherever they go. Their hearts have found true satisfaction in their heavenly Father's affection. This qualifies them to be carriers of this affection to others, exhibiting the Father's acceptance and compassion wherever they live and work.

I remember an incident after which this really hit home in my heart.

I was still in Stuttgart at the time and I was attending a Mind, Body, Spirit exhibition. I had set up a stand there to introduce spiritual seekers to Jesus.

A woman came up to the stand and started speaking to some of the team members who had come with me. She was dressed in black and wearing amulets.

'I hate your God! I hate your God!' she kept saying.

'You should speak to Stefan,' one of the team said.

'Thanks very much,' I thought.

The woman came up to me and started mouthing the same comments.

'Why do you keep sending such strange people to me?' I complained to God silently.

'I hate your God! I hate your God!' she continued.

I didn't know what to say. I was trained to speak about Jesus and share the Good News of his love but right now I was stuck for words.

But at the same time I felt this profound and immense love for the woman - a love that I knew was the Father's. I sensed this deep sadness in his heart for all the pain that she'd had to go through - a pain that was now pouring out of her mouth in the form of a rage against God.

'I hate your God!' she continued to shout.

'I'd rather go to hell,' she added.

When she said that, words began to flow from my mouth.

'You know what? That would be so sad because you are so precious.'

It's our decision where we eventually go, of course. But I sensed God saying to this wounded woman, 'I want you forever with me.'

In other words, I sensed his great love for her.

Hearing that she was precious to God, the lady was momentarily confused. She was expecting me to push back defensively. Maybe that's what she had become used to. But all she received was love - the Father's love.

So I prayed a simple prayer for her.

'Show this woman how much you love her, Father.'

I learned something vital that day.

God isn't against us. He's for us. And he is so sad at how unhappy and hurt we are.

The Family of God

If this is a true reflection of the heart of God, then everything has to change. For a start, those of us who are followers of Jesus will need to stop speaking about a religious God who is out to condemn us and start talking about a relational God who wants to be our loving Father.

Beyond that, not only do we need to change what we believe about God. We also need to change the way we understand the church.

For most people the word 'church' conjures up a whole host of negative thoughts and impressions. Some of these may be based on bad experiences. Others may be based on here say. Either way, the connotation of the word isn't positive. It almost always evokes a picture of a cold and formal institution. No one in their right minds wants to join that.

But to those who have been seized by the wonderful love of the Father, the church is no longer a cold and formal institution. It is now a warm and loving family. For if God is our heavenly Papa, then that means we have been adopted into his family as his sons and daughters. This then makes those of us who have chosen to follow Jesus adopted brothers and sisters. That means reality and relationship. It means fun and feasting. It means acceptance and affection.

This, I believe, is the church of the future.

In the future, denomination and institution will be less important than fellowship and family.

One of the signs of that will be the restoration of spiritual fathers and mothers in the church. Having experienced the revelation of the Father's love, these people will look to embrace younger believers as spiritual sons and daughters. When that happens, we will know that we have moved from the church as institution to the church as family.

This has in fact been one of the joys in my own life. When God became my true Father, I stopped looking for father substitutes in my life. But at the point when I no longer needed a father substitute, God sent a wonderful man called Giancarlo Elia into my life to be my spiritual father. He is now in his seventies and travels all over the world ministering God's love. He is a man who truly reflects the Father's love. He walks the talk and to me he has become the most amazing role model - an example of a man who has given up everything to share the Father's love, travelling with his wife Catherine from the icy land of Siberia to the blistering heat in the jungle of Borneo.

His impact has been so big that I have dedicated this book to him.

He is my spiritual father.

He is a grandfather to my children

Through him, I experience in a practical way what it means to be fathered.

I have also started to learn what it means to be a son.

That in itself is huge.

After all the pain I had been through, I had vowed never to trust anyone ever again.

But with Giancarlo's help, I began to change.

I began to rejoice in the privilege of being a son.

I began to trust in a new way.

Finding your Father

Perhaps you are looking for a father right now.

Maybe you were wounded by your father.

Maybe he abandoned you.

Maybe he wasn't there for you.

Maybe you hear the word 'father' but it has no meaning for you.

There came a day in my own life when I had to acknowledge that I knew how to write the word 'father' but I didn't really know what a father was. My stepfather had not fathered me well. How I used to wish that he – like other fathers – had come to the school on open day. How I wished that we could have done things together. That one wonderful Sunday morning when he took me to the pub was one of the rare occasions that we shared an experience. It is the only time I can remember. He was always sitting at the kitchen table, reading his newspapers and drinking his wine. We were not allowed to disturb him. If we got up to anything he would rap us on the head with his knuckles or hit us with his walking stick. If I had questions, he often said, 'ask your mother.'

As a teenager I hated it when he used to shout when he was drunk. One of my most terrible memories was when I was about seven years old and I saw my brother, my brother-in-law and my father in a brawl. I was so frightened. These were the people I loved. This was my family. Yet they were shouting at each other and hurting each other.

I stood there in horror until my mother took me away.

I swore to myself that I would never become like my stepfather.

At that time I still thought he was my real father.

So you seem if you have been poorly fathered, I can relate to that. But understand this.

You have a Father in heaven who watches over you without ever falling asleep.

He loves you and protects you.

He is crazy about you.

So whatever the deficit from your earthly father, he - and he alone - can make up for that.

The key is to get to know the Father.

How do you do that?

You do it by coming to Jesus, saying that you believe he's God's Son, confessing the things that you've done wrong, asking him to forgive you, and inviting him to come into your heart and fill you with the Father's love.

It's really that easy.

Then, when you have got to know Jesus, you start getting to

know this wonderful Father that you have in heaven. The reason for that is because Jesus came to reveal the Father heart of God. Everything he ever did and said was a reflection and revelation of the Father's love. That's why he said to a disciple called Phillip, 'he who has seen me has seen the Father' (John 14:8).

The more you get to know Jesus, the more you will be captivated by the Father.

As you grow in this revelation, one of the things that you may sense is that a key to experiencing your heavenly Father's love will be forgiving your earthly father.

This is not easy, I know. I came to a point in my life at Bible School when I realised I hated my biological father for abandoning me.

I was so full of anger at what he had done.

But what I can say is that when I forgave my biological father and indeed my stepfather, it brought indescribable breakthroughs in my heart.

I began to pray a prayer: 'Jesus, I have no idea what a father is like. Please show me what a father is like.'

Then God spoke to me.

'Stefan, stop searching. Stop searching for a father. You have a father. I am your Father.'

My seeking was over.

I had found the Father I had been looking for all my life.

What Should I Do Now?

If you relate to my story about 'Finding my Father', then the chances are you will be wondering how to respond.

Through the pages of this book you will have seen how lost I was before I found Jesus - or before Jesus found me. I was desperate for a father's love. I was a spiritual orphan, separated from my heavenly Father's love because of my own sin and rebellion.

Then one day I decided to end it all. Just as I was preparing to commit suicide, I heard the Lord say to me: 'you will live and everything will be fine.'

That was the beginning of a complete transformation of my life.

I am not saying that there haven't been any problems or challenges since I became a Christian. I have been through many trials. I have had my share of crises, including in my marriage. I have got very close to burn out by trying to work hard enough to gain God's approval, not realising for a long time that he is a dad who already approves of me.

So there have been difficulties and it would be wrong of me to suggest otherwise.

But at the same time I have come to see that I now have the best Dad in the universe. I have found in Jesus what I had been looking for since the day I was born.

I have found my heavenly Father.

And that is the source of the satisfaction I feel deep within my heart.

So to you, dear reader, God wants to say what he said to me.

'YOU WILL LIVE AND EVERYTHING WILL BE FINE.'

Why don't you come home now?

Choose to put an end to being a spiritual orphan.

Accept the invitation to become the adopted daughter or son of God.

Let me encourage you to say this prayer in your heart right now:

'Dear Lord Jesus, I believe that you are God's Son and that you came to reveal the Father. I confess that I feel separated from the

Father. Please forgive me for rebelling against God's love. I am truly sorry. Please forgive me for hating other people. I choose to forgive those who have hurt me right now, mentioning them by name. Thank you for the Cross and for opening up a way back to the Father. I turn from living life my way. I want to come home. Make me your adopted child and please fill me with the Father's love, in Jesus' name, Amen.'

If you prayed that prayer, then you are no longer a spiritual orphan. You are an adopted child of God.

Make it your aim now to find a church that looks like the family of God.

Tell someone about the prayer you've prayed and the decision you've made.

Tell them that you've found the Father.

If they understand what you mean, then you'll know you've found the right place.

And you will start the most amazing adventure of your life, helping orphans to find their Father.

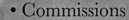